# Real-World Strategies for Implementing Quality and Safety From Hospital to Home Care

Badia Faddoul
https://orcid.org/0009-0007-2337-2658
*Johns Hopkins Medicine, USA*

IGI Global
Scientific Publishing
Publishing Tomorrow's Research Today

Vice President of Editorial Melissa Wagner
Director of Acquisitions Mikaela Felty
Director of Book Development Jocelynn Hessler
Production Manager Mike Brehm
Cover Design Jose Rosado

Published in the United States of America by
IGI Global Scientific Publishing
701 East Chocolate Avenue
Hershey, PA, 17033, USA
Tel: 717-533-8845 | Fax: 717-533-7115
Website: https://www.igi-global.com E-mail: cust@igi-global.com



Library of Congress Cataloging-in-Publication Data

LCCN: 2026931721 (CIP Data Pending)
ISBN13: 9798337364964
Isbn13Softcover: 9798337364971
EISBN13: 9798337364988
British Cataloguing in Publication Data
A Cataloguing in Publication record for this book is available from the British Library.

For the people who show up when the work is hard
and stay when the answers are not clear.
For those who care for others, often unseen,
and who keep learning in the spaces between certainty and doubt.
And for my daughters, **Amanee and Farrah**,
who remind me every day that presence matters,
that integrity is practiced in small moments,
and that how we care for one another is where all good work begins.

# Table of Contents

# Preface

As I move into the later years of my professional life, I find myself reflecting less on what I have accomplished and more on how I learned to see care. This book was written from that place. It is not an attempt to be comprehensive, nor does it introduce a new theory of quality or safety. Instead, it reflects how this work has lived in my hands over time, how I have practiced it, questioned it, taught it, and carried it across roles and settings as care moved from bedside to system and, increasingly, into people's homes.

Healthcare does not suffer from a lack of ideas. We are surrounded by frameworks, standards, checklists, and performance measures, all designed with the intention of making care safer and more reliable. Yet somewhere between the policy and the patient, between the training module and the lived moment of care, meaning can thin. What often remains is compliance without connection. This book grew out of that space. It was shaped by years of watching well intended initiatives lose relevance at the point of care, and by watching small, human decisions quietly prevent harm.

Much of my career has been devoted to translation. Not translation in a technical sense, but the everyday work of turning expectations into practice. Policies matter only when they make sense to the people asked to follow them. Dashboards matter only when they help someone notice risk sooner or respond with greater clarity. Safety becomes real not when it is defined, but when it shows up in routines, conversations, and choices made under pressure. Over time, I learned that improvement lives or dies in this space between intention and experience.

I write from the perspective of a nurse, a quality and safety leader, and a mentor. My approach evolved as my responsibilities expanded from direct patient care to organizational leadership. I share these experiences not because they are definitive, but because they are honest. Some lessons arrived quickly. Others emerged only through discomfort, missteps, or sustained reflection. Those moments shaped how I understand accountability, fairness, and learning, and they continue to influence how I approach the work today.

As my work moved across settings, I became increasingly aware of how easily good ideas lose their footing once they leave the page. An initiative can be sound in design and still feel misaligned in practice. A policy can meet every requirement and yet fail the moment it encounters the pace, pressure, and variability of real work. Over time, I learned to pay attention to where people hesitated, where work-arounds appeared, and where quiet compensation filled gaps no one had named. Those moments were not signs of resistance. They were signals that translation had not yet happened.

Translation requires proximity. It asks leaders to spend time where care is actually delivered, long enough to see how plans bend under ordinary conditions. It requires listening without rushing to fix and returning after the first change to see whether it holds. The most meaningful improvements I witnessed did not begin with a mandate. They began with a shared recognition that something felt harder than it should, or riskier than it looked on paper. When that recognition was taken seriously, people leaned in. When it was dismissed, effort thinned and trust followed.

Over the years, I learned that safety rarely announces itself through dramatic failures alone. More often, it whispers. It shows up as a near miss caught just in time, a question left unasked in a meeting, or a small sense of unease that someone carries home at the end of a shift. These signals are easy to miss when attention is pulled toward metrics alone. They become visible when leaders create space for conversation and when teams are encouraged to name uncertainty without fear. Reliability grows in those spaces, not because work becomes simpler, but because it becomes more honest.

This book reflects that understanding. It does not treat quality, safety, or service as programs to be launched or endpoints to be achieved. Instead, it approaches them as practices shaped by daily decisions, relationships, and local realities. The chapters that follow stay close to the work itself, tracing how conditions such as fatigue, judgment, trust, and clarity influence outcomes just as powerfully as formal processes do. My intent is not to prescribe a single way forward, but to offer a way of seeing that helps readers recognize risk earlier and respond with greater care and intention.

Many of the tools discussed in this book will be familiar to readers who work in quality and safety. Over the years, I have relied on improvement methods, safety frameworks, and change models to bring structure to complex problems. These tools matter. They help teams see patterns, slow thinking when urgency threatens to override judgment and create a shared language for learning. What may feel different here is not the choice of tools, but the way they are held.

Throughout my career, I have seen methods succeed or fail not because of their design, but because of the conditions surrounding their use. Variability, vulnerability, fatigue, judgment, and courage are not peripheral to improvement work. They are central to it. A process map does not reduce cognitive load on its own. A checklist does not create psychological safety. A framework does not ensure fairness. These outcomes depend on how tools are introduced, who is invited into the conversation, and whether people feel respected enough to tell the whole story.

Context shapes everything. The same improvement approach can feel constructive in one setting and constraining in another. A discussion held in a boardroom carries different weight than the same discussion held in a patient's living room. Time pressures differ. Power dynamics shift. The consequences of getting it wrong feel closer to the surface. Effective leaders learn to adjust their expectations and their methods to fit these realities, without losing sight of core principles.

For that reason, this book treats tools as supports rather than solutions. They are offered as ways of thinking, not as recipes to be followed without adaptation. Readers will see familiar methods paired with stories that reveal where those methods bend, where they hold, and where they need translation to remain useful. The goal is not fidelity to a framework, but fidelity to the people and situations the work is meant to serve.

To support this translation, the book makes deliberate use of visual storytelling. Diagrams, storyboards, and illustrations are used to help readers see how concepts move through real work rather than remain abstract. The ideas, narrative intent, and prompts underlying these visuals were developed by the author and grounded in lived experience. Artificial intelligence tools were used to generate visual representations of those concepts, serving as an illustrative aid rather than an author of content. The intent is clarity, not automation.

You can read these chapters straight through or return to them as questions arise in your own work. They are written to stand on their own, but they also build on one another, reflecting how understanding deepens over time rather than in a single pass. Together, they offer a way of thinking about quality, safety, and service not as end points, but as living practices shaped by everyday decisions, relationships, and local realities. I encourage readers to take what feels useful, question what does not, and adapt the ideas in ways that fit their organization, their community, and the people they serve.

Looking back, I am struck by how little of this work has been about discovering something entirely new. Most of it has been about noticing what is already present and choosing to act with intention. When improvement stalls, it is rarely because teams lack effort or insight. More often, it is because the conditions for learning have thinned. Time disappears. Conversations shorten. Curiosity gives way to urgency. This book returns again and again to the idea that reliable care depends on protecting those conditions, even when pressure is high.

If these chapters help connect a framework to a real moment, or a data point to a person's experience, then they have fulfilled their purpose. If they help a leader pause long enough to ask a different question or help a clinician feel less alone in naming a concern, they have done their work. In the end, quality, safety, and service are not initiatives to be launched or completed. They are ways of caring for patients, colleagues, and one another over time.

As the scope of my work widened, so did my appreciation for how differently care is experienced depending on where one stands. Clinicians feel risk in the immediacy of the moment. Leaders often encounter it later, through reports, metrics, or questions raised after something has already gone wrong. Patients and families experience risk in yet another way, through uncertainty, confusion, or the quiet fear of managing care once professional support steps back. This book is written with all of these vantage points in mind. It aims to narrow the distance between them.

This book exists now because the conditions under which care is delivered have shifted in ways that traditional improvement approaches do not always fully account for. Care has become more distributed, more technologically mediated, and more dependent on patients, families, and caregivers carrying responsibility once held by clinicians and institutions. At the same time, the pace of change has accelerated. New tools, policies, and expectations arrive faster than teams can absorb them, often layered on top of systems already under strain. In this environment, it is easy for improvement work to become fragmented, episodic, or reduced to compliance.

Many organizations are working harder than ever to improve quality and safety, yet clinicians and leaders alike report a sense of fatigue and disconnection. Metrics multiply. Dashboards fill. Training modules expand. Still, the feeling persists that something essential is being missed. This book responds to that unease. It is grounded in the belief that reliability does not emerge from volume of effort alone, but from alignment between intention, design, and lived experience.

The timing also reflects a growing recognition that harm is not always dramatic or immediate. It often accumulates quietly through delays, misunderstandings, inequities, and missed opportunities to intervene earlier. These forms of harm are harder to see and harder to measure, yet they shape trust, outcomes, and willingness to engage with care. Addressing them requires more than technical fixes. It requires attention to context, relationships, and the everyday conditions under which decisions are made.

The past several years have further exposed the fragility of systems that depend on constant adaptation without sufficient support. Workforce shortages, moral distress, and widening inequities have made clear that resilience cannot rest solely on individual effort. Systems must be designed to absorb strain without relying on heroics. This book offers a way of thinking about improvement that takes those realities seriously, not as temporary disruptions, but as defining features of modern care.

Writing now is also an act of stewardship. Many of the lessons described here were learned slowly, through repetition, error, and reflection. They deserve to be carried forward with care. Not as rules, but as ways of noticing. Not as answers, but as questions that travel across settings and roles. The hope is that by naming these patterns explicitly, others may recognize them sooner and respond with greater clarity and compassion.

Much of what follows is shaped by work that extended beyond hospital walls. As care moved into homes, community clinics, infusion centers, and virtual spaces, the limits of traditional safety thinking became more visible. In these settings, standardization alone is not enough. Conditions vary widely. Resources differ. Patients and families take on roles once held by professionals. Risk becomes more personal and often less visible to the system. These realities demand approaches that respect context, support judgment, and recognize that safety depends as much on relationships and communication as it does on protocols.

Home based care, in particular, reveals the strengths and fragilities of our systems. A home visit can uncover risks no policy anticipates: unreliable power for medical equipment, language barriers that complicate instructions, or caregiving responsibilities that collide with treatment plans. These are not deviations from care. They are care. When systems are designed only for ideal conditions, the burden of adaptation falls on patients and frontline staff. This book argues for a different stance, one that treats adaptation as a signal for redesign rather than as an expectation to endure.

The audience for this book is intentionally broad. It is written for clinicians who want practical structure without losing the human center of their work. It is written for leaders who are responsible for conditions they may not directly experience, yet whose decisions shape daily risk. It is written for educators and mentors who are helping others develop judgment, not just technical skill. And it is written for anyone who senses that improvement work must do more than meet standards. It must make care feel safer and more trustworthy to the people who depend on it.

Throughout the chapters, readers will encounter moments of tension. Stories where the right path was not immediately clear. Situations where policies conflicted with reality. Decisions made under constraint, with imperfect information. These moments are included deliberately. They reflect the texture of real work and resist the temptation to smooth complexity into certainty. Learning happens in these spaces, when teams are supported to pause, reflect, and adjust rather than to rush toward closure.

The book also reflects a sustained commitment to mentorship and teaching. Over the years, I have learned as much from students, new graduates, and early career leaders as I have from formal training. Their questions often surface assumptions that more experienced clinicians have stopped noticing. Their hesitations reveal where systems are brittle or unclear. Teaching, like safety, is a relational practice. It depends on trust, patience, and the willingness to admit what we do not yet know.

As you move through the chapters, you will see recurring themes. Presence matters. Fairness matters. Listening changes outcomes. Data gains meaning when paired with story. Transitions deserve special attention. Readiness shapes whether change endures. These ideas appear in different forms across settings and roles, reflecting how they adapt to context rather than remaining fixed.

The chapters are not meant to be read as proof of expertise, but as an account of practice. They reflect choices made, questions asked, and lessons learned over time. Some examples describe successes. Others reveal limitations. Both are necessary. Improvement work that hides its uncertainty loses credibility. This book takes the position that transparency, when paired with responsibility, strengthens trust and supports learning.

Before the chapters begin in earnest, it is important to explain why this book starts where it does. We begin at the bedside not because it is the most visible place in the system, but because it is where the consequences of every decision are ultimately felt. Policies, technologies, staffing models, and performance targets all converge in that moment. The bedside is where clarity matters, where uncertainty surfaces, and where trust is either reinforced or quietly eroded. Starting there keeps the work grounded.

Beginning at the bedside also honors how many people enter health care. Most of us did not arrive thinking in terms of systems. We arrived wanting to help, to be useful, and to do right by the person in front of us. The early chapters return to that orientation deliberately. They do not romanticize frontline work, nor do they minimize its strain. Instead, they treat bedside experience as a source of intelligence about how systems succeed or fail. What clinicians notice in the flow of work often precedes what appears in reports or dashboards.

From that starting point, the book gradually widens its view. Later chapters trace how bedside signals move, or fail to move, through teams, departments, organizations, and communities. They explore what happens when early warnings are amplified and acted upon, and what happens when they are lost to hierarchy, time pressure, or competing priorities. This progression mirrors how I learned the work myself, first by noticing what felt off, and later by learning how to shape the conditions that made those moments more or less likely.

The closing reflection of this Preface returns to a simple idea. Reliable care is not achieved through vigilance alone. It is created when systems are designed to support ordinary people doing complex work under imperfect conditions. It is sustained when leaders remain close enough to see where effort is compensating for design, and when teams are given permission to speak honestly about what makes work hard.

As you move into the chapters that follow, I invite you to read with both attention and generosity. Attention to the details that resemble your own setting, and generosity toward the people whose decisions and constraints may differ from yours. The aim is not agreement on every point, but a shared commitment to learning from the work as it is lived.

I return, finally, to the quiet moments that have shaped my understanding of care. A pause before an order is signed. A question asked despite uncertainty. A handoff where someone stays long enough to be sure the plan is understood. These moments rarely appear in formal accounts of improvement, yet they are where safety is practiced most faithfully. When systems support these moments, reliability grows. When they do not, risk finds space to settle.

This book exists to keep those moments in view. To connect frameworks to experience, data to people, and intention to outcome. From bedside to system, and back again, the work is the same. To notice what matters, to act with care, and to build conditions where doing the right thing is not an act of heroism, but the expected path. With that, we begin. These practices do not require perfection or certainty. They ask for steadiness, humility, and attention to what unfolds in real time. When organizations make space for these qualities, learning becomes possible even in moments of strain. This is how improvement endures, not through grand redesigns alone, but through small, consistent acts that protect clarity, dignity, and trust.

The chapters that follow reflect how my understanding of quality, safety, and service widened over time, moving from the immediacy of bedside care to the broader responsibility of system design.

## CHAPTER OVERIVEW

**Chapter 1, *From Bedside to System: Why This Book Matters*,** grounds the work in lived clinical experience, showing how everyday conditions such as transitions, workarounds, and cognitive load shape risk more often than individual failure. Safety is framed as an organizational practice sustained through presence, fairness, and psychological safety rather than compliance alone.

**Chapter 2, *Boots on the Ground: Where Safety Lives*,** examines leadership presence at the Gemba and how disciplined observation, impact-based prioritization, and follow-through turn visibility into sustained improvement across settings.

**Chapter 3, *Culture First: Laying the Foundation with Just Culture and Team Engagement*,** explores how accountability and compassion coexist when Just Culture becomes a daily practice, shaping trust, engagement, and shared learning.

**Chapter 4, *Lean and Six Sigma in Real Life: Getting to the Root Without Getting Lost*,** brings improvement methods out of theory and into lived care, emphasizing curiosity, context, and human factors as essential companions to technical rigor.

**Chapter 5, *From Strategy to Story: Building Dashboards That Drive Change*,** shows how measurement becomes meaningful when data are designed to support understanding, curiosity, and learning rather than surveillance.

**Chapter 6, *Patient Voices at the Heart of Safety*,** reframes patient experience as a core safety signal, demonstrating how listening reveals early risk, deepens trust, and strengthens prevention across the continuum of care.

**Chapter 7, *Workplace Violence Prevention: Protecting Those Who Care*,** positions workforce safety as a foundational dimension of quality, showing how culture, environment, and leadership response determine whether harm is interrupted or normalized.

**Chapter 8, *Seeing Risk Before It Sees You*,** shifts risk assessment from retrospective explanation to forward-looking practice, illustrating how proactive approaches help organizations detect weak signals and design systems that hold under pressure.

**Chapter 9, *Building Bridges: Transitions of Care and Safety at the Edges*,** focuses on the fragile moments when responsibility changes hands, treating transitions as both technical processes and human relationships.

**Chapter 10, *Real Tools, Real Impact: Templates, Scripts, and Checklists*,** offers practical supports shaped by real work, helping teams speak up, notice drift, and turn experience into learning under unpredictable conditions.

**Chapter 11, *Assessing Organizational Readiness Through ADKAR*,** reframes change management as a human sequence, providing practical ways to assess readiness, address resistance, and sustain adoption beyond surface compliance.

**Chapter 12, *From Continuous Improvement to Enduring Impact: Sustaining Change Through Safety Stories*,** explores how narrative complements measurement, anchoring attention, accountability, and learning over time.

**Chapter 13, *When Policy Meets People: Translating Regulation into Safer Care*,** examines how policies function under real conditions of uncertainty, arguing that effectiveness depends on clarity, credibility, and alignment with how work actually unfolds.

**Chapter 14, *Equity in Every Step: Building Safer Systems Through Inclusion*,** positions equity as integral to safety, showing how disparities often surface as early signals of preventable harm, particularly in transitions and home-based care.

**Chapter 15, *The Likelihood to Recommend as a Signal of Safety*,** reframes patient experience data as an early indicator of risk and trust, demonstrating how listening enables earlier, more meaningful intervention.

**Chapter 16, *When Things Go Wrong: FMEA, RCA, and ACA*,** approaches analytic methods as acts of organizational sensemaking, showing how disciplined analysis can restore trust, support healing, and strengthen learning.

**Chapter 17, *Invisible Failures: Algorithmic Bias as a New Category of Safety Risk*,** frames algorithmic bias as a latent safety condition and adapts established safety science tools to support responsible, equitable use of AI in care delivery.

**Chapter 18, *Imagining Care Again: Returning Safety, Quality, and Service to Their Human Roots*,** closes the book with reflection rather than prescription, inviting readers to reconnect improvement work with judgment, relationships, and responsibility in an increasingly mediated healthcare landscape.

Together, these chapters trace a progression from bedside experience to system responsibility, offering a way of seeing quality, safety, and service not as endpoints, but as practices shaped by attention, presence, and care over time.

# Acknowledgment

No book is written alone, and this one reflects the influence of many people whose thinking, questions, and integrity shaped it over time.

The ideas in these chapters grew out of shared work with colleagues, mentors, and teams who were willing to engage deeply with the realities of care, including its uncertainty and complexity. I am grateful to those delivering and supporting care across hospitals, ambulatory clinics, and home care settings who allowed me to work alongside them during moments of learning, challenge, and vulnerability. I am especially thankful for the teams I had the privilege to mentor and guide in this space. Their curiosity, honesty, and willingness to engage with complexity strengthened my own thinking and shaped how the ideas in this book evolved. Teaching and learning in this work has always been reciprocal, and much of what appears in these chapters was refined through those shared exchanges.

I owe particular thanks to my mentors, whose guidance shaped how I understand leadership, accountability, and learning. They taught me that leadership is as much about listening as direction, and about creating conditions where people can speak honestly about what makes work hard. I am also grateful to the broader quality, safety, and regulatory communities whose ongoing dialogue and scrutiny continue to raise expectations for what care can and should be.

Finally, I thank my family, and especially my daughters, **Amanee and Farrah**. Their patience, perspective, and love grounded this work in ways that are difficult to name but easy to feel. They reminded me that presence matters, that leadership begins at home, and that how we show up for one another ultimately shapes how we care for patients.

# Introduction

Quality and safety in healthcare are often discussed through models, metrics, and improvement programs. In practice, they are shaped in quieter ways through handoffs that feel rushed, decisions made with incomplete information, workarounds that solve one problem while creating another, and moments when people hesitate to speak. Harm rarely appears as a single failure. It grows from everyday conditions that accumulate across settings, roles, and time. As care continues to move beyond hospital walls into clinics, homes, and digitally mediated environments, these conditions become harder to see and easier to normalize.

This book begins with that reality. It is written from the perspective that safety is not a destination or a scorecard outcome, but a way of working that must be continually designed, observed, and renewed. Drawing on lived experience across hospital, ambulatory, and home-based care, the chapters explore how systems shape behavior, how culture influences reliability, and how leaders can detect risk before it becomes harm. Rather than treating safety as a technical exercise, the book approaches it as a human practice that depends on presence, trust, fairness, and the willingness to learn under pressure.

The chapters move deliberately from practice to system. Early chapters focus on the conditions that make safety possible where care is delivered, emphasizing leadership presence, Just Culture, and psychological safety as foundations rather than add-ons. Leadership is examined not as visibility alone, but as disciplined attention, follow-through, and the ability to translate what is seen at the frontline into meaningful change. Culture is treated as something that forms through daily interactions and decisions, not through statements or policies. Accountability and compassion are presented not as opposing forces, but as mutually reinforcing when applied with clarity and care.

Improvement methods such as Lean, Six Sigma, and analytic reviews are addressed as ways of noticing rather than fixed toolkits. Their value lies less in technical mastery than in how they help teams stay curious long enough to understand why work unfolds the way it does. When these methods are applied without attention to human context, they can flatten experience and narrow learning. When paired with respect for cognitive limits, role clarity, and lived conditions, they help reduce friction and support shared understanding. The chapters draw on real situations to show how improvement becomes meaningful when it keeps people visible within the data.

Patient and family voices are positioned as central to safety, not as proxies for satisfaction. Listening is treated as a form of risk detection and a signal of trust. Stories from patients and families often reveal breakdowns long before they appear in dashboards or event reports. When these narratives are integrated into governance and daily practice, they broaden how organizations understand harm and prevention. Safety, in this framing, is strengthened not only through analysis, but through attention to what people experience, fear, and need.

Workforce safety receives equal attention. The well-being of those who deliver care is presented as inseparable from quality itself. Exposure to violence, moral strain, and chronic overload erodes reliability in ways that are often invisible until they surface as turnover, disengagement, or error. The chapters examine how leadership response, environmental design, and cultural norms determine whether harm is interrupted or quietly repeated. Protection is framed not as compliance, but as a measure of whether people feel valued and supported to do their work well.

Transitions of care are examined as moments where responsibility shifts and relationships matter most. These are the edges where systems often fail to connect, even when documentation is complete. The book argues that continuity is both a technical and a relational process. Presence, verification, and empathy at the moment of handoff do more to protect safety than additional checklists alone. Across settings, transitions are shown as opportunities to reinforce shared responsibility rather than procedural endpoints.

As the book progresses, attention turns to the tools and structures that help organizations hold steady when conditions are unpredictable. Scripts, checklists, dashboards, and readiness assessments are presented as supports for speaking up, closing the loop, and sustaining attention. These tools are not offered as static templates, but as living guides shaped by real voices and refined through use. Change management is approached through a human lens, recognizing that adoption depends on awareness, motivation, capability, and reinforcement over time. Resistance is treated not as opposition, but as information.

Stories play a central role in sustaining improvement. Metrics remain essential, but they lose meaning when detached from lived experience. Safety stories translate data into context, influence leadership attention, and preserve the intent of improvement efforts across transitions. When used ethically and consistently, storytelling complements measurement by keeping focus anchored on people rather than aggregates. Sustained improvement emerges when structure and narrative work together.

Later chapters widen the lens to policy, equity, and emerging risk. Policies are examined as promises that must function when work becomes uncertain. Their strength is measured not by alignment alone, but by whether people reach for them when clarity matters most. Equity is reframed as a core dimension of safety, with disparities understood as signals of preventable harm rather than abstract gaps. Through practical examples, the book shows how inequities often surface as early warning signs, particularly in transitions and home-based settings.

The book also addresses the growing influence of artificial intelligence in healthcare. Algorithmic bias is framed as a latent safety condition, subtle and distributed, yet capable of distorting judgment and reproducing inequity without triggering traditional alarms. Rather than treating AI as a separate domain, the chapters adapt established safety science approaches to digitally supported workflows, emphasizing governance, transparency, and human accountability.

The final chapter pauses for reflection. Over time, safety, quality, and service have become closely tied to metrics, incentives, and digital systems. These efforts have reduced harm and driven progress. They have also reshaped how care is understood and practiced. The book closes by asking what safety might look like if guided first by care and responsibility rather than performance alone, and how leaders can protect judgment, relationships, and accountability as healthcare continues to evolve.

Together, the chapters offer an experience-based guide for leaders, clinicians, and quality professionals working across the continuum of care. The aim is not to provide definitive answers, but to strengthen the conditions under which organizations can see more clearly, learn more honestly, and act more responsibly in service of patients, families, and the workforce.

# Chapter 1
# From Bedside to System:
## Why This Book Matters


## ABSTRACT

*This chapter reflects on quality, safety, and service as inseparable elements of care, grounded in the author's lived experience transitioning from bedside practice to system leadership. Rather than treating safety as a standalone function, it explores how quality, service, and safety are co-produced in everyday work. Drawing on clinical practice, organizational learning, and safety science, the chapter demonstrates how risk more often arises from routine conditions such as workarounds, transitions, cognitive overload, and communication gaps than from individual failure. Narrative vignettes are integrated with principles from Just Culture, Lean, and human factors to illustrate how systems shape behavior and outcomes. Presence, fairness, curiosity, and psychological safety are presented as essential conditions for reliability. Equity is framed as integral to safety and service, with disparities viewed as signals of preventable harm and opportunities for system redesign.*


## INTRODUCTION

### Beginnings at the Bedside

I did not enter nursing thinking about systems, metrics, or policy. I entered because I wanted to be useful when people needed care, clarity, or reassurance. I learned first through presence. I learned to read a room before I learned to read a report. I trusted what I noticed in patients before I had words for risk, reliability, or human factors. Safety did not appear as a heading on our shift assignments. Sometimes it was the pause before a medication. Sometimes it was a second look at an order that did not feel right. Sometimes it was staying in the room a few minutes longer

DOI: 10.4018/979-8-3373-6496-4.ch001

because a quiet detail needed space to surface. We did not call this safety science. We called it being careful.

We relied on one another. We learned, often quietly, who would listen and who would not. Care felt close. I remember the night shift light, monitors softening the room, the phone ringing down the hallway. I remember the pull between what the protocol asked and what the person in front of me needed. Nothing was theoretical at two in the morning when someone was short of breath, or when a family stood in the doorway with a question that did not fit the chart. The decisions did not feel grand. They were small and continuous. That is where safety grows.

## Conceptual Distinction Between Quality and Safety Competencies

As my work expanded beyond the bedside, I began to see that those same moments depend on different forms of support. Some structures aim to improve consistency and performance. Others aim to anticipate and manage risk when work does not unfold as planned. Quality improvement and patient safety overlap but remain distinct. Quality improvement focuses on standardization, measurement, and optimizing known processes. Patient safety focuses on anticipating, absorbing, and adapting to risk in complex, human-centered systems.

Throughout this book, they appear together by design and not to blur them, but to reflect how reliable care rests on pairing technical improvement methods with safety science, human factors, and cultural conditions that support speaking up and learning. That mirrors how I lived them. These domains did not arrive as separate packages. They emerged together, shaped by daily decisions, relationships, and the realities of care as it actually unfolded.

Quality and safety are not treated here as isolated programs or endpoints. They are interdependent forces that move across settings from hospital to home and find their fullest expression through service, where clinical reliability, human experience, and design meet. This perspective is not theoretical for me. It comes from years alongside clinicians, patients, and families, working through practical realities and the unintended consequences of well-intended systems. I have watched quality and safety improve not only through plans, but through everyday interaction: pausing to listen during a handoff, redesigning a workflow after a near miss, adjusting expectations when the home reveals risks no policy anticipated.

At times, quality, safety, and service were so tightly interwoven that they could not be separated: a safety intervention that improved trust; a quality metric that missed patient experience; a service recovery that exposed a deeper vulnerability. These quiet moments recur throughout the book. They ground the frameworks and tools and keep the work close to real decisions, emotions, and constraints. The strategies are drawn from methods and from lived experience, where humility, attentiveness, and willingness to learn at the point where systems meet human lives are essential.

## When Systems Remain Invisible

In those early years, the system around me was largely invisible. I did not think of the pharmacy as a node in a network, the electronic record as a complex socio-technical tool, or staffing as a risk variable. The system announced itself only when it failed. A missing medication; a lab result that did not post; a transfer delayed without a clear reason.

Routine hid risk. We normalized workarounds because they got us through. We improvised because patients could not wait. We smoothed rough edges in quiet ways and then forgot the edges existed. As we got better at the work, the system faded from view, held together by labor that never appeared in a chart. I took comfort in that invisibility. It felt like craftsmanship. I knew who to call on a hard night. Which physician took concern seriously. Which respiratory therapist would come quickly. Which nurse would watch a patient for me while I managed a new admission. None of it was written down. All of it mattered.

## The Error That Reframed Care

About thirty years ago, I made a medication error that resulted in harm. I offer this as context, not confession. It did not happen because I did not care. It did not happen because I ignored responsibility. It happened in a system where complexity outpaced safeguards and silence replaced clarity. We had no shared language beyond personal fault. No structured way to ask how the system contributed.

The aftermath was tangled. Grief. Shame. Anger. The wish to hide. The urge to defend. The longing to move one decision to a different hour. I remember the patient's face. I remember my own hands. I also remember the quiet afterward. We lost a chance to understand. We talked about vigilance and responsibility. We did not talk about workload, label similarity, floating to another unit during a staffing shortage, a shift change colliding with a complex schedule, or interruptions that fractured thin attention.

That moment changed how I understood care. Not to instill fear, but to deepen attention. I began to see how harm often comes not from a single mistake but from ordinary conditions that align. Workarounds that become normal. Assumptions that go unchallenged. Transitions where responsibility blurs. A memory guides me still. Weeks after the error, I stood outside a patient's room with a new graduate nurse. She paused and whispered that something felt off. Vitals were stable. The plan was clear. She could not yet name the problem, so she stayed a few minutes longer. A gentle question uncovered a medication mismatch that no dashboard would have shown. The pause was ordinary. It was also the difference between risk and safety.

## Learning to See Risk

As my focus shifted from individual patients to teams and from units to organizations, risk began to look like something the system shapes. Not a property of a person who failed. A predictable outcome of conditions. Some risks are obvious. Others stay latent. The most dangerous are often subtle: silence where questions should be; steady reliance on heroics; the quiet normalization of strain. And then there are the busy days when interruptions stack so high that attention itself becomes scarce.

Seeing risk is a discipline. Curiosity helps more than fear. The central question becomes: what in the context made this likely for a conscientious person? The same human strengths that let us improvise can hide the need for structural change. When people repeatedly compensate, leaders must ask what the compensation covers. When the workaround becomes the workflow, it is time to redesign.

This did not pull me away from the bedside. It drew me closer. Patterns repeating across units made sense. Good people felt trapped by the same constraints. Improvement that rests on individual effort alone does not last. Systems return people to their usual grooves unless the system itself changes.

## From Units to Organizations

As my view widened, I saw that patients experience care as a continuum while organizations often live as fragments. A hospitalist makes a plan a skilled nursing facility cannot implement. A clinic sends a message that gets lost between inboxes. A discharge summary answers questions no one asked and misses the ones that matter. Documentation can look complete while the experience feels unfinished.

Presence matters. Not only executive rounds, but the kind of attention given to the place where work actually happens. Leaders who show up with intention and stay long enough to close the loop change the conversation. Observation without action breeds frustration. Listening without follow-through erodes trust. When leaders return with the results of what they heard, reliability improves. When they do not, people stop speaking up.

A wider view also brought humility. Systems are intricate. Change in one area creates new constraints in another. A staffing change that makes one unit more resilient may reduce flexibility elsewhere. A policy that aims for clarity can create confusion once it meets real workflow. Improvement is not only about tools. It is about relationships between people and work. It is about closing the distance between intention and outcome.

## Presence, Leadership, and the Work Between

Leadership did not mean leaving the bedside behind. It meant seeing the system without losing sight of the people inside it. It meant standing where consequences are felt first. It meant asking simple questions and staying for the full answer. It meant returning to the same place after the first effort to see whether the change holds on a busy Tuesday. Presence is a practice. Time is always scarce, so it has to be built into the week. Short rounds with a clear focus. A listening session with one question. Huddles that honor what was learned yesterday and ask what is at risk today. Presence is not surveillance. It is solidarity. It signals that leaders are accountable for conditions, not only for results.

There is a phrase I return to: the work beneath the work. The plan on paper is one layer. The way the plan meets reality is another. When leaders stand long enough in that second layer to understand why the plan bends, they earn the right to ask for change. Without that understanding, requests feel like demands from far away. Safety improves when the distance between decision and consequence gets smaller.

## The Language That Helped Us Name What We Knew

As I learned the language of quality, safety, and service, frameworks gave names and structure to what frontline clinicians knew intuitively. Just Culture created room for honest discussion about accountability. It did not erase responsibility. It placed it in context. It distinguished human error, at-risk behavior, and reckless behavior. It asked leaders to respond with fairness and consistency. Fairness makes it easier to speak up. Learning becomes possible when people feel safe enough to tell the whole story, not only the flattering parts.

Lean and Six Sigma gave structure to curiosity. They framed problems as products of process rather than personality. They honored the people who do the work by asking them to map it. They invited teams to see variation and to test small changes quickly. They reminded us that waste is not only material or time, but the loss of purpose when effort is spent on steps that do not help patients.

Root cause analyses and failure mode reviews shifted focus from who failed to how systems allow failure. Done well, these methods reveal patterns across events that look unrelated. A confusing label in one area is also confusing in another. Gaps at discharge resemble the gaps during transfer from the emergency department. These tools do not replace clinical judgment. They sharpen it by placing it in the flow of work.

The risk is to turn tools into rituals. A tool without curiosity becomes a checkbox. A meeting without honest tension becomes a ceremony. The skill is to hold structure and inquiry together. Ask what the data suggests, then test it against what people experience. Let a method guide the conversation without allowing the method to become the conversation.

## Data and the Distance of Numbers

Data arrived as both light and shadow. Dashboards promised clarity. They also carried risk. Numbers can illuminate. Numbers can distance us from the human experience of care. When teams feel judged rather than invited to learn, they protect themselves. They wait. They explain away variation rather than explore it. Over time, I learned that the most meaningful measures invite dialogue. Measures gain power when paired with stories. Patient experience becomes a safety signal rather than an afterthought. Teams see themselves in data when the conversation begins with their reality, not with a graph alone.

One unit's falls rate improved steadily, then stalled. The dashboard could not say why. The team had implemented standard interventions. In a short huddle, a nurse mentioned that chairs with simple alarms had been replaced during a facilities refresh, and the new alarms took longer to set. The delay led to workarounds. Risk returned quietly through that gap. A small equipment change altered the process enough to cause the plateau. The solution was not more education. It was to fix the mismatch between tool and workflow.

Patient comments told a similar story. A clinic with strong clinical outcomes received lukewarm Likelihood to Recommend scores. No adverse events were recorded. Patients described confusion after visits and uncertainty about next steps. They were signaling risk that incident reports do not capture. The team restructured the end of visits to include a two-minute review with teach-back and a clear written plan at checkout. Trust improved. So did safety, because people knew how to follow the plan.

## Listening That Changes the Work

Patients and families reshaped my understanding of harm. They described moments of confusion, fear, or lack of confidence during transitions. These were early warnings. They pointed to risks not yet visible in any report. When someone hesitates to recommend care to a person they love, something feels unreliable even if no adverse event has occurred.

The listening that changes the work is specific. It asks for the story behind the score. It looks for details a person outside the experience might miss. A discharge packet read by an exhausted patient. A phrase that sounds reassuring to clinicians and dismissive to a family. An instruction that requires a device a patient does not own.

Patient and family advisors became part of the safety team. They saw what we could not. They helped rename problems. They reminded us that the unit's success is finally measured by the person who carries care home. When patients described the confusion of multiple phone numbers or uncertainty when a test result never arrived, they were describing reliability failures. Our terminology shifted, but the aim did not. Safety remained the practice of keeping people from harm, and the most reliable way to do that is to know their experience well.

## Workforce Safety Is Patient Safety

The conditions that place patients at risk also place caregivers at risk. Fatigue, moral distress, and exposure to violence erode the ability to provide safe care. We are not separate from the system we try to improve. We are shaped by it and sometimes injured by it. Protecting staff is not separate from protecting patients. It is foundational.

Psychological safety is a phrase we use often. It can be reduced to a workshop. It is harder to build into daily work. Psychological safety is present when people can ask basic questions without apology. When a student speaks first and a senior clinician changes course. When a person involved in an error is treated with fairness and respect, which is the precondition for telling the truth about what happened.

Emotional recovery matters. Health care holds difficult moments. Grief and moral injury are practical realities that shape attention, decision making, and teamwork. Time for debrief. Access to peer support. Leaders who acknowledge the emotional cost of the work. These are not luxuries. They are prerequisites for reliability. Physical safety is no less urgent. Threats of violence, unsafe patient handling, and exposure to hazards are not only occupational concerns. They affect outcomes directly. A workforce that feels unsafe cannot be fully present. A unit that normalizes risk to staff normalizes risky work. This is safety science. Central, not peripheral.

## Risk That Hides in Plain Sight

Risk does not always announce itself. It sometimes arrives disguised as efficiency. A calendar too full to allow a pause. A culture that praises speed more than clarity. Dependence on a few high performers whose effort cannot be sustained. Some risks live inside assumptions that rarely get named. A completed form is taken to mean understanding. A closed loop is taken to mean that the next question was possible to ask. A new technology looks like it will simplify a step and we do not see the steps it makes harder.

Subtle signals help. The absence of questions in a meeting where questions should be. The phrase it has always been done this way offered as a full explanation. A trendline that improves for a quarter and then sinks back. A checklist gathering dust. These are not signs of indifference. They are signs of strain. They are invitations to ask what is missing.

In one emergency department, sepsis screening improved after a checklist was introduced. Months later, performance slipped. Direct observation revealed the reason. The checklist lived on a clipboard near triage. During peak hours, that clipboard was often in use. Improvement was gated by a piece of plastic. Printing a copy for every bay restored performance. Commitment was not the problem. A small constraint was.

## Transitions Tell the Truth

If you want to see the system, watch a transition. Handoffs, discharges, and moves between settings show how easily responsibility diffuses. Structured tools help only when paired with genuine connection. Patients need to feel known, not processed. Technology can support coordination. Human presence sustains it.

One afternoon, a medicine team delivered a meticulous sign out. The format was perfect. The receiving team had the story, the plan, and anticipated problems. The patient still arrived on the new unit with important questions unanswered. The difference was not in the content. It was in the relationship. The voice that carried the plan did not belong to anyone the patient recognized. A brief warm handoff would have changed the tone of the transition and prevented an avoidable night call when a predictable issue arose.

Discharge tells a similar truth. Strong summaries matter little if the person carrying the plan home does not understand it, cannot act on it, or cannot reach someone when the plan meets real life. A callback within forty-eight hours can surface issues early. A pharmacy review can intercept mismatched instructions. Community partners can bridge the space between clinic and living room. We often treat discharge as the end. Patients experience it as the beginning of a different kind of care that needs connection more than documentation.

## Readiness Before Rollout

Change management confirmed what experience had already taught me. Readiness matters. People rarely adopt what they do not understand, do not want, or do not feel able to sustain. When change skips these steps, it creates compliance without commitment. Durable improvement depends on how change is experienced, not only how it is launched.

Readiness is not a mood. It is a set of conditions. A clear why that resonates with the people who will live the change. Time to learn. A way to ask for help that does not feel like failure. Leaders who adjust the plan when early signals show a mismatch. When these conditions exist, people who felt exhausted by prior initiatives can find energy for a new one. When these conditions are absent, even good ideas feel like burdens.

A clinic adopted a new communication tool to reduce phone tag and missed messages. The rollout date was fixed. Training modules were posted. On the morning of launch, the front desk was short staffed and two clinicians were out sick. The go-live proceeded. Anxiety rose. Workarounds multiplied. The tool became a story about disruption rather than relief. A brief delay, daily practice sessions, and a super user at each station produced a different outcome. The point was not about software. It was about pacing change to the reality of work.

## The Work of Policy

Policy can guide rather than constrain when it is written with intention. The best policies reflect how work actually happens. They reduce guesswork in moments of uncertainty. They support memory in complex processes. They help a person do the right thing when time is short and attention divided. The worst policies exist to satisfy regulation, not to support care. They pile up into layers no one can follow without stopping the work. They create risk by forcing people to choose between compliance and common sense. Cynicism follows. People sign the form and carry on as before, but with less trust.

A question helps: does this policy earn its place? Does it solve a problem that continues to cause harm? Does it remove ambiguity in a process that will remain complex even when well designed? Does it match the cognitive load of the moment in which it will be used? Most of all, does it include the voices of the people who must use it? If clinicians keep a second, unofficial playbook to survive a shift, revise the policy until the unofficial one becomes unnecessary.

## Equity as a Condition for Safety

Equity reframed everything. Disparities are not only unfair. They are signals of preventable harm distributed unevenly. They show where the system fails in patterned ways. Averages conceal. Stratified data reveals. Listening to patients and communities exposes barriers systems have normalized. Once inequity is seen as a safety signal, it is hard to unsee. Missed follow-up appointments are not only scheduling issues. They may reflect transportation, caregiving responsibilities, or language access. Blood pressure control that looks acceptable overall may conceal large gaps across neighborhoods or languages. Such gaps point to harm that can be prevented by redesign, not reminders to try harder.

Equity work is practical. Is information readable in the language and at the level of the person who needs it? Do clinic hours fit people who cannot take time off during the day? Are devices and diet recommendations possible in the home where someone lives? Do algorithms used to allocate services include variables that reduce access for the very groups that need them?

A heart failure program noticed that readmissions clustered in a few zip codes. Instead of increasing education alone, the team partnered with community organizations for home visits, ensured scales were available, simplified sodium guidance with culturally relevant examples, and created a phone pathway without multiple menus. Readmissions fell. Trust improved. Safety improved because care met life as it is, not as policies assumed it to be.

## Algorithms and the Return of Deference

Health care stands at another threshold. Artificial intelligence and algorithm driven decisions bring new forms of risk. The pattern is familiar. Deference to authority, now digital. Confidence without transparency. The temptation to accept output without validation. The language has changed. The lesson has not. Tools do not replace responsibility. Judgment still matters.

I have watched what happens when a model's score is treated as weightier than a clinician's assessment. People hesitate to speak up. They distrust their judgment. The model becomes an authority that cannot be questioned. Leadership must be clear. Tools support decisions. They do not make them. Data science must be accountable to clinical science and to patient experience.

The concern is not only wrong output. It is invisible inequity built into some models. When training data reflect prior access patterns, predictions mirror the bias of history. When proxies for need are proxies for utilization, vulnerable patients can receive less attention precisely because they accessed care less in the past. The safeguard is not rejection of new tools, but insistence on transparency, validation, and the right to say no when output conflicts with what the team sees and what the patient says.

A simple test helps. Can the team explain in plain language what the tool does, what it does not do, and how it might be wrong? Can they describe how it was validated for the population they serve? Do they know how to escalate concerns when the tool and reality diverge? If not, the tool is not ready for bedside use. Safety remains a practice grounded in human judgment.

## Stories That Sustain

Improvement often plateaus. Initiatives lose urgency. Work can feel like pushing a heavy door that barely moves. In those seasons, stories preserve purpose. They remind teams why improvement matters. They stitch together the human meaning behind measures. I keep a small notebook. A nurse who caught a near miss because she trusted her concern enough to ask for a second look. A family who described a discharge call that saved them a trip to the emergency department. A unit clerk who noticed a confusing scheduling phrase and suggested a change that reduced missed appointments. Not headline stories. Daily proofs that reliability grows where people are invited to notice and to act.

Stories also teach. Context is the hidden variable in every intervention. A small change works in one unit and fails in another because the path from plan to action is different. Stories help us close the gap between report and room.

## Why This Book Exists Now

This book grows out of the space between intention and outcome. It is written for those who sense that health care is more than compliance, and improvement more than a series of projects. It speaks to clinicians who want structure without losing the human center of their work, and to leaders who seek presence that changes conditions, not only morale. It is for teams who need language to name what they already know and tools that respect the complexity of care as it is lived.

The chapters that follow do not ask readers to choose between narrative and method. They offer both. Each begins close to the bedside and traces outward to operations, leadership, and policy without leaving the room where care happens. Frameworks are guides, not rituals. Data starts a conversation, not a verdict. Equity sits within the definition of safety, not beside it. Technology is met with curiosity and caution. The work assumes good intent while insisting on clarity, responsibility, and learning.

This book does not promise a destination. Reliable care is not a place we arrive. It is a practice built through presence, fairness, listening, and the courage to learn. It grows through small, everyday decisions and the willingness to name what is fragile. It grows when leaders earn trust by returning with the outcomes of what they heard. It grows when teams see themselves honestly, in data and in the stories of their patients. It grows when policies match the way work actually happens. It grows when we attend to risks that hide in plain sight, when worker well-being is treated as essential to care, and when equity is integral to quality and service.

A memory brings this into focus. Late one evening, a patient grew anxious during a transfer. The handoff was thorough. Equipment worked. Staff were prepared. The patient still felt uneasy. A nurse placed a hand on the bedrail and introduced the night team by name. She explained the plan again, slowly, and asked the patient to repeat it back. She wrote down the name of the person who would answer the call light. The patient exhaled. The room changed. No new policy. No new tool. Something essential returned: presence, clarity, connection.

This is where reliable care begins. In the courage to slow down for what matters. In the discipline of asking why a process bends under real conditions. In the willingness to learn from harm without humiliation. In the respect that treats experience as a signal, not an inconvenience. From bedside to system, this is the work. This is why this book exists.

## Beginnings at the Bedside, Revisited

I end where I began because the beginning still anchors the wider view. If the system does not serve the moment in the room, it does not serve. Indicators can look good. Reports can be clean. If the person in the bed feels unknown or uncertain, the work is not finished. The system will remain complex. Constraints will remain. Improvement will stay a slow art.

There is good news. Small, honest changes compound. When a unit replaces a brittle workaround with a reliable process, people feel the difference. When a leader returns with an answer to a concern raised on rounds, the next concern surfaces sooner. When a team treats a patient's story as a signal rather than a summary, risk comes into view before harm arrives.

That is the spirit of what follows. Not a prescription. Not a promise of a smooth path. An invitation to practice. To hear quiet signals. To see patterns. To bring curiosity to places where blame once lived. To build reliability in ways that respect the complexity of care. The bedside taught me that safety lives in small decisions. The system taught me that small decisions can be designed to go right most of the time. Together, they form a practice that honors the person in the room and the many people who make the room safe.

## What You Can Expect

Each chapter weaves lived experience with structured tools. You will find brief stories that surface specific hazards and practical checklists used as thinking aids rather than substitutes for judgment. The methods diagnose failure in ways that clarify responsibility while protecting dignity. Guidance appears on measuring what matters and pairing numbers with narrative. Throughout, a consistent throughline keeps equity, workforce well-being, and patient experience within the definition of safety.

You will also encounter limits. At times, the guidance will sound like it depends or start here, then test. That is not indecision. It is the humility complex work requires. Context shapes outcomes. What works in one setting often needs translation in another. The goal is not a universal blueprint. It is a way of seeing and working that travels well.

## The Commitments That Hold the Work

If there is a set of commitments that runs through the chapter, it is this:

- Presence as practice. Show up where the work bends, not only where it is presented.
- Fairness with accountability. Hold people to standards while placing action in context.
- Curiosity before certainty. Start with the question that has not been asked yet.
- Data with story. Let numbers matter most when anchored in lived experience.
- Transitions as tests. Watch the handoffs; they reveal the system's seams.
- Readiness before rollout. People take up change when they understand it and can live it.
- Policy as support. Good policy reduces guesswork; revise what creates it.
- Equity as safety. Where patients fall through, the system shows where it needs repair.
- Technology with judgment. Tools support decisions; they do not substitute for them.
- Stories to sustain. Small moments of noticing are what keep the work alive.

These commitments are not complex. The challenge is to live them when time is short and pressure is high. That is why leadership matters. Leaders are responsible for conditions. They are stewards of time, attention, and trust. When leaders protect these resources, teams can practice safety as more than a slogan.

## A Final Word Before We Begin

I often think of the student nurse who paused at the door because something felt off. In many ways, the field asks us to cultivate that pause at scale. A system that makes room for good pauses. A system that notices early signals. A system that treats confusion as a clue. A system that prizes clarity more than speed when the two diverge.

When we do this together, we learn to see risk before it arrives. We build processes that honor attention. We write policies that support judgment. We measure what matters. We bring equity into the center. We use technology with care. We sustain the work with stories. We make health care safer in ways people can feel, not only in ways that look good on paper. That is the hope. That is the work. That is where we will begin.

## CONCLUSION

For me, quality, safety, and service are one story, not three. In health care, they rarely emerge from a single intervention or a single role. They develop through interaction. They depend on one another, and when they fall out of balance, trust and reliability erode quickly. I think about quality and safety as complementary halves of a whole, much like a yin and yang (Figure 1). Each shapes the other. Quality without safety feels incomplete, even performative. Safety without quality becomes narrow and brittle. Service moves between them, not as a boundary, but as a living current. It is the force that translates technical reliability into something patients and families can actually feel. When one element weakens, the others do not remain untouched. The strain travels.

This chapter traced a path from bedside experience to system leadership to show how closely safety, quality, and service are tied together, both personally and structurally. They live in a nurse's pause before administering a medication, in the moment of hesitation that asks whether something feels right. At the same time, that pause is shaped by policies, workflows, staffing levels, and culture that either support it or quietly work against it. What looks like an individual choice is often a system signal in disguise.

The frameworks and stories in this chapter point to a simple truth. Systems shape behavior, and leaders shape systems. When presence, fairness, curiosity, and equity guide decisions, reliability becomes possible. When those commitments thin out, risk moves in to fill the space. The work ahead is not to perfect the system. It is to stay attentive to its pressures, responsive to its signals, and faithful to the people who depend on it, especially when care moves beyond the walls of a single setting.

As shown throughout, quality improvement methods and patient safety principles remain distinct in focus, yet deeply interdependent in practice. This interdependence becomes even more visible as care crosses settings, where risk is shaped less by protocols alone and more by context, transitions, and human experience (Figure 1).

*Figure 1. Quality, safety, and service*

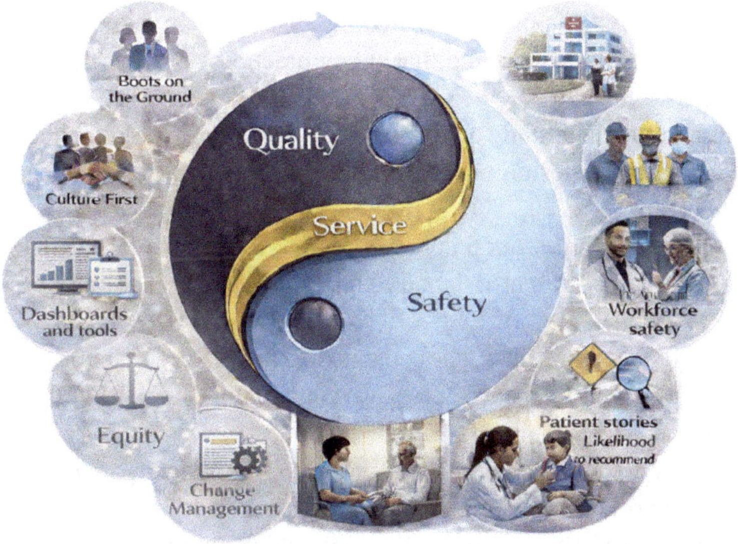

## KEY TERMS AND DEFINITIONS

**Equity in Safety:** The practice of treating disparities in outcomes or access as signals of system failure, ensuring that safety practices address structural barriers and unequal risk.

**Human Factors:** The study of how people interact with tools, technologies, and environments, used to design processes that support cognition, reduce workload, and prevent error.

**Just Culture:** A framework that balances accountability and learning by distinguishing human error from at-risk and reckless behaviors, enabling fair responses and honest reporting.

**Organizational Reliability:** The capacity of a health care system to deliver consistent, high quality performance across varying conditions by aligning processes, culture, and learning structures.

**Patient Safety:** The discipline focused on preventing harm to patients by designing systems that support reliable care, anticipate risk, and reduce vulnerability to error.

**Psychological Safety:** A team condition in which individuals feel safe to speak up, ask questions, acknowledge uncertainty, and report concerns without fear of humiliation or reprisal.

**Readiness for Change:** A set of conditions including clarity of purpose, capability, and psychological availability that determine whether teams can adopt and sustain new practices effectively.

**Systems Thinking:** An approach that examines how structures, processes, relationships, and organizational conditions interact to shape behavior and outcomes in complex health-care environments.

**Transitions of Care:** Points in the care continuum such as handoffs or discharges where information, responsibility, and relationships shift, creating heightened vulnerability to error.

**Workarounds:** Informal or improvised practices developed to bypass constraints within the system; useful in the moment but often indicators of underlying design flaws.

# Chapter 2
# Boots on the Ground:
## Where Safety Live


## ABSTRACT

*This chapter examines how leadership presence at the Gemba, the place where care occurs, strengthens safety, reliability, and trust across healthcare systems. The purpose of this chapter is to demonstrate that effective presence extends beyond visibility and requires disciplined observation, curiosity, emotional intelligence, and follow through. Drawing on influences from nursing, quality improvement, and production systems, the chapter illustrates how leaders who observe work, ask thoughtful questions, and show respect can identify risk earlier than formal reporting systems alone. Through practical examples, the chapter shows how attentive presence reveals system vulnerabilities, supports frontline judgment, and transforms near misses into learning opportunities. Presence is presented as both a systems practice and an ethical commitment, grounded in equity, inclusion, and psychological safety. To translate observation into action, the chapter introduces an impact-based Eisenhower Matrix to help teams prioritize meaningful work and close feedback loops.*


## INTRODUCTION: THE POWER OF PRESENCE

When I first stepped into healthcare leadership, I believed safety was about oversight, more audits, more checklists, more dashboards. Over time, a quieter lesson arrived: showing up. Oversight confirms compliance. Presence builds trust. And when leaders are present, what we think we know changes. Abstraction becomes empathy.

I have watched scorecards help. I have also seen reliability turn brittle without relationships. When care goes sideways, it is usually not for lack of data. It is that no one was close enough, early enough, to notice. The Toyota Production System

DOI: 10.4018/979-8-3373-6496-4.ch002

reframed that stance with a simple discipline: go see, ask why, show respect. In healthcare, that means stepping out of meeting rooms and into corridors, clinics, and homes to listen and learn. The mantra 'go see, ask why, show respect' reframed accountability from blame to curiosity (Liker, 2004).

Presence is not a drive by. It is staying curious, noticing small signals, resisting quick judgment, and staying long enough to learn. Staff report more trust, less burnout, and stronger engagement when leaders make a habit of showing up, asking good questions, and closing the loop (Foster et al., 2023). The effect is not magic. It is psychology and practice. When people feel seen, they speak up earlier, surface near misses, and help craft solutions.

Presence is also a systems tool. Watching work as it happens exposes collisions between policy and workflow and shows how environment and staffing shape choices. Numbers gain texture; stories return to the data. Up close, inefficiency rarely looks like indifference. It looks like fatigue, competing priorities, or a process that does not work. Presence interrupts judgment before it hardens. It turns "Why did they do that?" into "What made that the reasonable choice then?" That shift sits at the heart of Just Culture (Marx, 2001).

In a world of dashboards and alerts, showing up can feel like a quiet rebellion. Technology extends reach, but it cannot replace the meaning made in a careful conversation at the bedside. Organizations where senior leaders are visibly present consistently show stronger teamwork, more open communication, and fewer punitive responses to error (Singer & Tucker, 2014). Especially, when visibility is paired with dialogue and follow up. Prescence builds trust (Sexton et al., 2018). Presence tells you what dashboards miss. It is predictive. The good news: presence requires no new budget line. It asks for time, humility, consistency, and the courage to leave the desk, stand in uncertainty, and listen.

The objectives of this chapter are to:

- Emphasize that safety begins with leadership support and visible presence as the foundation for trust and reliability.
- Position Gemba as a disciplined leadership practice that moves beyond observation to intentional prioritization, action, and accountability.
- Introduce practical frameworks, including an impact based Eisenhower Matrix, to help leaders translate frontline observations into shared priorities and sustained improvement.

With these objectives in mind, the chapter moves from concept to lived leadership practice. Rather than presenting Gemba as an abstract theory, the discussion unfolds through the story of Mrs. Green, whose care journey illustrates how leadership presence combined with thoughtful prioritization and follow through, can surface hidden risks, align teams around what matters most, and drive meaningful operational improvement.

## A LINEAGE OF PRESENCE: FROM NIGHTINGALE TO DEMING

The idea that proximity improves safety is not new. I've always felt connected to Dossey's description of Florence Nightingale during the Crimean War, moving through the wards at Scutari, combining rigorous hygiene practices with deep compassion and transforming simple observation into actionable care (Dossey, 2010). A century later, Deming urged leaders to drive out fear so problems surface early (Deming, 1986). I carry both lenses. One human, one analytic. Toyota later wove them together. When healthcare adopted these ideas, we were not inventing something new. We were remembering something old: the bedside lamp and the process chart belong to the same story.

## HISTORICAL ROOTS OF GEMBA

Gemba ("the real place") was born out of scarcity, precision, and respect. Post-war Toyota leaders realized rigid hierarchies were too slow for complex problems. Solutions lived where value was created (Ohno, 1988). Taiichi Ohno called it Genchi Genbutsu: "go and see for yourself." Not just to look, but to engage, ask quiet questions, and listen. The aim was not to catch mistakes but to understand what made them likely. As these ideas spread, organizations began to see efficiency not as speed but as learning. Quality improved when people felt understood and supported; as Toyota leaders put it, 'go see, ask why, show respect' (Liker, 2004). Two pillars emerged: continuous improvement and respect for people. Both depend on presence.

Healthcare paid attention. To Err Is Human made clear that most errors live in systems, not in bad people. Borrowing from aviation and production, we adopted high reliability methods grounded in transparency, standardization, and continuous learning (Weick & Sutcliffe, 2015). Leadership walk rounds took shape: go to where care happens, ask what gets in the way, and respond. The best encounters are relational, not regulatory.

Organizations like the Institute for Healthcare Improvement and Joint Commission translated this into practice through leadership walk rounds, executives visiting care areas, asking what gets in the way of safety, and responding (Frankel et al., 2003). I've used those same plain questions myself: "What's worrying you today?" "If you could change one thing, what would it be?" The best encounters are relational, not regulatory.

By the 2010s, “Gemba Walk” had become common language in healthcare. Regulators even named leadership visibility as essential to safety culture (Joint Commission, 2019; World Health Organization, 2023). Still, I have seen the meaning thin out, ceremonial walkthroughs with no follow up or over engineered checklists that squeeze out curiosity. The programs that thrive hold the middle: structured enough to learn, flexible enough to stay human. A 2023 review found that curiosity driven walk rounds correlate with stronger safety climates, but only when leaders close the loop (Foster et al., 2023). Without visible action, presence risks feeling performative.

To me, Gemba is less an imported industrial tool than a return to healthcare’s oldest ethic: the discipline of noticing. Nightingale practiced it by lamplight; today I practice it in medication rooms, waiting areas, and living rooms. The lesson has not changed: solutions live where the work happens.

## Gemba Walk Observation and Action

As illustrated in the Gemba Walk Observation and Action Template (Figure 1), a reliable walk uses a simple sequence:

1) Define the purpose. Be clear about what you hope to learn. Align to a theme such as safety, flow, or readiness. Let staff know the walk is about learning, not inspection.
2) Standardize observation. Go see, ask why, listen, avoid assumptions. Watch work as it happens. Use open questions to understand context and variation.
3) Execute the routine. Keep a predictable structure so teams know what to expect. Notice physical cues, workflow patterns, workarounds, and barriers. Learn first; resist fixing in the moment.
4) Close the actions. Convert observations into clear, owned, timebound tasks. Share “you said, we did” updates to reinforce credibility. Move small system fixes quickly to maintain momentum.
5) Measure results. Track simple indicators that show whether changes improved safety or flow. Share results and refine the next cycle.

Some days the walk yields no tidy categories. That is still learning

*Figure 1. Gemba walk observation and action process*

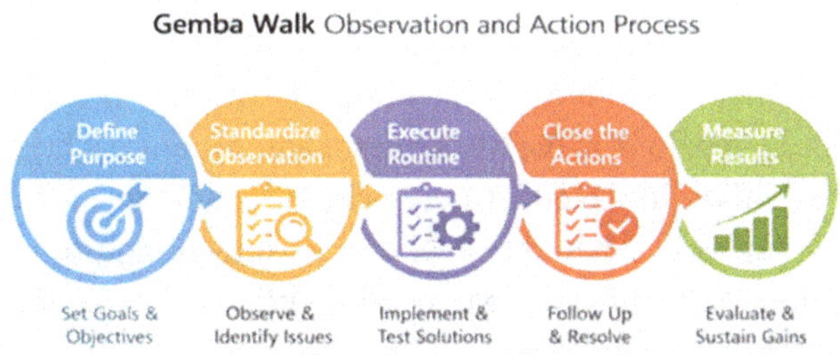


## Making Gemba Fun: Why Joy Matters in Improvement Work

Gemba is serious work. Safety, reliability, dignity live here. Serious does not mean cold. When the tone is curious and warm, people surface near misses earlier. In one unit, a two minute "Gemba wins" wall drew out fixes no form ever captured. Light rituals such as a quick thanks, a hallway laugh, a bright spot jar lower the emotional temperature so truth can enter the room.

## Bringing Joy into Gemba

Once, after a hard night, we arrived with clipboards and good intentions. Staff read the visit as inspection. We paused the checklist, asked two questions, and came back the next shift with coffee and a single action we could close that day. Trust recovered, slowly. Warmth is not decoration. It is a tool.

The goal isn't to turn Gemba into entertainment. The goal is to honor the humanity of the work. Small strategies help:

- **Celebrate small wins intentionally**: a restocked cart, a faster handoff, a tiny process fix that made someone's shift easier.
- **Use visual joy**: boards, stickers, color, simple symbols that create energy.
- **Invite staff to shape the tone:** ask what would make Gemba feel meaningful or fun for them.
- **Share gratitude out loud**: not as a formality, but as recognition of real effort.
- **Bring curiosity instead of critique**: the fastest way to make Gemba feel safe.

These small gestures build the emotional infrastructure that keeps improvement alive.

## Joy Is a Leadership Discipline

Joy is not frivolous; it is strategic. It supports attention, strengthens relationships, and fuels learning the three things Gemba requires most. When leaders show that connection and delight belong in the work, they create a culture where people can not only speak up but thrive. In the end, safety is built by humans, not checklists. And humans do their best work when they feel part of something positive, purposeful, and yes even joyful. While the Gemba process outlines how leaders learn, its true value emerges in the everyday realities it reveals. Mrs. Green's story shows how presence and inquiry translate that process into meaningful action.

## MRS. GREEN'S STORY: WHERE SAFETY LIVES

I will not forget Mrs. Green, eighty-two, retired teacher, a wool blanket around a small frame. Two nights earlier she fell reaching for a kettle. The fracture hurt. Losing independence hurt more. The room gave off oxygen hiss and the soft rhythm of shift change. Her walker sat a few inches too far. She leaned toward it. We moved it closer. Seconds, not minutes, and the room shifted. The nurse added a fall risk tag, moved the walker, updated the mobility plan. A near miss turned into a learning moment because someone paid attention. It was not what I said. It was what I saw.

On the third day, her daughter stood by the door, whispering that the stairs at home were impossible. A rounding supervisor, on her way out, stopped to listen. Within an hour, a care coordinator and physical therapist were at the bedside mapping discharge. Grab bars went in. A shower chair arrived. Responsiveness, not bureaucracy. Listening like that creates psychological safety. It is an early warning system. When people feel heard, they raise concerns sooner.

In clinic, a week later, the waiting room felt crowded and still. No spare chairs. Mrs. Green leaned on a cane, her posture listing. A medical assistant noticed the small tremor in her hand and brought a chair with a cushion. "Let's get you comfortable." Small act, big meaning. A dashboard might show average wait. It cannot show this.

At home, the porch light flickered. Inside, one lamp lit a circle of table and supplies. Mrs. Green reached too far to change a dressing. The nurse moved a small table closer and adjusted the chair. Tension eased. The intervention was not medical. It was practical. Small environmental changes shift independence. We removed barriers rather than adding more services. By the end, she completed her care on her own, unhurried and proud. That small act, organizing, captured something I've always believed about quality and safety: sometimes the greatest interventions are the simplest ones. It reminded me of the CAPABLE program (Community Aging in Place, Advancing Better Living for Elders), developed by Sarah Szanton and colleagues at Johns Hopkins University, which empowers older adults by making small, practical changes that restore independence (Szanton et al., 2011; 2016). Instead of focusing solely on clinical care, CAPABLE looks at the person in their full environment how a grab bar, a better chair height, or a reachable shelf can mean the difference between dependence and autonomy.

## THE ANATOMY OF OBSERVATION

Observation is not standing in a corner with a clipboard. It is building understanding through quiet conversation. "I notice open vials. Can you walk me through how this usually works?" invites explanation, not defense. Presence plus curiosity equals learning. Learning shared becomes safety.

Three lenses help:

- Physical. Lighting, layout, clutter, proximity. I once saw three similar medication tubes in faint print, side by side. In a hurry, anyone could reach wrong. We fixed the labels and the organization.
- Cognitive. "Walk me through what you were thinking." Redundancies that live in experience, not in manuals, often prevent harm.
- Emotional. Tone and silence carry information. In one hospice program, unease at night in the medication room traced back to poor lighting and an unreliable motion sensor. Better bulbs and a timed switch lowered anxiety and errors.

## EMOTIONAL INTELLIGENCE AND PRESENCE

Observation reveals what is visible. Emotional intelligence opens dialogue. Four capacities anchor how leaders enter, respond, and connect.

- Self awareness. Check your presence before you speak. People sense hurry and tension. A breath at the doorway resets tone.
- Relationship management. Empathy only matters if it becomes action. "You said the cart is unsafe" followed by a fix within a week builds trust.
- Self management. Rounds surface discomfort. Choose responses that help, not just ones that solve. Stay silent long enough to learn context.
- Social awareness. Invite the quietest voice: "What is your view?" Problems surface earlier when people feel heard.

At its best, is steady ground. After a medication error, a night shift team braced for reprimand. We sat. "I can see how hard you are trying." The tension fell. No memo. Just steadiness. Admitting uncertainty; "I do not have all the answers yet"; does not weaken credibility. It deepens it. Accountability and learning can coexist. Vulnerability is the bridge.

Seeing is the start. But how leaders show up determines what people share, what they hide, and whether learning becomes safety. That is where emotional intelligence comes in. To understand how these dynamics unfold in practice, it helps to look at a real moment of care that illustrates how observation moves from concept to lived experience. Figure 2.2 illustrates observation as a layered practice that extends beyond what is immediately visible. The physical layer captures what the eyes see, the cognitive layer reflects how individuals interpret and make decisions within context, and the emotional layer attends to what the heart notices, signals of trust, fear, confidence, or strain. Together, these layers emphasize that meaningful observation in care settings requires seeing, thinking, and feeling to fully understand how work is experienced and where safety, quality, and service are shaped.

*Figure 2. Anatomy of observation. depicts illustration of the physical, cognitive, and emotional layers of observation, highlighting what is seen, how it is interpreted, and what is felt*

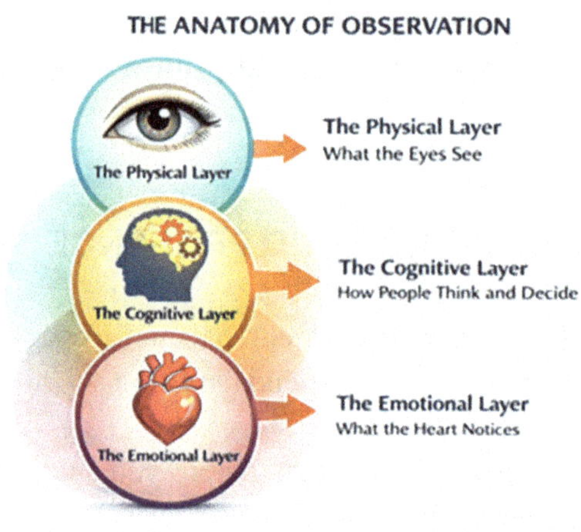

## EMOTIONAL INTELLIGENCE AND THE LEADER'S PRESENCE

Goleman (2022) emphasizes that observation may reveal what is visible, but emotional intelligence is what opens authentic dialogue. It is not an optional skill; it forms the foundation of effective leadership presence. The way leaders show up shapes what people say, what they withhold, and how they feel about their work. To translate this principle into practice, emotional intelligence unfolds through specific capacities that guide how leaders enter, respond, and connect in real time. These capacities begin with self-awareness and extend to self-management, social awareness, and relationship management, each reinforcing presence as a stabilizing force.

### Self-Awareness: Setting the Tone Before Speaking

Before entering any space, leaders must check their own presence. Am I rushing? Tense from the last meeting? People sense that energy before a word is spoken. A hurried walk or folded arms can unintentionally communicate judgment. Pausing at the doorway, taking a breath, and reminding oneself, *I'm here to learn, not to fix,* shifts the tone immediately. Conversations open (Hatfield et al., 1994).

### Self Management: Responding with Intention, Not Impulse

Rounds often reveal uncomfortable truths, broken processes, strained staff, and gaps between ideal and real. Early in my career, I tried to correct everything on the spot. Over time, I learned that self management means choosing responses that help, not just ones that "solve." Sometimes it means staying silent long enough to understand context. Asking, *What made this the best choice at the time?* opens problem-solving without blame (Marx, 2001).

### Social Awareness: Listening for What Isn't Said

In every team, some voices fall to the background, often carrying the most insight. Looking for the quietest person and asking, *What's your view?* has changed my understanding more times than I can count. Listening this way is not just kind; it's strategic. When people feel heard, they surface problems earlier and fewer surprises follow (Goleman, 2022).

### Relationship Management: Turning Empathy into Action

Empathy matters only when it leads to follow up. When a nurse says the supply cart is unsafe and it is fixed within a week, that's not just improvement; it is trust.

Over time, "you said, we did" moments accumulate into credibility. Relationship management is not about being liked; it is about being reliable (Sexton et al., 2018).

## Presence as Steady Ground

Presence, at its best, is emotional regulation in real time, helping teams move from fear to focus and from defensiveness to dialogue. I once joined a night shift team shortly after a medication error. The staff were anxious, bracing for reprimand. I sat and said, *"I can see how hard you're trying.* The tension shifted. No memo followed; just the sense that leadership could mean empathy. That night taught me: calm is contagious (Hatfield et al., 1994). When leaders show up grounded, others find their footing too. Emotional intelligence opens honest dialogue; vulnerability keeps it open and makes learning possible (Edmondson, 2018). For a long time, I believed leaders had to project certainty, answers, direction, poise. Experience softened that belief. Confidence without honesty feels distant; honesty without humility feels brittle. The balance is vulnerability (Edmondson, 2018). After a complex transition went poorly, the team waited for my verdict. Instead, I began with, *I do not have all the answers yet. I need your help understanding what happened.* The tone shifted immediately. People spoke freely, not fearfully. I learned that admitting uncertainty does not weaken credibility; it deepens it (Edmondson, 2018).

The same lesson surfaced one evening when a nurse wept after a long term patient's unexpected death. I sat beside her, silent. There was nothing to fix and nothing to document, only presence. When she finally said, *thank you for staying,* I realized leadership is not always about saying the right thing; it's often about staying with the hard thing (Goleman, 2022). I have seen vulnerability modeled upward, too. A senior leader opened a safety summit by sharing a personal mistake, though not catastrophic, but formative. The room changed in seconds. People stopped performing and started reflecting. When leaders tell the truth about their humanity, others find permission to be human (Edmondson, 2018).

In Just Culture work, we say accountability and learning must coexist. Vulnerability is what bridges them. It signals you are safe to tell the truth, and the truth makes us stronger (Marx, 2001). Over time, pairing vulnerability with follow-up: "*you said, we did*", builds credibility and strengthens safety culture (Sexton et al., 2018; Singer & Tucker, 2014). Now, when I teach new leaders about presence, I say: *It is okay not to know. It is not okay not to care.* Uncertainty shared with sincerity builds more credibility than perfection ever could (Edmondson, 2018). Truth telling and trust-building only work if our presence reaches the entire system. That demands equity in visibility (Joint Commission, 2019; World Health Organization, 2023).

## EQUITY IN VISIBILITY

Presence must be distributed fairly across shifts, roles, and places. Early on, my own visibility mapped to daytime and to the most visible disciplines. Night and weekend rounds revealed a different reality; quiet, candid, sometimes lonely. Tracking our time showed imbalance. Nurses saw leadership often; environmental services and warehouse teams rarely did. I changed the pattern. Each week, every discipline at least once. Safety insights live everywhere: in a driver's icy driveway, a scheduler's duplicate referral, a janitor's trip hazard. Inclusion begins with where attention lands.

## CULTURAL AWARENESS AND INCLUSION

Equitable presence means removing barriers that keep voices out. During a hospice huddle, aides stood quiet. They spoke Spanish among themselves, then switched to English when leaders arrived. We tested bilingual huddles with live translation. Participation nearly doubled. Inclusion is not a guest pass to a meeting. It is the removal of what silences people.

## THE ETHICS OF PRESENCE

With time, presence has come to feel like an ethic. To see someone fully, especially when the work is hard and unseen; is a form of respect. To walk by and not notice is its own kind of neglect. Recognition should not wait for crisis. It should meet people in the steady rhythm of what they do right every day. Ethics begin earlier than data: in the way we notice, listen, and follow through.

## PRACTICE IMPACT

Where presence is practiced as a discipline and paired with follow through, measurable changes appear fewer process delays, stronger safety culture indicators, and fewer rework events and escalations. In one implementation, we tracked walk frequency, action closeout time, missing supplies, and staff access to tools. Over time, indicators improved and credibility rose as actions closed faster and duplicate escalations fell. Not everything moved. One metric; turnaround time on cross shift restocks; stalled for two cycles. The fix required a small calendar change and a late evening handoff check. Once we protected that slot, restocks stabilized. Sharing both wins and stalls with the frontline kept trust intact.

## THE IMPACT BASED EISENHOWER MATRIX

These outcomes make one point clear: presence creates visibility, but action creates change. Without a structured way to prioritize what leaders observe, even the best intentions can dissolve into reactive firefighting. To bridge that gap, organizations need a disciplined approach that converts observation into impact. We prioritize with an Eisenhower lens: 'what is important is seldom urgent, and what is urgent is seldom important'. In clinical operations, that means defending work, the small system fixes that stop tomorrow's escalations (Tronier, 2025; Bell, 2025). The Eisenhower Matrix (Figure 3), originally based on President Dwight D. Eisenhower's principle that "what is important is seldom urgent, and what is urgent is seldom important," provides a structured framework for prioritization. It categorizes tasks into four quadrants, helping leaders distinguish between immediate action and strategic investment (Bell, 2025):

**Quadrant I** (High Impact / High Urgency): Work that is both urgent and consequential, requiring immediate leadership ownership and action. These are critical issues that cannot wait such as safety hazards or compliance breaches.

**Quadrant II** (High Impact / Lower Urgency): Work that meaningfully strengthens systems, culture, and reliability over time and must be deliberately protected even when it does not demand immediate attention. This is where operational effectiveness and long term resilience are built (Berwick, 1989; Tronier, 2025).

**Quadrant III** (Low Impact / High Urgency): Work that feels pressing but does not materially improve outcomes. These tasks often create noise and should be delegated, streamlined, or questioned to prevent distraction from higher value priorities.

**Quadrant IV** (Low Impact / Low Priority): Activities that add little or no value and can be eliminated to create capacity for higher impact priorities. Removing these tasks frees time for strategic work (Bell, 2025).

We approach the model not as a simple productivity tool, but as a leadership discipline. Together, we sort what we observed into these four categories during debrief sessions. This shared exercise allows us to reach consensus quickly and objectively. Rather than debating opinions or deferring to hierarchy, we anchor decisions in impact and urgency. The Eisenhower model gives us a structured way to agree on what deserves leadership attention now, what must be protected for later, and what can safely be deprioritized (Tronier, 2025; Bell, 2025).

The Eisenhower (Impact–Effort) Matrix illustration (Figure 2.3) provides a practical framework for prioritizing work by distinguishing between what is urgent, what is important, and what truly drives impact. By visually mapping tasks across four quadrants, the matrix helps leaders and teams focus immediate attention on high-impact, time-sensitive issues that require action now, while deliberately protecting time for important but non-urgent work that prevents future failures and builds long-term reliability. It also clarifies which activities should be delegated or streamlined and which low-value tasks should be minimized or eliminated altogether. In quality and safety work, this approach supports disciplined decision-making, reduces reactive overload, and ensures that effort is aligned with outcomes that matter most to patients, staff, and the organization.

*Figure 3. Eisenhower (impact–effort) matrix illustrating how to prioritize work based on urgency, importance, and impact*

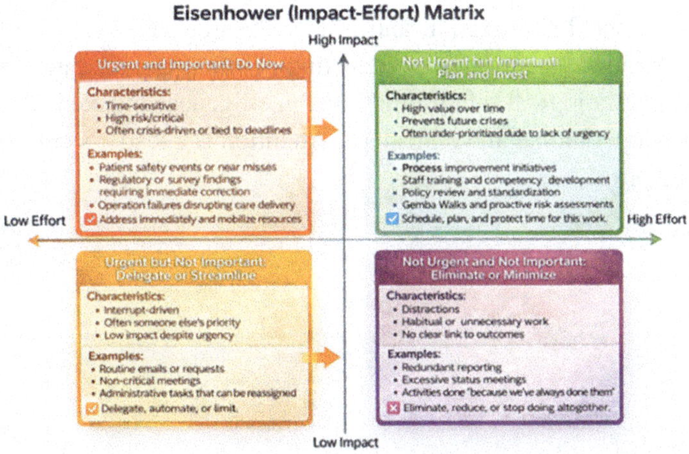


## BRINGING IT HOME: LEADERSHIP REFLECTIONS

Mrs. Green's journey from bed to clinic chair to kitchen table mirrored the continuum of care. Safety is not a department or a checklist. It is a relationship among people and places, renewed each day. Presence connects those places. It turns isolated systems into a network of trust. Dashboards can rise. Compliance can improve. What sustains both is the consistent act of showing up, asking, listening, and acting with integrity.

Lessons I carry:

- Presence is prevention. The earlier you see it, the sooner you can change it.

- Listening is leadership. Sometimes silence is the intervention.
- Equity is visibility. Safety either belongs to everyone or it does not hold.
- Action closes the loop. "You said, we did" is the backbone of trust.
- Calm travels. When leaders are steady, teams find courage.

## CONCLUSION

Leadership visibility in healthcare is not a symbol. It is a discipline. Safety and reliability emerge when leaders move beyond oversight and show up with purpose; observing, listening, and acting where care happens. The details that often matter most are small and human: a walker within reach, a pause to listen, a light adjusted in a night room, a table moved within arm's length. Observation alone does not drive improvement. Prioritization and follow through do. The Eisenhower lens helps teams defend system fixes while acting on what cannot wait. Grounded in Just Culture, psychological safety, emotional intelligence, and equity, presence becomes both an operational and ethical act. Attention is a leader's currency. Follow through is the proof.

## REFERENCES


Bell, S. (2025, July 25). Eisenhower's urgent/important principle. *Mind Tools*.

Berwick, D. M. (1989). Continuous improvement as an ideal in health care. *The New England Journal of Medicine*, *320*(1), 53–56. DOI: 10.1056/NEJM198901053200110 PMID: 2909878

Deming, W. E. (1986). *Out of the crisis*. MIT Press.

Dossey, B. M. (2010). *Florence Nightingale: Mystic, visionary, healer* (2nd ed.). Springer.

Edmondson, A. C. (2018). *The fearless organization: Creating psychological safety in the workplace for learning, innovation, and growth*. Wiley.

Foster, M., Shultz, B. M. A., & Mazur, Ł. (2023). Impact of leadership walkarounds on operational, cultural, and clinical outcomes: A systematic review. *Journal of Patient Safety*, *19*(6), 455–462. DOI: 10.1097/PTS.0000000000000992 PMID: 37827728

Frankel, A., Grillo, S. P., Baker, E. G., Huber, C. N., Abookire, S., Grenham, M., Console, P., O'Quinn, M., Thibault, G., & Gandhi, T. K. (2003). Patient safety leadership walkrounds at Partners HealthCare. *Joint Commission Journal on Quality and Safety*, *29*(1), 16–26. https://pubmed.ncbi.nlm.nih.gov/12520830. DOI: 10.1016/S1549-3741(03)29003-1 PMID: 12528570

Goleman, D. (2022). *Emotional intelligence: Why it can matter more than IQ* (25th anniversary ed.). Bantam.

Hatfield, E., Cacioppo, J. T., & Rapson, R. L. (1994). *Emotional contagion*. Cambridge University Press.

Joint Commission. (2019). *High reliability in healthcare: Creating the culture and improving the process*. Joint Commission Resources.

Liker, J. K. (2004). *The Toyota way: 14 management principles from the world's greatest manufacturer*. McGraw-Hill.

Marx, D. (2001). *Patient safety and the "Just Culture."*. Columbia University.

Ohno, T. (1988). *Toyota production system: Beyond large-scale production*. Productivity Press.

Sexton, J. B., Adair, K. C., Leonard, M. W., Frankel, T. C., Proulx, J., Watson, S. R., Magnus, B., Bogan, B., Jamal, M., Schwendimann, R., & Frankel, A. S. (2018). Providing feedback following Leadership WalkRounds is associated with better patient safety culture, higher employee engagement and lower burnout. *BMJ Quality & Safety*, *27*(4), 261–270. DOI: 10.1136/bmjqs-2016-006399 PMID: 28993441

Singer, S. J., & Tucker, A. L. (2014). The evolving literature on safety WalkRounds: Emerging themes and practical messages. *BMJ Quality & Safety*, *23*(10), 789–800. DOI: 10.1136/bmjqs-2014-003416 PMID: 25228779

Szanton, S. L., Wolff, J. W., Leff, B., Thorpe, R. J., Tanner, E. K., Boyd, C., Xue, Q., Guralnik, J., Bishai, D., & Gitlin, L. N. (2011). CAPABLE trial: A randomized controlled trial of nurse, occupational therapist, and handyman to reduce disability among older adults: Rationale and design. *Contemporary Clinical Trials*, *32*(6), 1–9. DOI: 10.1016/j.cct.2011.05.003 PMID: 24685996

Szanton, S. L., Wolff, J. W., Leff, B., Thorpe, R. J., Tanner, E. K., Boyd, C., Xue, Q., Guralnik, J., Bishai, D., & Gitlin, L. N. (2016). CAPABLE program: Outcomes of a randomized trial of community aging in place. *Health Affairs*, *35*(9), 1558–1565. DOI: 10.1377/hlthaff.2016.0140 PMID: 27605633

Tronier, R. (2025, December 29). The Eisenhower Matrix: How to prioritize your to-do list. *Asana Resources*.

Weick, K. E., & Sutcliffe, K. M. (2015). *Managing the unexpected: Sustained performance in a complex world* (3rd ed.). Wiley. DOI: 10.1002/9781119175834

World Health Organization. (2023). *Global patient safety action plan 2021–2030: Towards eliminating avoidable harm in health care*. WHO Press.

## KEY TERMS AND DEFINITIONS

**Gemba:** The physical or virtual location where work is performed and value is created.

**Just Culture:** An organizational framework that balances system accountability with individual responsibility by distinguishing human error from reckless behavior.

**Psychological Safety:** A shared belief that individuals can speak up with ideas, questions, or concerns without fear of negative consequences.

**High-Reliability Organization (HRO):** An organization that operates in complex, high-risk environments while maintaining consistently low rates of serious failure.

**Eisenhower Matrix:** A decision-making framework that prioritizes tasks based on urgency and importance.

**Operational Effectiveness:** The ability of an organization to perform processes efficiently by minimizing waste and maximizing quality.

**Genchi Genbutsu:** A principle emphasizing direct observation at the source of work to understand processes and problems.

**Sensitivity to Operations:** An HRO principle characterized by continuous awareness of frontline activities and system conditions.

**Cultural Humility:** A lifelong commitment to self-reflection and self-critique that recognizes the limits of one's own cultural perspective.

## APPENDIX I

The appendix below include practical tools and examples that extend the chapter's discussion and support real-world application of the concepts presented.

### Gemba Walk: Five-Step Observation and Action Framework

Use this framework to turn real world observations into reliable action, strengthen visibility, and build trust; one walk at a time (Figure 4).

1. Define the Purpose
    - Clarify *why* you are walking and what you hope to learn.
    - Align the purpose with a specific theme (e.g., safety, flow, readiness).
    - Communicate the intent so staff know the walk is about learning, not inspection.
2. Standardize Observation
    - Use a consistent method: **go see → ask why → listen → avoid assumptions**.
    - Observe work as it actually happens, not as it appears on paper.
    - Ask open-ended questions to understand context and variation.
3. Execute the Routine
    - Follow a predictable structure so teams know what to expect.
    - Notice physical cues, workflow patterns, workarounds, and barriers.
    - Focus on learning, not fixing in the moment.
4. Close the Actions
    - Convert observations into clear, owned, time-bound actions.
    - Share "**you said, we did**" updates to reinforce credibility.
    - Implement small system fixes quickly to maintain momentum.
5. Measure Results
    - Track simple indicators that show whether changes improved safety or flow.
    - Share results transparently and refine processes based on what you learn.
    - Use insights to guide the next cycle of Gemba work.

*Figure 4. Gemba walk: Five-step observation and action framework*

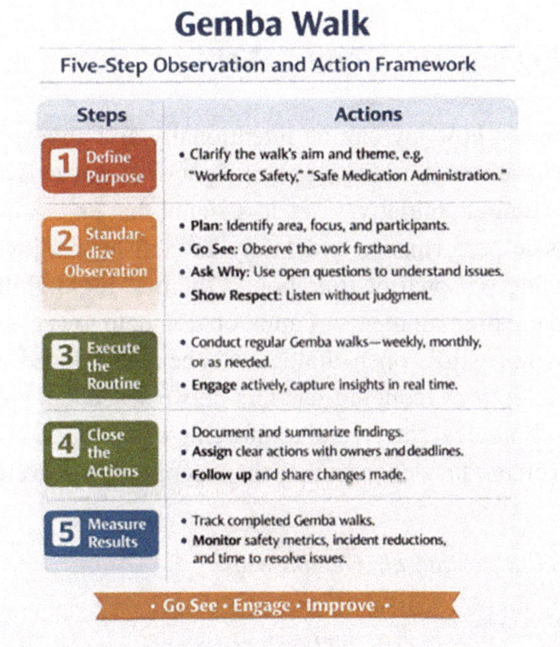

## APPENDIX II

### Introducing Joy into the Gemba Walk

Figure 5 illustrates how joy can be intentionally and appropriately integrated into Gemba Walks without diminishing their rigor or purpose. By anchoring "fun" to organizational strategic initiatives, leaders signal that engagement and learning are valued alongside performance and safety. Establishing a joy theme linked to strategic goals, using seasonal or time bound themes, highlighting "great catch" safety stories, and creating moments of appreciation help lower anxiety, encourage participation, and normalize open dialogue. When introduced thoughtfully, joy serves as a leadership tool reducing barriers between leaders and frontline staff, strengthening psychological safety, and reinforcing that continuous improvement is a shared, human centered endeavor rather than a compliance exercise.

*Figure 5. Introducing joy into the Gemba walk*

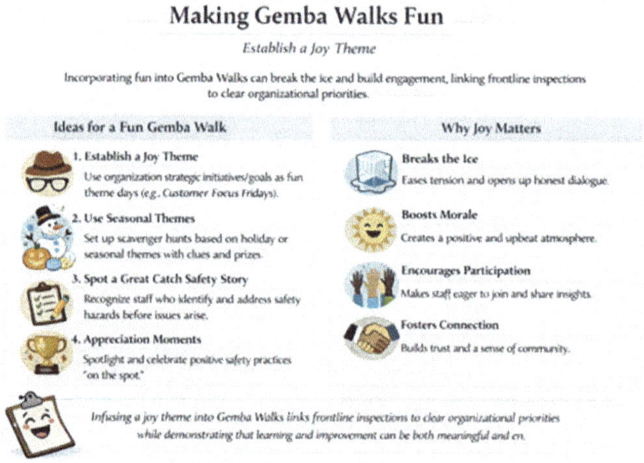

# Chapter 3
# Culture First:
## Laying the Foundation With Just Culture and Team Engagement


## ABSTRACT

*This chapter examines how a durable culture of safety is shaped less by rules alone and more by relationships grounded in trust and fairness. The purpose of this chapter is to illustrate how Just Culture evolves from a conceptual framework into a daily practice that balances accountability with compassion. Drawing on real situations across hospitals, clinics, and home care settings, the chapter demonstrates how leadership presence, purposeful visibility, and emotional intelligence influence engagement and reliability. Practical tools, including the Just Culture Algorithm and an implementation guide, are presented to support consistent and equitable decision making. By integrating improvement science, systems thinking, and human factors, the chapter outlines a practical approach for embedding psychological safety and shared learning into everyday work, emphasizing that safety is strengthened when leaders and staff address challenges together with attention, empathy, and integrity.*


## INTRODUCTION. WHERE CULTURE BEGINS

In healthcare, risk rarely announces itself cleanly. It tends to surface in the seams between shifts, between screens, between what policy assumes and what work actually looks like. We respond with structure: policies, dashboards, metrics. All of that matters. Still, when something goes wrong, the first thing people register is not a data point. It is uncertainty. What happens next depends less on what exists on paper than on how leaders respond in that moment.

I learned this early, working a night shift in the ICU. A medication error came to light during change of shift. The patient was stable, yet the room felt tense in a

DOI: 10.4018/979-8-3373-6496-4.ch003

way numbers do not capture. The nurse explained what had happened; calm, careful, clearly choosing her words. I had seen similar situations handled differently, often moving quickly toward discipline because it signals control. That morning, the manager did something else. She slowed the conversation. She asked what the ordering screen looked like at six a.m., who was in the room, which alerts fired, and where the handoff became fragmented. The focus shifted not away from accountability, but away from the individual and toward the conditions shaping the decision. It was brief. It never appeared on a report. But people noticed. When a near miss occurred later, staff spoke up earlier. Experiences like that do not announce themselves as culture change, but they accumulate. Culture is written quietly, first in pencil, then in ink.

Just Culture offers a shared language for moments like these. It rests on a simple, often neglected premise: not all errors are the same. Human error, at-risk behavior, and reckless behavior arise from different contexts and intent, and they call for different leadership responses. When organizations collapse those distinctions, reporting tends to fall off and complexity gets reduced to blame. At the same time, Just Culture is not comfortable. Leaders may worry that it softens accountability. Staff may hold back, watching to see whether the framework holds when pressure rises. That unease is not incidental. It is part of the work. As the literature on safety culture and leadership WalkRounds suggests, credibility is built through repeated, aligned responses over time not through isolated initiatives or statements of intent (Singer & Tucker, 2014).

Engagement develops under similar conditions. When people believe that speaking up carries personal risk, engagement narrows into task completion and self protection. When fairness is experienced consistently, engagement widens into problem solving, peer accountability, and shared ownership. In practice, this often looks ordinary: a resident pausing to ask whether a dose makes sense, or a respiratory therapist flagging a ventilator that fails intermittently but predictably. These are small acts, but they matter. They signal what is safe to notice and what is safe to say.

This chapter argues for establishing Just Culture and team engagement early and doing so together. Either one on its own is unstable. Just Culture without engagement risks becoming procedural. Engagement without Just Culture lacks a reliable backbone for fairness and accountability. When aligned, the two allow teams to learn while continuing to move forward. Applied with discipline, Just Culture provides a framework for accountability that accounts for system design as well as individual choice (Dekker, 2016). Paired with genuine engagement, it creates the conditions where people speak sooner, interpret risk collectively, and take responsibility not only for their tasks, but for one another.

## Objectives of this chapter

- Explain why a sustainable safety culture begins with trust, fairness, and psychological safety rather than compliance alone.
- Define core Just Culture principles and show how they balance accountability with learning.
- Offer practical steps for embedding these principles in daily work using tools like the Just Culture Algorithm and engagement habits that strengthen reliability.

## WHAT IS JUST CULTURE?

As Marx (2001) notes, the strength of a Just Culture lies in its ability to distinguish between human error, at risk behavior, and reckless behavior, ensuring that each is met with a response that is both fair and proportionate. It is a way of leading that brings fairness, accountability, and learning into balance. Most safety events do not come from one person making one bad choice in a vacuum. They emerge from system pressures, design gaps, and human limits. The heart of Just Culture is classification with care:

- **Human error** calls for consoling and system redesign.
- **At-risk behavior** calls for coaching and better alignment of incentives and design.
- **Reckless behavior** calls for firm accountability.

This reframes the question from "Who is at fault?" to "What allowed this and how do we prevent it?" When staff trust that honesty will be met with curiosity before judgment, they surface weak signals and near misses earlier. That is when learning accelerates.

## BEHAVIORS IN A JUST CULTURE

### Human Error

Human error refers to slips, lapses, or mistakes unintentional actions that occur despite good intentions and reasonable effort. Marx (2001) reminds us that these errors are an inevitable part of human performance. They are best met with support and system review, not punishment. The leader's role is to look beyond the individual and examine the conditions that made the error possible: design flaws, workflow complexity, cognitive load, interruptions, and environmental factors. The work is not to assign fault, but to strengthen the system so the same mistake is less likely to occur again.

## At Risk Behavior

At-risk behavior arises when someone takes a shortcut or departs from expected practice because the risk appears low, familiar, or outweighed by competing demands. Marx (2001) describes this as behavioral drift; often shaped by production pressure or the gradual normalization of deviance rather than by ill intent. The appropriate response is coaching. That means helping individuals recognize hidden risk, addressing the pressures that make shortcuts feel necessary, and redesigning processes so the safer choice is also the easier one.

## Reckless Behavior

Reckless behavior involves a conscious disregard of a substantial and unjustifiable risk; an intentional choice that falls outside what a reasonable peer would consider acceptable. Marx (2001) notes that this category warrants remedial or disciplinary action, not to assign blame, but to uphold shared professional standards and protect organizational integrity. Within a Just Culture framework, recklessness is the only category in which punitive action is appropriate. Figure 3.1 illustrates the three Just Culture behavior categories: human error, at-risk behavior, and reckless behavior and the corresponding leadership responses of system improvement, coaching, and accountability in support of learning and safety.

*Figure 1. Three behavioral categories within a Just Culture framework based on Marx's Just Culture model*

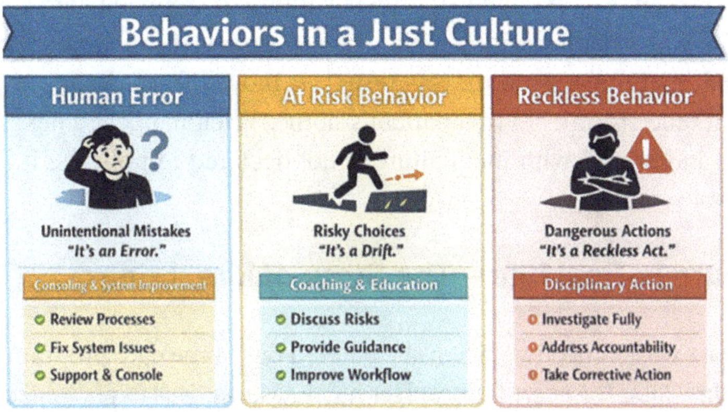
Behaviors in a Just Culture
Human Error
Unintentional Mistakes
"It's an Error."
Consoling & System Improvement
Review Processes
Fix System Issues
Support & Console
At Risk Behavior
Risky Choices
"It's a Drift."
Coaching & Education
Discuss Risks
Provide Guidance
Improve Workflow
Reckless Behavior
Dangerous Actions
"It's a Reckless Act."
Disciplinary Action
Investigate Fully
Address Accountability
Take Corrective Action

Understanding these distinctions stopped being a tidy theoretical exercise the day I watched a nurse shrink under a single question: *"Who was on duty?"* Until that moment, Just Culture made sense to me on paper. Marx's framework felt orderly; the clean separation of behaviors, the tailored responses, the emphasis on fairness (Marx, 2001). But in that instant, I saw how quickly a team could retreat into silence when accountability is framed as fault rather than context.

The categories Marx describes unintentional human error that calls for consoling, at-risk behavior that requires coaching, and the rare but real reckless behavior that warrants disciplinary action suddenly had faces, emotions, and consequences. I realized then that misclassifying behavior does more than lead to the wrong response. It changes the emotional temperature of the room. It determines whether people lean in or shut down. Just Culture became real to me not through policy or training, but through the look in a clinician's eyes when she was unsure whether honesty would be met with curiosity or judgment.

## A JUST CULTURE MOMENT

Early in my leadership journey, I sat in a safety huddle as a nurse nervously described a medication near miss. She spoke quickly; eyes fixed on the floor. When she finished, someone asked, *"Who was on duty?"* In that moment, the room shifted. Her shoulders stiffened, and the conversation ended before it could begin. That experience taught me that psychological safety is not about whether we hold people accountable: it is about how we do it. When accountability lacks empathy, people retreat. When empathy lacks accountability, standards erode. The work of leadership is holding both firmly and fairly.

That day reshaped how I understood Just Culture. It stopped being a framework and became a way of being with people when outcomes disappoint us. In the days that followed, that understanding was tested. It moved from theory into practice not in a conference room, but in a patient's home. What happened next reinforced a lesson that has stayed with me: culture is not declared in policies. It is revealed in moments of honesty.

## Just Culture in Real Life – The Story of Mrs. Lopez

Mrs. Lopez was eighty-two when she entered our home care program following a hospital admission for heart failure. Her nurse, Maria, was experienced and careful, the kind of clinician others naturally trusted. One morning, Maria called me. Her voice was unsteady. She explained that she had documented the previous day's weight instead of the current one. Overnight, the patient's weight had increased. Maria caught the error the next morning and acted immediately, but she was shaken.

*"I can't believe I missed that," she said. "I feel awful."*

There was a pause before I responded. Earlier in my career, I might have gone straight to the mechanics of the error; what step failed, where the process broke down. This time, the response began somewhere else.

*"You caught it, and you spoke up." That matters most right now," I said. "Let's learn from it together."*

We walked through the process and uncovered a design gap: the electronic record provided no alert when a patient's weight exceeded established parameters. Correcting that flaw was straightforward. What stayed with me was something smaller. I remember the look of relief on Maria's face when she realized she was being supported rather than judged.

Later, she told me, "That conversation made it easier for me to speak up again." That was when I truly understood the reach of a leader's reaction. Every response sets a direction. A careless comment can quiet a team for months. A moment of grace can sustain honesty for years.

## LEADERSHIP REFLECTION – THE CULTURE WE WRITE WITH OUR REACTIONS

Culture rarely shifts through sweeping reforms. It changes through single interactions. Policies create structure, but people give that structure character. A Just Culture is not built through modules or memos; it takes shape in the split second between hearing about a problem and deciding how to respond. When I pause before reacting, I almost always uncover something I would have otherwise missed; a system flaw hiding behind a human error, or fear disguised as silence. Each pause becomes a kind of mirror, revealing not only the issue at hand, but my own role in shaping the response.

Experience has shown me that trust does not grow from avoiding difficult conversations. It grows when those conversations preserve dignity. The aim is not to soften accountability, but to anchor it in fairness. People can accept consequences when they believe the process is just; what erodes trust is humiliation. As Marx (2001) reminds us, fairness is not the opposite of accountability; it is what makes accountability possible. When people stop fearing shame, they begin to tell the truth. That is where safety work truly begins.

The story of Mrs. Lopez may seem ordinary, and that is precisely what gives it weight. Most safety breakthroughs do not happen in boardrooms. They unfold quietly, in moments like hers; uncertain, unguarded, and profoundly human. In those spaces, a leader's tone can alter the entire trajectory of a team's learning.

I saw this again years later in a case involving a misplaced medication label. Instead of scolding, the manager sat beside the pharmacist and walked through the process step by step. Together, they noticed that the label printer sat across the counter, forcing staff to multitask mid process. Moving it closer reduced labeling errors by half within a month. The fix mattered. The mindset that made it possible mattered more.

Over time, it has become clear to me that culture is not built through slogans or campaigns. It is built through micro moments: the pause before judgment, the question asked with genuine curiosity, the consistency that proves promises are real. A checklist cannot protect a patient if the person using it feels unsafe to speak. The soil must be ready before improvement can take root.

supports what lived experience reveals. Teams that establish psychological safety show higher engagement, clearer communication, and lower turnover (Edmondson, 2018). When staff feel trusted, they report more near misses, not fewer. That increase signals vigilance, not weakness. It means the system is beginning to see what was once invisible.

## TRUST AS THE STRONGEST SAFETY SYSTEM

Once trust takes root, it becomes one of the most efficient forms of risk management a team has. When people trust their leaders, they stop performing for inspection and start performing for purpose. I've seen nurses stay late to debrief, not because they were told to, but because they believed someone would actually listen. I've seen technicians share quiet workarounds that made care safer, not faster. These are not compliance behaviors. They are belonging behaviors.

Leaders often remind their teams that culture is not written in manuals. It lives in hallways, when no one is watching. It shows up in the nurse who admits a near miss with a shaky voice, the aide who gently corrects a peer, and the leader who says, "I don't have all the answers, but I'm here." None of these moments appear on dashboards, yet their effect is unmistakable. A genuine Just Culture is not soft; it is disciplined. It requires precision in distinguishing human error from at-risk or reckless behavior (Frankel et al., 2006). It asks leaders to investigate context rather than people. One of the hardest habits I had to unlearn was solving too quickly. Real learning often lives in the discomfort of holding complexity a little longer before closing the loop.

Culture comes first because everything else rests on it. Without trust, tools turn into rituals. Without engagement, policies fade into wallpaper. Anything built on fragile culture eventually collapses under pressure. When trust is earned and visible, improvement becomes almost self-sustaining.

## LEARNING WITHOUT FEAR

At a hospital where I once worked, a pharmacist caught a chemotherapy dose entered at ten times the intended strength. Years earlier, that discovery might have triggered a tense root-cause meeting; chairs scraping, voices tight, eyes down. This time, the tone was different. The discussion did not begin with *Who entered it wrong?* But with *Where did the process fail?* Using the Just Culture algorithm, the team asked whether this was human error, at-risk behavior, or reckless disregard. They quickly noticed that the ordering screen displayed two nearly identical dosage options. Under pressure, the resident clicked the wrong one. The problem was not a careless person; it was careless design.

The pharmacist was publicly thanked for catching the error. Within a week, the IT team simplified the screen. Similar near misses dropped by half within a month. Yet the most meaningful change was not statistical. It was emotional. Staff began speaking with relief instead of fear. One nurse told me, "I used to double-check everything in silence. Now I just ask." That permission to ask out loud is the heartbeat of psychological safety. Fear isolates. Trust connects. When connection becomes habit, learning accelerates.

Edmondson (2018) describes this as the learning zone, where people feel both challenged and supported. In that space, accountability feels grounding rather than exposing. Of course, it is never simple. Leaders experience fear too, fear of metrics, scrutiny, or job security. During an internal review, one manager whispered to me,

"If our scores drop, my job is at risk. How do I stay curious when I'm scared?" That question reminded me that psychological safety has to flow upward as well. Leaders cannot model curiosity in environments that punish transparency. So, we changed how we trained. Instead of policy lectures, we practiced real conversations. We role-played difficult discussions after errors, paying attention not just to words, but to tone; the sigh that shuts someone down, the mistimed pause, the sharp phrase that lingers. The sessions were uncomfortable, sometimes awkward, and ultimately transformative. Language began to shift. "Why did you do that?" became "Help me understand what made that seem reasonable at the time." One question assumes guilt; the other invites context. Language, I've learned, is a kind of architecture. It shapes the emotional space people inhabit. When words carry respect, honesty has room to emerge. When they carry judgment, people retreat.

## When Fatigue Replaces Fear

In one cardiology clinic, fear was not the barrier; fatigue was. Staff viewed near-miss reporting as busy work. "We just move on," one technician said. "Nothing changes." Rather than pushing harder on compliance, the manager tried something simpler: a five-minute morning huddle with three questions written on a whiteboard.

*What went well yesterday?*

*Where did we almost have a problem?*

*Who deserves thanks today?*

The first meetings were stiff. By the third week, someone mentioned that an ECG machine froze mid-test. IT repaired it within hours. That quick follow-through changed the atmosphere. Within weeks, the wall behind the desk filled with sticky notes, small wins, near misses, moments of kindness. Laughter slowly returned. That transformation still moves me because it shows that improvement does not require fanfare. It requires attention. Asking, listening, and responding build engagement far more effectively than mandates. Within three months, near-miss reports increased by half. What struck me most was how often people looked up from their screens to talk. Safety had become social again.

Psychological safety often reveals itself not during crises, but in ordinary rhythms; how colleagues greet one another, how humor circulates, how silence feels. Some silences hum with focus. Others buzz with tension. Leaders who notice the difference know where culture needs care.

## CULTURE ON THE MOVE: LESSONS FROM HOME CARE

In home based care, culture has to travel. Staff work alone, often in unfamiliar spaces. Policies cannot walk through those doors, but values can. A home care nurse once told me she felt uneasy about mislabeled oxygen tanks from a vendor but hesitated to report it. "I didn't want to sound like I was blaming someone," she said. After attending a Just Culture session, she reframed the issue as concern rather than complaint. The review confirmed a vendor misprint affecting multiple patients. Fixing it required collaboration, not discipline. Weeks later, she told me, "It felt good to be heard."

That simple sentence captures what most frontline clinicians want. They do not expect perfection. They want evidence that honesty leads somewhere constructive. Trust moved in both directions that day. The agency strengthened vendor checks, and the vendor changed its labeling process. One voice protected dozens of patients. That ripple effect reflects what Weick and Sutcliffe (2015) describe as weak-signal amplification; noticing small anomalies before they escalate into harm. But voicing weak signals takes courage. When leaders asked home care staff how they decide whether to report concerns, one aide answered candidly, "It depends on who's asking. Some people listen; some just log it." Her words were a reminder that systems do not create trust. People do.

## PATTERNS THAT CONNECT

Across these stories; a pharmacist in a hospital, a technician in a clinic, a nurse on the road; a pattern emerges. None are heroic tales. All are human ones. In each case, safety grew because someone felt safe enough to speak a difficult truth, and someone else stayed steady enough to hear it. Culture is fragile precisely because it is relational. It does not live in policies. It lives in interactions. I often describe it as an invisible current beneath every conversation. You cannot see it, but you can feel when it shifts.

The best leaders I've observed share simple habits. They pause before reacting. They narrate their reasoning so others can follow. They invite feedback and accept it without defensiveness. These quiet behaviors send a powerful message: psychological safety is not declared; it is demonstrated. One executive became known for ending every staff forum with the same invitation: "If we miss something, tell us before it becomes harm." For weeks, no one spoke. Then, after a medication recall, a nurse finally said, "You keep asking us to tell you; so here it is." That moment triggered a system-wide review. A year later, that same nurse had become a Just Culture champion. Visibility had turned into leadership.

When I teach these principles, I emphasize that Just Culture is not a way to avoid accountability. It is accountability practiced with integrity. It separates mistakes from choices and choices from disregard (Frankel et al., 2006). Fairness fuels learning. People will accept correction when the process feels just; they resist even gentle coaching when it feels inconsistent or performative.

## KEEPING CULTURE ALIVE THROUGH ENGAGEMENT

Fairness alone cannot sustain culture. It needs engagement; the daily rhythms that keep trust breathing. Engagement is the oxygen that prevents decay. Some teams use brief pulse surveys. Others rely on storytelling. My favorite practice is a simple "thank you chain." Each week, a leader thanks one staff member for a specific act that made care safer. That person then thanks someone else the following week. Over time, gratitude begins to flow sideways instead of top-down. It is a small ritual, but it changes what people notice. Attention shifts toward what is working, not only what is broken.

Research echoes what experience has long suggested: psychological safety strengthens voice and speaking-up behaviors (O'Donovan, De Brún, & McAuliffe, 2021; Grailey, Murray, Reader, & Brett, 2021). What matters most, though, is how it feels. When people feel seen, they begin to see more themselves. At one facility, recognition rounds unexpectedly led to an increase in reports about supply shortages. "It's like we got braver together," someone said. Courage, it turns out, spreads when safety feels shared.

## PRACTICE IMPACT

Emerging research reinforces what experience has long suggested: implementing a Just Culture algorithm does more than change how conversations unfold; it strengthens safety systems in measurable ways. Healthcare organizations that adopt Just Culture principles, including structured decision algorithms and visible leadership engagement, consistently report gains in transparency and organizational learning.

One large tertiary care center, for example, documented a 37% increase in event reporting following implementation, along with improved staff perceptions of leadership response to error and overall safety culture (Davis et al., 2025). Similarly, a cross-sectional study found a strong positive relationship between perceptions of Just Culture and willingness to report near misses, accounting for more than half of the variance in reporting behavior (Dwidar et al., 2025). These findings affirm that fairness and psychological safety are not abstract aspirations. They function as practical levers for improvement. When staff trust the process, they speak sooner. When leaders respond with consistency and integrity, systems learn faster. Embedded this way, Just Culture is not simply a cultural preference; it is an evidence based strategy for reducing harm and amplifying vigilance across the organization (Kumah, 2025).

## CONCLUSION

Culture is not built through policies or slogans. It takes shape in everyday interactions; often small, often unremarkable that quietly define what is safe to say and how accountability is experienced. This chapter has shown how Just Culture offers a practical framework for balancing fairness with responsibility, shifting safety from a compliance exercise into a shared, lived commitment.

Through real-world stories spanning hospital units and home-based care, we saw how psychological safety enables people to speak up, learn from missteps, and prevent harm before it escalates. In each case, leadership mattered; not in abstract terms, but in reactions taken under pressure. A leader's response in a critical moment either reinforces silence or invites honesty.

The Just Culture algorithm provides a structured way to make those responses reliable. By distinguishing human error from at-risk and reckless behavior, it supports consistency, protects dignity, and keeps learning at the center of accountability. Evidence confirms its impact: organizations that embed these principles see sustained increases in event reporting and stronger perceptions of safety culture. Culture comes first because everything else such as tools, policies, processes; rests on it. When trust and engagement take root, improvement becomes durable, and safety shifts from a written promise to a daily practice.

Crucially, this approach extends beyond individual actions to surface system contributors. Reviews deliberately examine workflow design, policy usability, staffing and scheduling, and competing priorities, with the expectation that at least one system factor is identified in cases of human error or at-risk behavior. Responses are matched to behavior type, explicitly prohibiting punitive action when system contributors are present. Closing the loop with staff by sharing what was learned, what will change, and how recurrence will be prevented is treated as an essential step, not an optional courtesy.

Over time, these reviews are aggregated to reveal patterns: recurring system failures, pressure points, or inconsistencies in classification. Those insights feed directly into QAPI structures and safety dashboards, linking frontline experience to organizational learning. Taken together, these practices distinguish Just Culture not as a tool, but as a system; one grounded in calibrated leadership, auditable decisions, separation of behavior from outcome, and visible, sustained learning.

## REFERENCES


Davis, T. R., Straatmann, K., Snyder, N., Shiner, D., Evans, A., Caruso, C., & Alton, M. (2025). Promoting a culture of patient safety: Using the principles of just culture to improve transparency and risk reporting in the hospital setting. *Patient Safety, 7*(2). Advance online publication. DOI: 10.33940/001c.137737

Dekker, S. (2016). *Just culture: Restoring trust and accountability in your organization*. CRC Press. DOI: 10.4324/9781315251271

Dwidar, M. M., Fakhry, S. F., & Abdel-Hamed, L. A. (2025). Just culture and its influence on nurse interns' willingness to report near-miss events: A cross-sectional study in five Egyptian university hospitals. *BMC Nursing*, *24*(1), 1397. Advance online publication. DOI: 10.1186/s12912-025-03979-w PMID: 41233794

Edmondson, A. C. (2018). *The fearless organization: Creating psychological safety in the workplace for learning, innovation, and growth*. Wiley.

Frankel, A. S., Leonard, M. W., & Denham, C. R. (2006). Fair and just culture, team behavior, and leadership engagement: The tools to achieve high reliability. *Health Services Research*, *41*(4 Pt 2), 1690–1709. DOI: 10.1111/j.1475-6773.2006.00572.x PMID: 16898986

Grailey, K. E., Murray, E., Reader, T., & Brett, S. J. (2021). The presence and potential impact of psychological safety in the healthcare setting: An evidence synthesis. *BMC Health Services Research*, *21*(1), 773. DOI: 10.1186/s12913-021-06740-6 PMID: 34353319

Kumah, A. (2025). Adverse event reporting and patient safety: The role of a just culture. *Frontiers in Health Services*, *5*, 1581516. Advance online publication. DOI: 10.3389/frhs.2025.1581516 PMID: 40910122

Marx, D. (2001). *Patient safety and the "just culture."*. Columbia University.

O'Donovan, R., De Brún, A., & McAuliffe, E. (2021). Healthcare professionals' experience of psychological safety, voice, and silence. *Frontiers in Psychology*, *12*, 626689. DOI: 10.3389/fpsyg.2021.626689 PMID: 33679547

Singer, S. J., & Tucker, A. L. (2014). The evolving literature on safety WalkRounds: Emerging themes and practical messages. *BMJ Quality & Safety*, *23*(10), 789–800. DOI: 10.1136/bmjqs-2014-003416 PMID: 25228779

Weick, K. E., & Sutcliffe, K. M. (2015). *Managing the unexpected: Sustained performance in a complex world* (3rd ed.). Wiley. DOI: 10.1002/9781119175834

## KEY TERMS AND DEFINITIONS

**Adaptive Leadership:** Guiding teams through change by fostering learning and shared purpose.

**At-Risk Behavior:** Actions that increase risk unintentionally because the person believes they are safe or necessarily under pressure, addressed through coaching, not punishment.

**Change Management:** A process for helping people and organizations move through transitions.

**Continuous Improvement:** A mindset of ongoing testing, reflection, and refinement of work systems.

**Human Factors:** The study of how people interact with tools and environments to improve safety.

**Just Culture:** A fairness-based model that balances accountability and learning, focusing on what went wrong, not who did it.

**Measurement for Learning:** Using data to guide reflection and improvement rather than judgment.

**Operational Learning:** Turning everyday experiences and near-misses into system-wide lessons.

**Psychological Safety:** A shared belief that it's safe to speak up, ask questions, and report concerns without fear of blame or embarrassment.

**Systems Thinking:** Viewing errors as outcomes of system interactions, not individual failings.

# APPENDIX

## Practice What You've Read: Implementing Just Culture

This appendix provides a practical approach for translating Just Culture principles into daily leadership practice. The Just Culture Algorithm, developed by David Marx, supports fair and consistent responses to safety events by distinguishing human error from at-risk and reckless behavior while accounting for system influences. The tools and steps outlined below are intended to help leaders move from conceptual understanding to operational use.

## A. Implementation Plan

### Build awareness and shared language

Introduce the Just Culture Algorithm during brief safety huddles or team discussions. Use a real or recent scenario to illustrate how the algorithm differentiates types of behavior. Shared stories help establish a common understanding of fairness and learning.

### Example: Simplified Just Culture Algorithm

Figure 2 outlines a sequential, system-level approach to embedding Just Culture in daily operations, from establishing shared language and baseline understanding, through integrating coaching based accountability into routine work, to sustaining visible fairness through measurement, communication, and leadership reinforcement.

*Figure 2. Just culture implementation process*

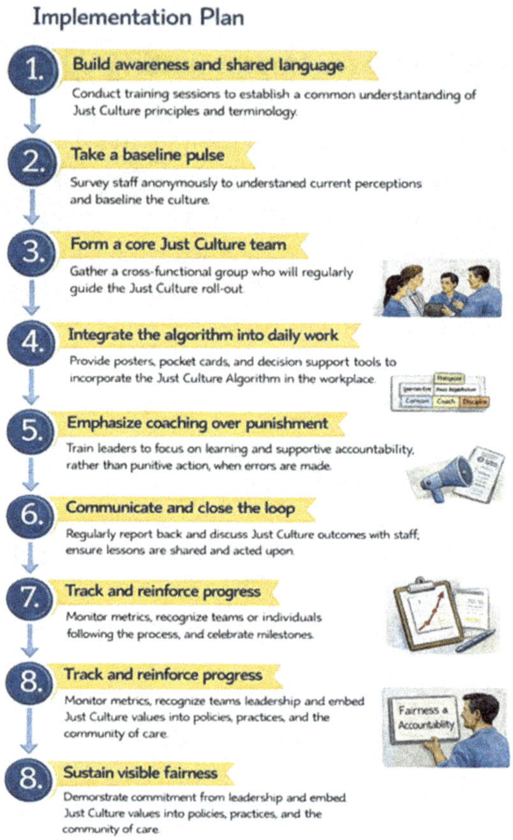
Implementation Plan
1.
Build awareness and shared language
Conduct training sessions to establish a common understantanding of Just Culture principles and terminology.
2.
Take a baseline pulse
Survey staff anonymously to understaned current perceptions and baseline the culture.
3.
Form a core Just Culture team
Gather a cross-functional group who will regularly guide the Just Culture roll-out.
4.
Integrate the algorithm into daily work
Provide posters, pocket cards, and decision support tools to incorporate the Just Culture Algorithm in the workplace.
5.
Emphasize coaching over punishment
Train leaders to focus on learning and supportive accountability, rather than punitive action, when errors are made.
6.
Communicate and close the loop
Regularly report back and discuss Just Culture outcomes with staff, ensure lessons are shared and acted upon.
7.
Track and reinforce progress
Monitor metrics, recognize teams or individuals following the process, and celebrate milestones.
8.
Track and reinforce progress
Monitor metrics, recognize teams leadership and embed Just Culture values into policies, practices, and the community of care.
Fairness & Accountability
8.
Sustain visible fairness
Demonstrate commitment from leadership and embed Just Culture values into policies, practices, and the community of care.

## B.2 Just Culture Algorithm Template

**Purpose:** To support fair, repeatable decision-making after safety events.
How to Use:

- Review facts objectively.
- Apply the decision questions in sequence.
- Match actions (console, coach, remediate) to the identified behavior type.

Template Overview:

- Intentional action? → Yes / No
- Human error? → Console and fix system

- At-risk behavior? → Coach and redesign process
- Reckless behavior? → Remedial action
- System contributors? → Address latent causes

## B.3 Behavioral Assessment Guide

This guide supports consistent classification during event reviews.

- **Human Error:** Unintentional slip or lapse

*Response:* Console and redesign systems
*Example:* Selecting the wrong medication due to similar names

- **At-Risk Behavior:** Unsafe shortcut believed to be acceptable

*Response:* Coach, educate, and remove barriers
*Example:* Skipping a checklist perceived as redundant

- **Reckless Behavior:** Conscious disregard of known risk

*Response:* Disciplinary or remedial action
*Example:* Ignoring a high alert warning without assessment

Figure 3 illustrates how leaders use a Just Culture algorithm to move from initial fact finding to fair behavioral classification, distinguishing at-risk behavior from reckless conduct, and resolving events through coaching and system improvement rather than blame, while reinforcing accountability and organizational learning.

*Figure 3. The Just Culture decision pathway in practice*

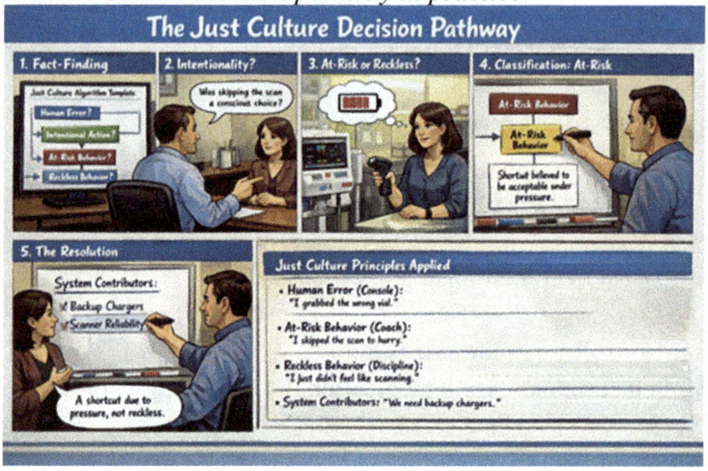
The Just Culture Decision Pathway
1. Fact-Finding
Human Error?
At-Risk Behavior?
Reckless Behavior?
2. Intentionality?
Was skipping the scan a conscious choice?
3. At-Risk or Reckless?
4. Classification: At-Risk
At-Risk Behavior
At-Risk Behavior
Shortcut believed to be acceptable under pressure.
5. The Resolution
System Contributors:
Backup Chargers
Scanner Reliability
A shortcut due to pressure, not reckless.
Just Culture Principles Applied
• Human Error (Console):
"I grabbed the wrong vial."
• At-Risk Behavior (Coach):
"I skipped the scan to hurry."
• Reckless Behavior (Discipline):
"I just didn't feel like scanning."
• System Contributors: "We need backup chargers."

## Vignette Applying the Just Culture Decision Tree

During a routine documentation review within a home infusion team, it was identified that an antibiotic had been administered later than scheduled. No patient harm occurred. Rather than focusing on the outcome, the Just Culture decision tree was applied to guide a fair and structured response that examined behavior, context, and system contributors (Figure 4).

*Figure 4. Applying Just Culture in practice*

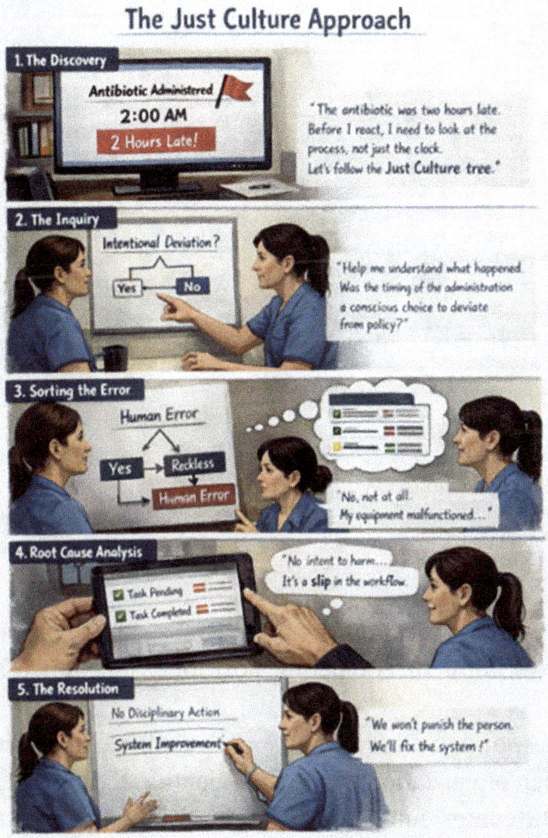


## Just Culture as an Integrated System

Figure 5 depicts how a nurse leader applies Just Culture as an organizational system identifying system contributors, calibrating non-punitive responses, closing the loop with staff, aggregating patterns over time, and integrating insights into QAPI dashboards ensuring decisions are consistent, auditable, and focused on sustained learning rather than individual blame.

*Figure 5. Just Culture as an integrated system*

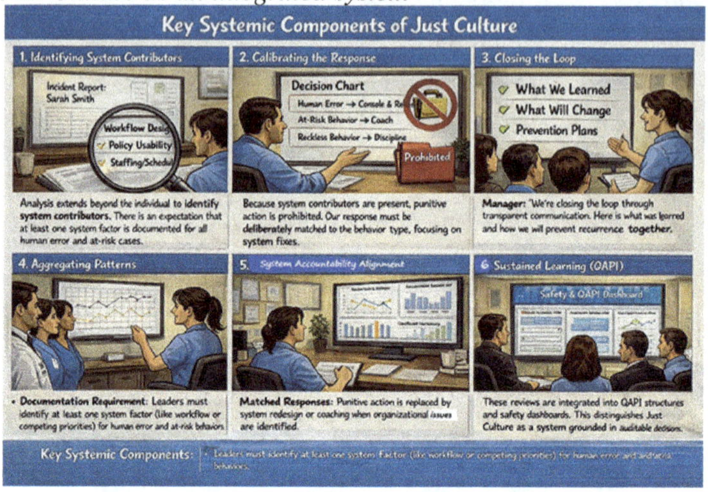


Key Systemic Components

- **Documentation Requirement:** Leaders must identify at least one system factor (like workflow or competing priorities) for human error and at-risk behaviors.
- **Matched Responses:** Punitive action is replaced by system redesign or coaching when organizational flaws are identified.
- **Auditable Outcomes:** Integration into **Quality Assurance and Performance Improvement (QAPI)** ensures that decisions are visible and lead to actual change.

## System Contributor Checklist

Use this during event reviews for Human Error and At-Risk cases. At least one factor must be documented. The checklist in table 1 supports structured identification of system contributors during reviews of human error and at-risk behavior, prompting leaders to examine workflow design, policy usability, staffing, equipment, training, and cultural signals, with the expectation that at least one system factor is documented to drive learning, redesign, and prevention rather than individual blame.

## System Factors Assessment Table

*Table 1. System contributor checklist for Just Culture event reviews*

| Category | Assessment Questions |
|---|---|
| **1. Workflow & Process Design** | [ ] Does the current workflow naturally lead to the error?<br>[ ] Is there a mismatch between how the policy is written and how work is actually performed?<br>[ ] Are there unnecessary steps or bottlenecks that encourage workarounds? |
| **2. Policy & Documentation Usability** | [ ] Is the relevant policy easily accessible and clear?<br>[ ] Was the policy usable under the specific conditions of the event (e.g., crisis, rush)?<br>[ ] Does the documentation system (EHR/Log) provide adequate safety prompts or warnings? |
| **3. Staffing & Scheduling** | [ ] Were staffing levels appropriate for the patient acuity at the time?<br>[ ] Were there excessive "competing priorities" that forced a choice between safety and speed?<br>[ ] Did fatigue or long shift hours play a potential role? |
| **4. Equipment & Environment** | [ ] Did equipment failure or unreliability (e.g., dead batteries, slow connections) trigger the behavior?<br>[ ] Were the necessary tools/supplies physically available and in working order?<br>[ ] Did enviro |

# Chapter 4
# Lean and Six Sigma in Real Life:
## Getting to the Root Without Getting Lost


## ABSTRACT

*This chapter takes Lean and Six Sigma out of the classroom and into the everyday work of care. Rather than treating these methods as certifications or fixed toolkits, it approaches them as ways of noticing barriers, asking better questions, and solving problems together. The discussion follows how technical frameworks become shared ways of seeing practices that keep people visible within the data. Using the case of a patient readmitted after pneumonia, the chapter illustrates that the hardest part of improvement is rarely detecting a defect. It is staying curious long enough to understand why it occurred. When attention is paid to both system design and human context, Lean and Six Sigma help teams reduce friction, clarify roles, and develop a common language for learning one that improves reliability without losing sight of patients or the staff who care for them.*


## INTRODUCTION

In healthcare, Lean and Six Sigma are often mentioned together, though they attend to different dimensions of improvement. Lean, rooted in the Toyota Production System *(Liker, 2004; Ohno, 1988)*, focuses on work that adds no value and creates drag in daily practice waiting, excess motion, rework, and handoffs that stall rather

DOI: 10.4018/979-8-3373-6496-4.ch004

than support care. The intent is easy to state and harder to live out: make it easier for patients and staff to move through care without unnecessary stops or confusion.

This chapter begins where checklists tend to fall short and lived experience takes over. A readmission or delay is not an abstract defect. It is someone's disrupted recovery, a family's anxiety, and a quiet erosion of trust. For that reason, the chapter does not offer a step-by-step tutorial; the appendices already address practical application. Instead, the focus is on the human work of using these methods well; how they shape attention, conversation, and learning.

Six Sigma complements Lean by addressing variation and defects through measurement and the DMAIC sequence: Define, Measure, Analyze, Improve, and Control. Its discipline is particularly useful when consistency matters, which in healthcare is most of the time. Many organizations combine the two approaches, using Lean to understand the flow of work and Six Sigma to understand why outcomes drift. The methods endure not because they are fashionable, but because they help teams see what is actually happening and act on it together.

*Figure 1. Comparison of lean and six sigma approaches*

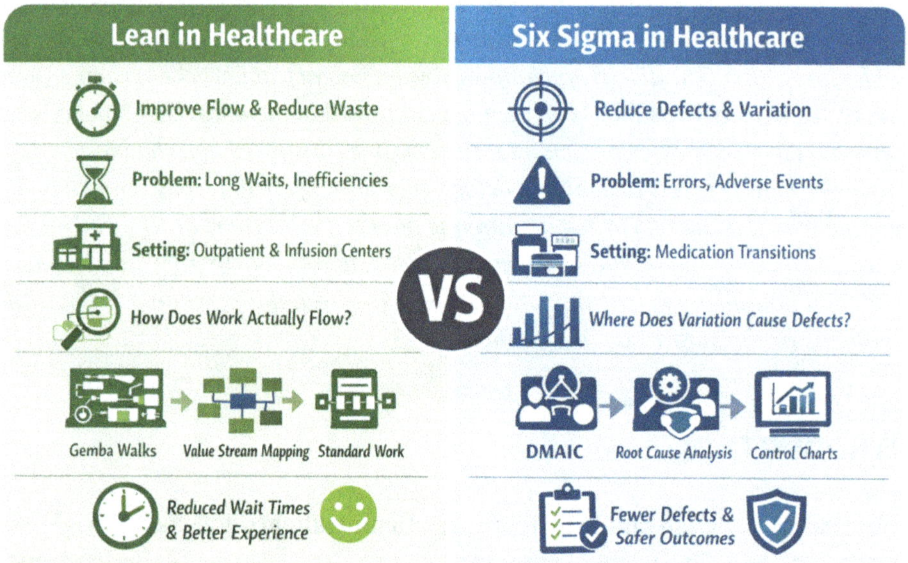


## Objectives of the Chapter

This chapter aims to:

- Demonstrate how Lean and Six Sigma move beyond theory to become practical, human-centered methods for solving real world problems that patients and staff directly experience.
- Emphasize curiosity and root cause thinking, encouraging teams to understand why problems occur rather than stopping at defect detection.
- Promote a culture of continuous improvement and empathy-driven design that aligns processes with patient and staff needs, supporting collaboration and shared accountability.

## Seeing the System through Mr. Davis's Story

Mr. Davis, a quiet man in his seventies, was discharged home after treatment for pneumonia. Two weeks later, he returned. His daughter met me outside his room and said, almost apologetically, "He never really got better. The home nurse said his oxygen wasn't working right." I remembered his discharge clearly. The forms were complete. The instructions were signed. Medications had been reconciled. Every indicator of a "good process" was present. And yet he was back. In Lean terms, this might be labeled a defect in the transition of care. In human terms, it was a gap between what we documented and what he actually lived with at home.

## Following the Flow of Care

We traced Mr. Davis's discharge backward, treating it like a moving process map rather than a static checklist. On paper, the summary held together. The oxygen order was placed. The vendor delivered on time. Nothing in the documentation raised concern. The home nurse, however, described a different scene. The oxygen tubing had been coiled tightly and kinked behind his recliner. Mr. Davis believed the equipment was set up correctly, but the flow was inadequate. That small, almost invisible detail changed the story. We had optimized paperwork and missed the environment he returned to. What appeared as clean throughput became, in practice, a hidden safety risk.

## The Moment the Data Spoke Back

We brought together the discharge planner, respiratory therapist, bedside nurse, and a representative from the oxygen vendor to walk through the event. The conversation stayed focused on the system rather than on individual fault. As we sketched the steps, a pattern surfaced. Education about home oxygen use was delegated inconsistently, delivered unevenly, and rarely documented. The vendor assumed the nurse would check the setup. The nurse assumed the vendor had already done so. Between those assumptions, patient safety relied on chance.

Using the Five Whys in a conversational, unforced way, each question surfaced a small piece of the picture. Eventually, a nurse said quietly, "We don't really share a clear picture of what 'ready for discharge' means." That comment landed. The process had been designed to confirm completion of tasks, not readiness for life at home. That distinction subtle on paper, decisive in practice marked the true gap in the system.

## What Lean Really Means When You're Standing in the Hallway

After that case, Lean felt less like a collection of tools and more like a discipline of attention. Process maps still mattered, but mostly when they carried us out of conference rooms and into hallways, bedrooms, and supply closets, places where the work revealed its friction. Numbers pointed to trends. Walks showed us what those trends felt like in real time.

Earlier in my improvement work, teams often rushed toward solutions. Another form. A reminder. One more checklist. Standing alongside staff as interruptions stacked up and workarounds became routine slowed that reflex. Most missteps were not neglect. They were improvisations under pressure. More often than not, it was the process and not the person that needed repair.

## When Curiosity Becomes Design

We tested a change with a small group before making it standard. Discharge teaching for home oxygen shifted to a brief visual checklist paired with teach back. Within a month, the 30-day readmission rate for that group dropped by roughly a third. The change itself was modest, but it aligned expectations. Everyone shared a clearer sense of what "done" meant for this patient, in this home. That shared picture traveled better than reminders ever had.

## When the Numbers Don't Tell the Whole Story

There was a time when I believed measurement alone would carry us to answers. Experience tempered that belief. Data works best when it provokes a conversation we might otherwise avoid. In Mr. Davis's case, the metrics looked reassuring. Turnaround times were acceptable. Documentation rates were high. Orders were placed correctly. Yet the story did not hold together until we looked at his chair, his living room, and the kinked oxygen line. The numbers pointed. The walk explained.

DMAIC helped by giving structure to our work, but it also demanded restraint. Tools are most useful when they help us discover, not defend, a conclusion.

## Defining the Real Problem

Many improvement projects begin with aggressive targets: *cut errors in half, reduce turnaround by 20 percent.* Targets can be useful, but they often draw attention to symptoms rather than causes. A strong Define phase keeps the problem anchored to the people living with it.

Before opening a spreadsheet, we asked:

- Who is most affected when this does not work?
- What does a good day look like for you?
- When did this process last go smoothly, and why?

Those questions surfaced realities that charts rarely capture.

## Measuring What Matters

During a project on medication delivery delays, the median turnaround time was 42 minutes. The target was 30. Timestamps suggested a bottleneck. Observation filled in the rest. A technician was answering calls, labeling syringes, double checking barcodes, and waiting for a pneumatic tube that jammed regularly. She glanced up with a half smile and said, "The numbers don't show this part, do they?" They did not. That moment shifted the work from "delay" as a metric to "waiting" as a daily strain. Once people felt seen, they offered solutions we had not anticipated.

## Analyzing without Blame

The Analyze phase can be uncomfortable. Patterns emerge that challenge assumptions. In one review of missed home visits, the data pointed to "scheduling errors." Process mapping told a different story. One scheduler carried nearly triple the patient load of another region. We had been holding individuals accountable for outcomes the system made improbable. Once that became visible, the tone changed. Fairness entered the design conversation. No control chart can compensate for work that cannot reasonably be done.

## Improving by Listening First

The urge to act is strongest during Improve. Quick wins feel satisfying and often fade. During a handoff project, nurses described what made shift change feel risky. One said, "It's not the time. It's that I don't feel heard when I raise a concern." We did not redesign the form. We redesigned the first minute. Every handoff began with one question: *Is there anything you're worried about?* That single change shifted tone, pacing, and trust. Within months, near-miss reports increased while preventable errors declined. The process map mattered. Listening mattered more.

## Controlling without Losing Curiosity

On paper, Control is about sustaining gains. In practice, it is about humility. Conditions change. So, after major rollouts, we returned to two questions:

- Is this still working as intended?
- What new problems did we create?

Control did not mean freezing the system. It meant building a habit of checking reality against design.

## What I've Learned Along the Way

Looking back, the most durable outcomes were not counts of projects completed or defects reduced. They were the ways teams learned together. Engineers taught nurses how to read control charts. Nurses taught engineers how to listen to the patient in front of them. Dashboards became conversations, and conversations shaped policy.

Lean and Six Sigma did not strip emotion from the work. They helped restore purpose to it. When used well, they hold data and dignity in the same frame.

## When Improvement Becomes a Culture

Over time, the methods changed how people noticed their work. Once a team learns to see waste, friction that once blended into the background becomes hard to ignore. When "why" replaces "who," defensive meetings soften into shared exploration.

A group of pharmacists mapped their compounding workflow and discovered more handoffs and checks than they intended. "We designed this for safety," one said, "but we slowed safety down." Within weeks, they reorganized the workspace, clarified handoffs, and cut verification time nearly in half. The most striking shift was energy. Staff brought forward ideas daily without waiting for a formal project. Improvement stopped being an event and became part of the workday.

## The Hard Part: Staying Curious When You're Tired

Some days the system feels heavy. Metrics accumulate. Deadlines press. The language of improvement starts to sound mechanical. That is when curiosity thins and leadership presence matters most. Data fatigue is real. Before a major presentation, we tried a simple practice. We asked aloud, *"Whose story does this data represent?* When people recognized their own experience in the numbers, engagement returned. The chart felt less distant, more useful.

## From Root Cause to Shared Purpose

The longer I practiced Lean and Six Sigma, the more I understood that "root cause" is rarely a single point. It is an entry into the habits and choices that shape a system. In one debrief, a nurse was convinced she had failed a patient. We mapped her environment instead; the interruptions, missing supplies, turnaround times no one could meet. By the end, she said, "It wasn't just me. The system set this up." After a pause, she added, "I can help change it." That shift from blame to contribution is part of the healing.

## Redesigning for Humanity

Process maps deepen when they include how people feel as they move through them. When we asked staff to describe each step with a single word, patterns emerged: *sprint*, *guessing game*, *hurry, then wait*. Placing those words beside the flow diagram made problems visible in a new way. We simplified steps, reduced confusion, and returned control to the people doing the work. The result was not only smoother flow, but a better day for the team.

## What I Carry Forward

If this chapter has a through line, it is respect; respect for patients' circumstances, for staff effort, and for what data can and cannot show. Lean and Six Sigma provide structure. People give that structure meaning. Progress in healthcare rarely arrives as a single breakthrough. More often, it shows up through steady attention and the willingness to test, learn, and try again.

## PRACTICE IMPACT

When applied in real clinical settings, Lean and Six Sigma have shown tangible gains in efficiency, safety, and patient experience. These gains are not abstract. They appear as fewer stalled handoffs, clearer roles, and processes that hold together under everyday pressure. Lean tools such as value stream mapping and waste identification help teams surface where work slows or fragments, particularly during transitions of care. In hospital settings, these methods have been associated with improved process capability and reduced variability, supporting more reliable delivery of care (Chyon et al., 2020).

Lean Six Sigma approaches have also demonstrated practical value in ambulatory and outpatient environments, where flow and waiting are often the most visible sources of patient dissatisfaction. By pairing measurement with root cause analysis, teams have been able to streamline clinic operations and shorten wait times without increasing staff burden (Kam et al., 2021). In these settings, improvement depended less on sophisticated analytics than on aligning daily work with a shared understanding of what "good flow" looks like for patients and staff.

Six Sigma's DMAIC framework contributes most when consistency and reliability are at risk. Its structured approach to defining problems, testing assumptions, and sustaining changes has been shown to reduce defects in complex healthcare processes, particularly where variation quietly undermines safety (Ilin & Bohlen, 2023). Used well, DMAIC does not replace professional judgment. It gives teams a disciplined way to pause, examine patterns, and decide where standardization helps and where flexibility must remain.

Across settings, the strongest results emerge when technical tools are paired with human-centered design and collaborative problem solving. Improvement efforts succeed not because teams follow methods perfectly, but because the methods create space for shared learning. When staff can see their experience reflected in the data, they are more willing to engage, adapt, and sustain change. In that sense, the practical impact of Lean and Six Sigma lies less in the tools themselves and more in how they help organizations learn together.

## CONCLUSION

In practice, Lean and Six Sigma work best when treated as disciplined ways of seeing and learning rather than as rigid programs. Mr. Davis's readmission made that distinction clear. The documentation was complete. His reality was not.

The methods helped us ask better questions, trace work in context, and design changes that endured. DMAIC, process mapping, and the Five Whys served as guides rather than scripts. Data pointed toward the problem. Dialogue and observation completed the picture. When improvement becomes a habit of attention, reliability grows—and the work becomes more humane for both patients and staff.

## REFERENCES


Chyon, F. A., Ahmmed, M. S., Shuvo, M. K. A., Suman, M. N. H., & Hossain, M. M. (2020). Measuring process capability in a hospital by using lean tools. *International Journal of Health Care Quality Assurance, 33*(7), 543–555. DOI: 10.1108/IJHCQA-09-2019-0096

Ilin, M., & Bohlen, J. (2023). Six sigma method. In *StatPearls*. StatPearls Publishing.

Kam, A. W., Gunja, N., & Seow, C. H. (2021). Using lean six sigma techniques to improve efficiency in outpatient clinics: Root cause analysis and clinic flow redesign. *BMC Health Services Research, 21*, 1105. DOI: 10.1186/s12913-020-06034-3

Liker, J. K. (2004). *The Toyota way: 14 management principles from the world's greatest manufacturer*. McGraw-Hill.

Ohno, T. (1988). *Toyota production system: Beyond large-scale production*. Productivity Press.


## KEY TERMS AND DEFINITIONS

**Control Chart:** A graph tracking process performance over time to distinguish normal variation from true changes.

**DMAIC:** A structured Six Sigma cycle: Define, Measure, Analyze, Improve, Control—a roadmap for problem-solving.

**Five Whys:** A questioning technique that uncovers root causes by asking "why" repeatedly.

**Human Factors:** The study of how people interact with systems, ensuring design fits human needs.

**Kaizen:** A Japanese term for "change for better," emphasizing small, continuous improvements.

**Lean:** A continuous improvement philosophy focused on eliminating waste and simplifying workflows for safer, easier work.

**Process Mapping:** A visual tool to outline process steps and identify inefficiencies or safety gaps.

**Process Variation:** Differences in process outcomes, often targeted in Six Sigma to improve consistency.

**Six Sigma:** A data-driven method to reduce variation and defects, ensuring consistency and reliability.

**Standard Work:** The best-known method for performing a process safely and consistently, serving as a baseline.

**Weak Signal Detection:** The ability to spot subtle early signs of potential problems before harm occurs.

# APPENDIX

## Applying Lean and Six Sigma in Daily Work

*Table 1. Lean vs. six sigma application in healthcare*

| Dimension | Lean in Healthcare | Six Sigma in Healthcare |
|---|---|---|
| **Primary Aim** | Improve flow and eliminate waste | Reduce defects and process variation |
| **Problem Type** | Delays, inefficiencies, workarounds | Errors, inconsistencies, adverse events |
| **Typical Setting** | Outpatient clinics, infusion centers, inpatient units | Medication management, diagnostics, transitions of care |
| **Trigger for Use** | Patients wait too long; staff spend time searching or reworking | Outcomes vary; defects occur unpredictably |
| **Core Question** | *How does work actually flow today?* | *Where and why does variation create defects?* |
| **Primary Methods** | Gemba walks, value stream mapping, standard work, visual management | DMAIC, root cause analysis, statistical measurement, control charts |
| **Data Orientation** | Observational and operational | Quantitative and statistical |
| **Frontline Role** | Co-designing better workflows | Following standardized, controlled processes |
| **Example Outcome** | Reduced wait times and improved patient experience | Fewer medication discrepancies and adverse events |
| **What Improves** | Reliability of daily work | Consistency and safety of critical processes |

The following figures show how Lean and Six Sigma principles translate into everyday problem solving through a real example of a delayed pain-medication delivery. A Five Whys analysis (Figure 2) traces a 45-minute delay from a missing order receipt to the upstream conditions that made it likely, including competing clinical demands, uneven admission distribution, and a short-staffed shift after an unexpected call-out. The DMAIC framework (Figure 3) connects those insights to targeted actions, from defining the problem and measuring key indicators to testing small changes and holding the gains with standard work. A learning and capability model (Figure 4) emphasizes transparency, reflection, and staff empowerment as the foundation for sustained improvement.

## Example: Using the Five Whys to Understand a Medication Delay

*Figure 2. Five whys analysis of a medication delay*

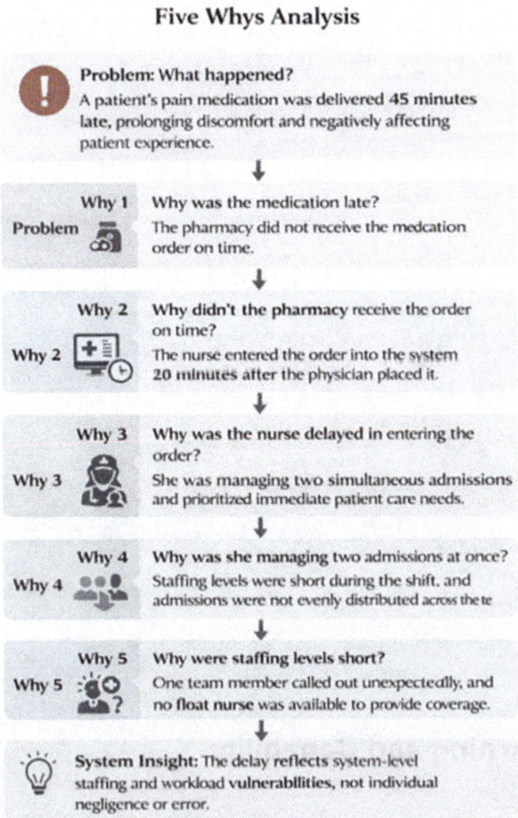


The visual shows how a delayed pain medication originally attributed to a late pharmacy receipt was shaped by upstream workflow and capacity constraints rather than individual error.

## Applying DMAIC and Sustaining Improvement

**Figure 3.** Applying the DMAIC framework to a medication delay, integrating operational analysis with a human-centered lens to guide Define, Measure, Analyze, Improve, and Control, while protecting patient comfort, staff reliability, and system performance.

*Figure 3. Applying DMAIC and sustaining improvement*

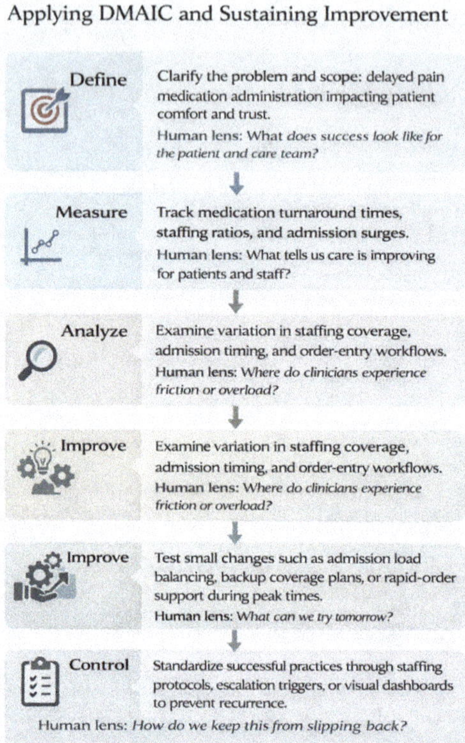


## Sustaining Learning and Capability

Figure 4. Three practices help sustain improvement, making progress visible, reflecting on learning, and building staff capability. Transparency, shared reflection, and empowerment strengthen organizational memory and support team-led improvement over time.

*Figure 4. Sustaining learning and capability.*

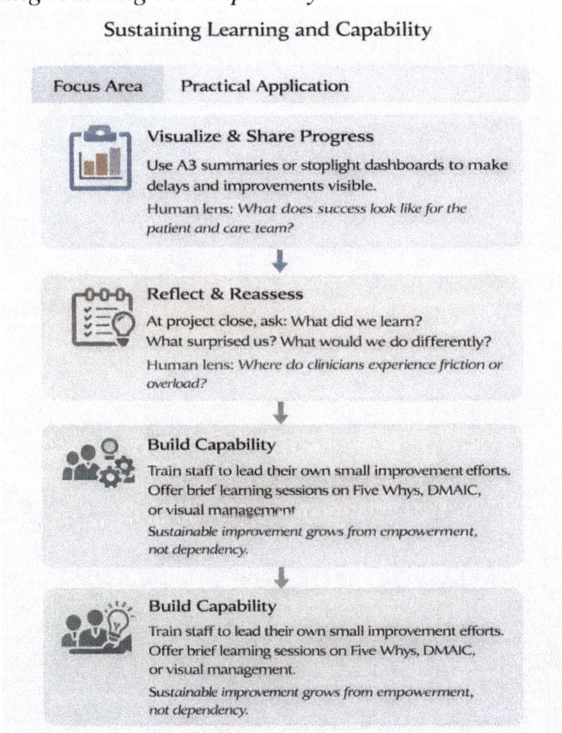

# Chapter 5
# From Strategy to Story:
## Building Dashboards That Drive Change

## ABSTRACT

*Numbers alone never tell the full story. Yet without them, the story is incomplete. This chapter examines how dashboards, Key Performance Indicators (KPIs), and behavioral design principles translate strategy into everyday action. It explores the space where measurement meets meaning, tracing how healthcare dashboards can evolve from compliance artifacts into tools that spark curiosity, alignment, and learning. Through real world examples including a missed patient follow up and an overcrowded dashboard the chapter shows how clarity and empathy transform data into insight. By attending to both technical structure and human interpretation, it offers a framework for designing dashboards that connect performance with purpose, where metrics function less as microscopes that magnify error and more as mirrors that support understanding.*

## INTRODUCTION

The widespread adoption of dashboards in healthcare emerged alongside national policies that required standardized reporting of quality and safety indicators. In the early 2000s, hospitals developed enterprise wide dashboards largely to meet accountability expectations. These early efforts often emphasized volume over usability, presenting dense collections of quantitative measures that were difficult for varied audiences to interpret or act upon (Weggelaar-Jansen et al., 2018).

By the 2010s, advances in electronic health records and incident reporting systems accelerated dashboard use, shifting organizations from retrospective summaries toward real time monitoring that made emerging safety patterns more

DOI: 10.4018/979-8-3373-6496-4.ch005

visible (Performance Health, 2025). Yet as dashboards multiplied, design lagged behind adoption. By the mid-2020s, research increasingly pointed to the absence of consistent design principles. Many dashboards suffered from cluttered layouts, unclear indicator definitions, and weak alignment with how people actually work. This gap prompted calls for best-practice guidance addressing not only content, but behavior, adoption, and integration into daily routines (Health Service Executive (Health Service Executive, 2025).

Across this evolution, dashboards mirrored a broader shift in healthcare from compliance driven reporting toward tools intended to support learning, communication, and continuous improvement. Still, intention and reality did not always align. As dashboards became routine, their use often settled into a mechanical rhythm: scrolling through rows of indicators, noting red or green cells, and moving on. In many organizations, early practices reinforced this pattern. Large inventories of metrics, assembled for accountability rather than understanding, made it easy to focus on color rather than consequence (Weggelaar-Jansen et al., 2018). Even real time safety dashboards, designed to surface patterns and prompt earlier intervention, were sometimes reduced to passive displays that flagged incidents without inviting reflection on the human experiences they represented (Performance Health, 2025).

In that environment, a missed follow up became a red cell, a fall became a trend line, and a near miss became a count stripped of the context, emotion, and narrative that give data meaning. Tools meant to illuminate the system instead obscured the lives they were intended to protect, a tendency reinforced by early dashboard designs that privileged quantitative accountability over interpretation (Weggelaar-Jansen et al., 2018).

Looking back, I recognize that this pattern did not live only in systems or committees. It lived quietly in me. The ease with which dashboards reduced human experience to colored cells mirrored the ease with which I once accepted those abstractions. I rarely asked what was missing, or whose day sat behind each number. I told myself I was leading with data, but often I was navigating by distance. It took time and a few uncomfortable realizations to see how easily dashboards can separate leaders from the people they intend to serve.

Early in my leadership work, I fell into the same trap. Dashboards felt like proof of progress, polished visuals that offered the comfort of control. Over time, it became clear that what gives a dashboard power is not how it looks, but how it is used. Data, like language, gains meaning only in conversation (Brown & Patel, 2021). Dashboards can either distance leaders from reality or draw them closer to it. The difference lies in intention. I have watched meetings where metrics were used as instruments of blame, and others where the room shifted when someone asked, *what is this data telling us about our patients, our staff, our system?*

Alignment begins there and not with technology, but with curiosity. Every improvement effort I have seen gain traction began when teams stopped reporting numbers *for* someone and started interpreting them *with* someone. That is the moment measurement turns into meaning (Weiner et al., 2020). In one ICU, a critical care pulmonologist changed the rhythm of morning rounds in a way that stayed with me. Instead of asking residents to report only the CLABSI rate, he insisted they begin with the patient behind the infection. He would pause at the doorway and ask, "Who was this line connected to? What was happening in their day, their illness, their care?"

The shift was subtle, but the effect was immediate. What had once been a statistic counted, logged, trended became a story with a name, a trajectory, and a moment of vulnerability. As residents described the circumstances surrounding each CLABSI, the conversation moved from reporting defects to understanding them. The metric retained its importance, but it gained a human anchor. In that anchor, the team found clearer accountability, deeper empathy, and stronger motivation to improve.

## Objective of the Chapter

This chapter is intended to help healthcare leaders design dashboards that move beyond compliance and become drivers of meaningful change. Specifically, it aims to:

1. Align metrics with mission by translating organizational strategy into actionable insights that connect performance with purpose.
2. Humanize data through stories and behavioral design principles that make dashboards intuitive, engaging, and emotionally resonant.
3. Foster a culture of learning and psychological safety in which dashboards invite curiosity, support improvement, and sustain progress through dialogue rather than fear.

## Mrs. Rivera's Story: The Metric Behind the Miss

Mrs. Rivera, a sixty-three-year-old patient with diabetes and heart failure, missed her post discharge appointment. The system recorded it as one of hundreds of "missed post-acute visits." When a manager called her home, the explanation was simple. She had never received a reminder. The automated message had gone to an outdated phone number. That detail reframed the issue. What initially appeared to be a scheduling failure was, in fact, a breakdown across discharge planning, scheduling workflows, and patient communication. In the next review meeting, the question shifted from *Why did she miss the appointment?* to *What made it easy for her to miss it?*

The red cell for "missed appointment" stopped being an abstract indicator. It became Mrs. Rivera's experience. Behind every metric sits a human moment, and the work of improvement begins by uncovering it. That reframing led to concrete redesign: same day scheduling, text confirmations, and a nurse callback within forty-eight hours. Within a single quarter, follow-up compliance increased by nearly 20 percent, and readmissions declined. The lesson was straightforward. Metrics matter only when they reconnect us to the people they represent (Damberg et al., 2014).

## From Counting to Caring: Making Metrics Meaningful

Many organizations are rich in dashboards and poor in meaning. I have seen scorecards with hundreds of indicators that still failed to answer a basic question: *How safe are we today?* At one clinic, we reduced more than forty measures to ten, each explicitly tied to strategy: patient safety, access, experience, workforce engagement, and equity. We then asked each team to select one "story metric", a measure that blended performance with purpose. Examples included:

- **Access:** Average days from referral to visit
- **Experience:** Percentage of patients who felt their care team listened carefully
- **Equity:** Diabetes control rates stratified by race and ZIP code

As staff began to recognize their own work in the data, engagement changed. Morning huddles shifted from reporting to learning. One medical assistant said, "When I saw that our listening score improved, I felt proud. Patients noticed." Alignment does that. It turns data from something we submit into something we feel. And when data evokes emotion, it has the power to move people toward action (Farias & Van de Walle, 2025).

## The Dashboard Nobody Looked At, Until It Found a Face

Dr. Singh's clinic had a dashboard that impressed analysts and exhausted clinicians. It held fifty metrics spread across multiple tabs, dense with trend lines and filters. "It's too much noise," he said, looking past the screen. When we asked which measures actually changed care, the response came without hesitation: A1c control, blood pressure control, flu vaccination, visit timeliness, and patient satisfaction. We rebuilt the dashboard around those five. One page. Color coded. Refreshed weekly. Green meant sustain. Yellow meant discuss. Red meant act.

Then Mrs. Rivera appeared on that screen. Her A1c flashed red. Next to it sat a patient comment: *"I felt rushed."* In that moment, the red cell stopped being abstract. It became a person. The team moved quickly, a same day lab, a visual medication plan, a pharmacist check-in. Two weeks later, her A1c shifted to yellow. A month later, it turned green. Dr. Singh later told me, "The data earned my trust when it started telling me something useful." That shift from information to intuition is well described by Coiera et al. (2025), who note that dashboards become credible only when they support timely, actionable decisions rather than passive review.

## Design Choices That Matter

The clinic's progress did not come from sophistication. It came from restraint. A small set of design choices carried the change:

- **One screen, one story.** No hidden tabs. Everyone saw the same version of the truth.
- **Color with purpose.** Green to sustain, yellow to discuss, red to act.
- **Behavior before data.** Each metric carried an explicit "If red, then..." cue.
- **Transparency.** A visible timestamp confirmed updates and rebuilt trust.

These principles echo what research continues to confirm that clarity drives action. Over time, the dashboard became part of the clinic's rhythm. Metrics sparked conversation. Red cells became invitations to learn.

## The Anatomy of Alignment

A dashboard is not a spreadsheet. It is strategy in motion. When measures reflect mission, alignment follows without force. In one health system, we mapped every dashboard metric to the organizational mission: safety, experience, equity, and efficiency. Each domain held no more than two or three indicators, and frontline teams defined what "good" looked like in their own work. The result was noticeable. Ownership grew. Improvement felt invited rather than imposed. One nurse manager said, "I stopped dreading the dashboard when I realized it was my story too." When dashboards are linked to purpose, they organize attention and transform compliance into curiosity (Symplr, 2024).

## Designing Dashboards That Drive Behavior

Seeing the system requires looking beyond individual sites. Data may live in dashboards, but people move across settings. A metric that looks strong in the hospital can unravel at home. I once observed three dashboards projected side by side: one from inpatient nursing, one from outpatient clinics, and one from home health. Each used different formats and color schemes. Hand hygiene compliance read 95 percent in one, 93 percent in another, and 92 percent in the third. A leader asked, "If we can't agree on what safe looks like, how can we measure it?"

The issue was not accuracy. It was alignment. The breakthrough came with the creation of *bridge metrics* shared indicators that spanned transitions of care. Instead of isolated departmental goals, teams tracked measures that followed patients across settings: medication reconciliation, communication timeliness, avoidable readmissions. When the home health dashboard turned red for medication discrepancies, it triggered an automatic alert and not an accusation to the ambulatory team. Joint case reviews revealed a common source: conflicting medication lists across systems. Within three months, reconciliation errors fell by 30 percent. The finding reinforced what research has long suggested: dashboards improve care not by displaying data, but by aligning human behavior around shared purpose (Farias & Van de Walle, 2025; Dolan et al., 2018).

## The Danger of Data Fatigue

Every healthcare leader eventually encounters it; the dashboard that grows until meaning thins out. At one organization, the quality council reviewed 120 metrics each month. Meetings ran for two hours, and by the end, no one could name a clear action. Someone finally asked, "Which of these numbers, if improved, would actually make a patient's life better?"

The answer was about ten.

We created what I now think of as *the vital few dashboards*: three to five measures per service line, balancing outcomes, processes, and experience. Each measure came with two prompts:

1. What story does this number tell?
2. What behavior should it drive?

The conversation shifted almost immediately. People stopped defending performance and started designing improvement. When an infection rate dipped, a preventionist said, "Let's not celebrate yet; what staffing changes happened last month?"

That was the moment reporting turned into reflection. Reducing data volume did not reduce insight. It sharpened it.

## Making Data Human Again

Numbers gain weight when they are connected to faces, not just figures. One organization placed a small silhouette representing ten real patients in the corner of each chart. Staff said it made them pause before scrolling. Another replaced labels like *deficiency* with *learning opportunity*. The language shift changed tone almost overnight.

Every dashboard also included a single patient quote; positive or negative; displayed beside the metrics. Reading *"The nurse stayed until I understood"* next to a trend line reframed improvement as compassion in action. These elements were not decorative. They were behavioral. They reminded staff that dashboards exist for people, not points (Coiera et al., 2025); National Patient Safety Foundation (NPSF, 2015)). A good dashboard feels like a conversation with values. If it only reports, it is incomplete. If it listens, it is alive.

## Behavioral Design: Turning Red Cells into Reflection

Dashboards that shape behavior do more than visualize performance. They guide response. To make data actionable, we applied what I call the *If Red, then...* rule:

- Red A1c → add same-day point-of-care testing
- Red timeliness → adjust appointment hours for working patients
- Red patient satisfaction → discuss communication tone in huddles

This approach aligns with implementation science: people act more quickly when the path from data to decision is explicit (Broughton et al., 2025). We also standardized traffic light cues: green to sustain, yellow to discuss, red to act, gray for missing data across all dashboards. When "red" meant the same thing everywhere, staff no longer had to decode signals. They could respond. That simplicity built trust.

## When Leaders Model Curiosity

During a systemwide safety meeting, a director noticed a sudden rise in delayed home infusion deliveries. Instead of asking, "Who's responsible?" she asked, "What's the pattern?" That single word shifted the room. Within minutes, staff identified a routing change that had added forty minutes to each trip. The fix was straightforward. The lesson was cultural. Curiosity, not control, drives improvement (Edmondson, 2018).

Leaders who model calm inquiry turn dashboards into learning tools. Over time, teams stop hiding problems and begin surfacing possibilities. Transparency takes shape not through exposure, but through trust built by inquiry.

## Building a Balanced Dashboard: Seeing the Whole Picture

A well designed dashboard balances precision with compassion. At one organization, siloed reports were replaced with a Balanced Scorecard spanning six domains: safety, experience, access, workforce, equity, and efficiency. Each domain included one or two meaningful metrics with clearly identified owners:

- **Safety:** Falls per 1,000 patient days (Owner: Nurse Manager)
- **Experience:** Likelihood to Recommend (HCAHPS) (Owner: Service Director)
- **Access:** Days from referral to visit (Owner: Scheduling Lead)
- **Workforce:** Employee Engagement Index (Owner: HR Partner)
- **Equity:** Preventive screening rates by ZIP code (Owner: Health Equity Liaison)
- **Efficiency:** Cost per episode of care (Owner: Finance Partner)

Meetings changed. Instead of "scroll and stare," leaders asked:

- What's improving, what's at risk, and what needs discussion?
- Which red cells reflect process problems rather than performance failures?

Dashboards work best when they clarify rather than impress (Tufte, 1997). Simplicity is not minimalism. It is mastery.

## Data as a Language, not a Ledger

Dashboards should teach organizations how to think, not just what to count. Over time, data has come to feel less like a record and more like dialogue; the system speaking back.

When a harm dashboard showed a subtle rise in pediatric readmissions, no single case stood out. Through discussion, the cause emerged. It was not clinical. It was logistical. Families lacked transportation for follow-up visits. Adding a ride support line reduced readmissions by one third. Dashboards reveal what numbers alone cannot: the story behind the slope. Listening to data requires the same discipline as listening to people; patience, humility, and a willingness to be changed by what you hear (Weick & Sutcliffe, 2015).

## From Measurement to Meaning

### The See–Share–Solve–Sustain Cycle

Over time, I learned that improvement rarely comes from staring at data. It comes from working through it together. What emerged was the See–Share–Solve–Sustain Cycle, a simple four-part rhythm that helped keep dashboards active rather than ornamental.

- **See:** Make performance visible as it is. No smoothing. No hiding.
- **Share:** Bring the data into the places where work actually happens, not only into boardrooms.
- **Solve:** Treat every red cell as a prompt for one concrete change idea.
- **Sustain:** Mark small wins in public, so learning does not quietly fade.

This rhythm changed the feel of review meetings. Monthly check-ins began to function as ongoing feedback loops. Teams started anticipating patterns instead of reacting to surprises, a hallmark of a health system learning (Weiner et al., 2020). Figure 1 shows the See–Share–Solve–Sustain Cycle as a clear, repeatable rhythm for keeping dashboards active rather than static. *See* makes performance visible; *Share* brings data into real work conversations; *Solve* turns concerning signals into concrete next steps; and *Sustain* reinforces progress so improvements stick. Although this exact four-step model does not appear in existing literature, it draws from the Toyota-influenced See–Solve–Share framework and echoes the iterative structure of the PDCA (Plan–Do–Check–Act) cycle widely used in continuous improvement. By adding the Sustain step, this adapted cycle emphasizes embedding improvements into daily practice, helping organizations shift from passive reporting to active, ongoing learning.

*Figure 1. See–share–solve–sustain cycle*

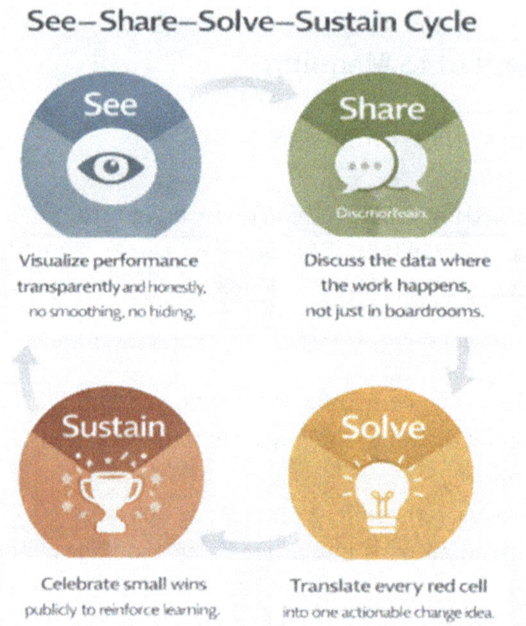


A four-step learning rhythm that keeps performance dashboards actionable and continuously improving.

## From Surveillance to Learning

In one department, early resistance softened when staff realized the dashboard was not a surveillance device but a mirror of progress. A respiratory therapist said, “At first, I thought you were checking on us. Then I saw the data helping us check on ourselves.”

That shift: from fear to ownership reflects what behavioral scientists describe as autonomy-supportive accountability: structures that guide behavior without shaming (Dolan et al., 2018). When people feel ownership of the data, they also assume ownership of improvement. This is why dashboards work best when they move beyond compliance and into coaching. Instead of spotlighting deficits, they surface opportunities to learn. Color becomes an invitation, not a verdict (Edmondson, 2018).

## The Role of Psychological Safety

Dashboards do their best work in environments where people can speak openly about what went wrong without fear of blame (Edmondson, 2018). In one case, a medication error appeared in red. Rather than asking, "Who made the mistake?" the leader asked, "What made the mistake possible?"

That single reframing shifted the discussion. The team redesigned a confusing electronic order screen, preventing dozens of near misses. Psychological safety is not softness. It is rigor practiced with respect. Dashboards make risk visible; leaders decide whether that risk can be discussed.

## Equity Through Data

Every dashboard carries moral weight. What we choose to measure determines who becomes visible. When outcomes were stratified by race, ZIP code, and language, inequities surfaced that had been hidden in aggregate views. Some areas showed higher readmissions not because of poor clinical care, but because of food insecurity, transportation barriers, and limited digital access.

Addressing those gaps required partnerships beyond the clinic walls. Metrics were linked to concrete supports through community agencies. Within six months, disparities in diabetes control narrowed by 15 percent. In that work, data became an instrument of fairness rather than simple comparison (Tervalon & Murray-García, 1998; Centers for Medicare & Medicaid Services, 2023). Equity shifted from a side analysis to a lens through which all metrics were interpreted.

## When Dashboards Tell Stories

At one quarterly review, I projected a slide showing three red bars turning yellow and then green over six months. A nurse leaned over and whispered, "Those bars are us." That moment was a reminder that dashboards are not about perfection. They are about progress. Numbers carry traces of effort, missteps, and learning. Each data point bears the imprint of people trying to do better work under real constraints (Wolf et al., 2021). Recognizing that sustains improvement long after attention moves elsewhere.

## Sustaining Through Recognition and Reflection

Sustainability depends on visibility. We began closing leadership huddles with a brief recognition, one story of how data had changed care. These moments reinforced that metrics were not abstractions but reflections of human outcomes.

Accountability and celebration began to coexist. We also published a short *Metrics That Matter* newsletter highlighting three things: what improved, what regressed, and what was learned. Over time, staff started submitting stories on their own. It was a small signal, but an important one. Measurement, when humanized, can energize rather than exhaust (Farias & Van de Walle, 2025).

### The Listening Leader

Eventually, I came to see that dashboards are less about numbers than about willingness to listen. When I approached them with humility, the data felt like an invitation, a quiet conversation waiting to unfold. When I approached them with fear, the same data hardened into judgment. Leadership, I learned, is not just reading the numbers. It is reading the room: the pauses, the tension, the flicker of curiosity that suggests people are ready to see something differently. In that light, a green cell became more than a marker of success; it signaled trust restored. A red cell, instead of failure, became an opening, an invitation to lean in, ask questions, and learn together. Data may start the conversation, but people give it meaning. That exchange, not any algorithm, is what carries improvement forward.

### Practice Impact

When dashboards align metrics with mission, humanize data, and support psychological safety, they can meaningfully improve care and organizational culture. Reducing data overload and focusing on a small set of strategically relevant indicators allows teams to act on insight rather than sort through noise. Behavioral design elements such as consistent color cues and explicit "If Red, Then…" responses shorten the distance between signal and action (Farias & Van de Walle, 2025).

Embedding patient stories and equity lenses within dashboards further shifts their role. Measures become tools for empathy and fairness, helping to surface and address disparities while strengthening trust (Tervalon & Murray-García, 1998; Centers for Medicare & Medicaid Services, 2023). When dashboards function as mirrors for learning rather than microscopes for blame, they encourage staff to raise concerns and co-create solutions, supporting durable gains in quality and safety (Edmondson, 2018; Weiner et al., 2020).

## CONCLUSION

Dashboards may begin as numbers, but they come to life only when leaders choose to look beneath them. This chapter traced a shift from compliance-driven reporting toward a practice grounded in curiosity, alignment, and human connection. Dashboards built solely to satisfy external demands flatten experience into red and green cells. Dashboards designed with intention, anchored in mission, guided by behavioral cues, and enriched by patient and staff stories become sources of insight rather than pressure.

What ultimately transforms a dashboard is not the sophistication of its visuals, but the posture of the people who use it. Metrics can sharpen focus. Thoughtful design can prompt action. Neither matters if leaders approach data with defensiveness or detachment. Meaning enters when inquiry replaces judgment and when teams feel safe enough to speak honestly about the patterns they see.

Throughout this chapter, one truth surfaced repeatedly: data draws its power from relationship with the people who interpret it, the patients whose lives it reflects, and the teams committed to improving the system behind it. When leaders honor that relationship, dashboards stop functioning as scorecards and begin to act as stories, stories of effort, vulnerability, resilience, and progress. As healthcare continues to evolve, dashboards will remain essential. Their impact, however, will depend less on the tools themselves and more on the conversations they invite. When measurement becomes a form of meaning making, dashboards cease to be destinations. They become invitations to look, to listen, and to lead with the clarity and compassion required to build safer, more equitable, more human systems of care.

## REFERENCES


Broughton, T., Weggelaar, A. M., & Sülz, S. (2025). From data to improvement: Social mechanisms as a key to understanding dashboard adoption. *American Journal of Medical Quality*, *40*(2), 31–37. DOI: 10.1097/JMQ.0000000000000225 PMID: 39910757

Brown, T., & Patel, N. (2021). Communicating with data: How meaning drives measurement. *Journal of Healthcare Management*, *66*(4), 215–223. DOI: 10.1097/JHM.0000000000000103

Centers for Medicare & Medicaid Services. (2023). *Value-based programs overview*. https://www.cms.gov/valuebasedprograms

Coiera, E., Chan, A., Brooke-Cowden, K., Rahimi-Ardabili, H., Halim, N., & Tufanaru, C. (2025). Clinical and economic impact of digital dashboards on hospital inpatient care: A systematic review. *JAMIA Open*, *8*(4), ooaf078. Advance online publication. DOI: 10.1093/jamiaopen/ooaf078 PMID: 40718761

Damberg, C. L., Sorbero, M. E., Lovejoy, S. L., Martsolf, G., Rybowski, L., & Meili, R. (2014). *Measuring success in health care value-based purchasing*. RAND Corporation.

Dolan, P., Hallsworth, M., Halpern, D., King, D., & Vlaev, I. (2018). *Influencing behaviour: The MINDSPACE approach*. Cabinet Office Behavioural Insights Team.

Edmondson, A. C. (2018). *The fearless organization: Creating psychological safety in the workplace for learning, innovation, and growth*. Wiley.

Farias, E., & Van de Walle, S. (2025). From dashboards to dialogue: Behavioural approaches to public performance management. *Public Administration Review*, *85*(2), 411–427. DOI: 10.1111/puar.13425

Health Service Executive. (2025). *Dashboards & data visualisation in healthcare: International best practices and design pillars*. https://www.hse.ie

National Patient Safety Foundation. (2015). *Free from harm: Accelerating patient safety improvement fifteen years after To Err Is Human*.

Performance Health. (2025). *Metrics that matter: Enhancing safety with healthcare dashboards*. https://www.performancehealthus.com

Symplr. (2024). *From pressure to progress: Healthcare operations & the path forward for clinical, operational & IT leaders (2024 Compass Survey Report)*. Symplr. https://www.symplr.com/press-releases/symplr-2024-compass-survey-shows-how-lack-of-alignment-impacts-us-healthcare-organizations

Tervalon, M., & Murray-García, J. (1998). Cultural humility versus cultural competence: A critical distinction in defining physician training outcomes in multicultural education. *Journal of Health Care for the Poor and Underserved*, *9*(2), 117–125. DOI: 10.1353/hpu.2010.0233 PMID: 10073197

Tufte, E. R. (1997). *Visual explanations: Images and quantities, evidence and narrative*. Graphics Press.

Weggelaar-Jansen, A. M. J. W. M., Broekharst, D. S. E., & de Bruijne, M. (2018). Developing a hospital-wide quality and safety dashboard: A qualitative research study. *BMJ Quality & Safety*, *27*(12), 1000–1007. DOI: 10.1136/bmjqs-2018-007784 PMID: 29950323

Weick, K. E., & Sutcliffe, K. M. (2015). *Managing the unexpected: Sustained performance in a complex world* (3rd ed.). Jossey-Bass. DOI: 10.1002/9781119175834

Weiner, B. J., Amick, H., & Lee, S. Y. D. (2020). Conceptualization and measurement of organizational readiness for change: A review of the literature. *Medical Care Research and Review : MCRR*, *77*(4), 379–392. DOI: 10.1177/1077558708317802 PMID: 18511812

Wolf, J. A., Niederhauser, V., Marshburn, D., & LaVela, S. L. (2021). Defining patient experience. *Patient Experience Journal*, *8*(1), 10–14. DOI: 10.35680/2372-0247.1594

## KEY TERMS AND DEFINITIONS

- **Dashboard: A visual management tool that displays prioritized performance indicators to support timely decision-making.:**
- **Key Performance Indicator (KPI): A quantifiable metric used to evaluate progress toward a defined objective.:**
- **Value-Based Care: A model linking payment to patient outcomes and efficiency rather than volume.:**
- **Bridge Metric: A measure that connects multiple care settings to reveal system-level performance gaps.:**
- **Balanced Scorecard: A structured framework aligning measures across safety:** quality, experience, equity, and finance.

• **Psychological Safety: A team climate where people feel safe to speak up with ideas or concerns without fear of retribution.:**

• **Behavioral Design: The intentional use of cues:** color, and structure to influence decision-making and promote desired actions.

• **Equity Lens: The practice of stratifying and interpreting data to identify and close disparities in outcomes.:**

• **Learning Health System: A continuously improving organization that uses data feedback loops to generate and apply knowledge in real time.:**

• **See–Share–Solve–Sustain Cycle: A practical framework for maintaining improvement momentum through visibility:** collaboration, and reinforcement.

## APPENDIX I

### Sample Dashboard View: Bridge Metrics

#### Visual Snapshot

The Bridge Metrics dashboard combined three data streams into one system view:

- A **line chart** tracked each domain across settings, visually highlighting where gaps widened (e.g., home health lagging 3% behind).
- A **heatmap** displayed cross-site variation by color intensity, deep green for alignment, yellow for variation beyond 5%.
- A **narrative column** captured *why* each variance existed, turning data into shared learning rather than silent comparison.

Figure 2 presents selected quality and safety measures across inpatient, outpatient, and home health settings, using a system level bridge metric to highlight variation, alignment, and targeted actions that support safe, reliable transitions of care.

*Figure 2. Cross-setting quality metrics with system bridge view*

| Domain | Metric | Inpatient | Outpatient | Home Health | Bridge Metric (System View) | Comments/Action |
|---|---|---|---|---|---|---|
| Infection Prevention | Hand Hygiene Compliance | 95% | 93% | 92% | 93% (System Average) | Aligned measurement definition across sites. |
| Medication Safety | Double Check on High-Alert Meds | 97% | 94% | 90% | 94% | |
| Patient Education | Documented Teach-Back Rate | 88% | 90% | 82% | 87% | Initiated joint simulation and coaching sessions |
| Readmission Risk | 30-Day Return Rate | 7% | 6% | 8% | 7% | Redesigned education template with standarized scripts. |
| Readmission Risk | 30-Day Return Rate | 7% | 6% | 8% | 7% | Redesigned education template with standarlized scripts. |
| Readmission Risk | 30-Day Return Rate | 7% | 6% | 8% | 7% | Shared case review board formed to analyze transitions. |

# APPENDIX II

## Practical Template: "Leader View" Dashboard Add-On

Use this template as a **repeatable structure** for integrating qualitative insights into any clinical dashboard.

1. Section Title

Leader View: What the Team Noticed This Week

This should appear at the bottom or top corner of the dashboard, visible but unobtrusive.

2. Weekly Reflection Prompt (Choose One)

Rotate prompts every week:

- *What made care safer this week?*
- *Where did we see teamwork make a difference?*
- *What moment reminded you why your work matters?*
- *What challenge taught us something important?*
- *What patient interaction stayed with you?*

3. Collection Method (Simple & Low-Effort)

Choose any of the following:

- 1–2 sentence submission via QR code
- Sticky notes collected at huddle
- One reflection shared verbally and typed in by the charge nurse
- Quick text box in your EHR-linked rounding tool

Ensure entries are anonymous unless staff choose otherwise.

4. Dashboard Display Format

Display only **one entry per week** with:

- **A short title** (e.g., "Preventing a Harm," "A Moment of Listening")

- **A 1–2 sentence description**
- Optional: **unit photo**, silhouette icon, or a soft color different from the main metrics

The tone should feel **human, hopeful, and grounded**.

5. Leader Practice Guide: How to Use It in Huddles

During each dashboard review:
Step 1 — Start with the Reflection
Read the weekly entry aloud before reviewing metrics.
This sets a human tone before discussing performance.
Step 2 — Connect Reflection to a Metric
Example:
"This moment ties directly to our CLABSI prevention work because…"
Step 3 — Ask a Curiosity Question
Examples:

- "What helped this happen?"
- "What can we learn from this moment?"
- "Where might we build on this next week?"

Step 4 — Close with Appreciation
Name the behavior, not the person, unless they volunteered attribution.

6. Example Insert for a Dashboard

Leader View: What We Noticed This Week
"A resident caught a contaminated line early. Instead of a CLABSI, it became a teaching moment and a reminder that vigilance prevents harm."
**Prompt Used:** *What made care safer this week?*
**Theme Identified:** Shared accountability & early detection

Figure 3 illustrates Leader Reflection Insert for Performance Dashboards. A structured, low-effort reflection panel that captures frontline observations, supports weekly learning, and integrates human insight into routine performance review and huddle discussions.

*Figure 3. A dashboard that integrates weekly staff reflections to humanize data*

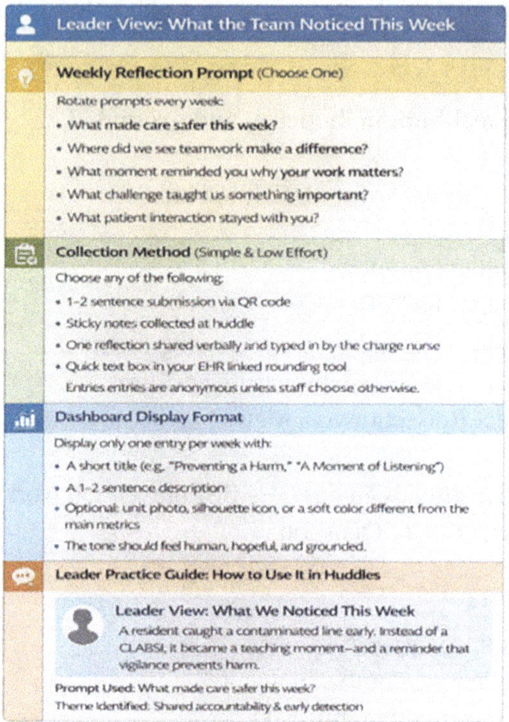

# Chapter 6
# Patient Voices at the Heart of Safety


## ABSTRACT

*Patient experience is often mistaken for hospitality. In practice, it is a central driver of safety. This chapter examines how attentive listening and meaningful engagement shift care from a sequence of tasks to a relationship grounded in trust. Drawing on research on family reported events and insights from frontline practice, it reframes experience as both a source of early risk detection and an expression of shared humanity. Through real world encounters and team-based learning, the chapter shows how patient and family narratives broaden understanding of harm, communication breakdowns, and prevention across the continuum of care. Safety strengthens not only through analysis of data, but through understanding what people feel, fear, and need. The chapter concludes with a practical structure for embedding patient and family voices into governance, daily practice, and event review so that empathy becomes measurable and engagement becomes a proactive safety strategy.*


## INTRODUCTION

For decades, patients and families noticed early signs of error long before health systems were prepared to hear them. A mislabeled medication. A subtle change in condition. A rushed answer that left someone unsure. These signals were often visible to those closest to the bedside yet rarely captured in the formal record.

One of the most widely cited examples is the experience of Sue Sheridan, who repeatedly raised concerns about her newborn son's visible jaundice. Her concerns were dismissed or left unaddressed (Patient Safety Learning. (2024). A critical bilirubin test was not performed, and her son was discharged, resulting in permanent neurologic injury. Years later, Sheridan encountered a similar failure when her husband's pathology results indicating cancer were not effectively communicated

DOI: 10.4018/979-8-3373-6496-4.ch006

or acted upon. In both cases, warning signs were present. Concerns were voiced. Yet the systems designed to hear families did not register what was being said.

Historically, safety events were handled quietly through internal memos and closed door reviews within cultures that viewed disclosure as risky and family involvement as optional. Harm was treated as an internal problem to be corrected by professionals rather than examined in partnership with those who experienced it. Families who spoke up were often labeled anxious or disruptive, their observations dismissed as subjective rather than recognized as credible signals of risk.

Over time, research began to confirm what families like the Sheridans had long understood. Patients and caregivers are frequently the first to recognize when care deviates from what feels safe. Early studies showed that families identify medication discrepancies, communication gaps, and care delays with notable accuracy, often before staff recognized that an event had occurred (National Patient Safety Foundation, 2015; Institute for Healthcare Improvement, 2022). This growing evidence challenged the assumption that safety could be engineered solely through professional surveillance and helped catalyze a broader shift. Patient and family voices came to be seen not as interruptions, but as essential sources of safety intelligence.

A pivotal moment came with research that systematically examined family reported safety events. One influential study demonstrated that families detected errors at rates far higher than traditional systems captured and identified preventable harm that would otherwise have gone unrecognized (Khan et al., 2017). This work reframed family input as data, not anecdote. It gave empirical weight to what many clinicians had observed informally: the patient and family perspective is a critical component of early risk detection.

Today, patient and family voices are increasingly woven into safety work. They participate in rounds, contribute to event reviews, and help design communication processes intended to reduce harm. The shift from secrecy to openness has altered how organizations understand error, not as an individual failing, but as an opportunity for shared learning. This chapter extends that evolution by examining how listening becomes data, how engagement becomes prevention, and how transparency reshapes trust across the continuum of care.

## Objectives of This Chapter

This chapter positions patient and family voices at the center of safety by reframing experience as a core element of harm prevention and trust-building. Listening is treated not as a courtesy, but as a clinical skill that transforms care into partnership. The objectives are to:

- Reframe patient experience as a safety function, emphasizing emotional and psychological security as foundations for trust and harm prevention rather than measures of satisfaction alone.
- Show how integrating patient and family voices into safety systems reshapes care into collaborative practice, using evidence and lived stories to illustrate the impact of listening on outcomes.
- Offer a practical framework for embedding family reporting and shared decision-making into governance and event analysis, so empathy becomes measurable and engagement evolves into a proactive prevention strategy.

## How Disclosure Builds Trust

Disclosure strengthens trust because it replaces uncertainty with clarity at moments of vulnerability. When organizations explain what happened, what is known, and what steps are underway, they signal respect and accountability. Silence or partial information invites suspicion. Transparency communicates partnership.

In the United States, regulatory frameworks have reinforced this shift. The Patient Safety and Quality Improvement Act of 2005 (PSQIA) created a national structure for reporting safety events, granting confidentiality protections to patient safety work product and authorizing Patient Safety Organizations (PSOs) to analyze events for learning rather than punishment. These protections enable clinicians and organizations to discuss errors, near misses, and contributing factors more openly, without increasing liability risk. The PSQIA establishes federal privilege and confidentiality protections intended to encourage voluntary reporting of patient safety events, supporting learning rather than punitive response (U.S. Department of Health & Human Services, n.d.).

Additional expectations for transparency arise through CMS regulations implementing Section 1311(h) of the Affordable Care Act. These require Qualified Health Plan issuers to contract only with hospitals that use patient safety evaluation systems and implement evidence-based initiatives engaging patients and families in safety and quality improvement. In this way, transparency is linked to reimbursement relationships and positioned as a core element of patient-centered care (Centers for Medicare & Medicaid Services, n.d.). Together, these structures establish disclosure not only as an ethical practice, but as a supported and expected component of contemporary safety work.

## Patient and Family Advisory Councils (PFACs) as Pillars of Patient Safety

As transparency expanded, Patient and Family Advisory Councils (PFACs) evolved from voluntary committees into core governance structures. Their growth paralleled regulatory expectations for patient engagement. Federal safety standards increasingly emphasize the integration of families into improvement efforts, particularly through quality improvement mechanisms and reporting systems that elevate the family voice. CMS standards require hospitals to demonstrate patient and family engagement in safety planning and discharge processes, aligning naturally with PFACs as organized forums for surfacing risk, communication gaps, and lived experience (Centers for Medicare & Medicaid Services, n.d.).

At the same time, PSQIA protections allowed organizations to discuss safety events within structured settings, including PFAC consultations, without exposing those discussions to legal risk. This regulatory safety net enabled PFACs to move beyond experience advisory roles and into active partnership in harm prevention strategies (U.S. Department of Health & Human Services, n.d.).

What followed was a structural shift. PFACs became embedded in the architecture of safety rather than positioned at the margins. In many organizations, PFAC representatives now participate in:

- safety walk rounds
- review of plain language policies
- redesign of communication processes
- evaluation of safety materials and discharge tools
- feedback loops tied to organizational quality metrics

Their presence ensures that patient and family perspectives are not consulted episodically but integrated continuously. Over time, PFACs have become mechanisms of accountability and trust, structures that make it easier for families to speak up before harm occurs.

As organizations wove patient and family voices into safety work, another insight emerged. What families shared was not commentary, but information about how care is experienced moment by moment. Their observations revealed not only errors, but the conditions that allow errors to form: the rushed exchange, the unanswered question, the hesitation that signaled something felt wrong. These human signals, often emotional, often subtle, began to illuminate patterns traditional metrics missed. Experience itself came to be recognized as a form of clinical intelligence.

## From Transparency to Predictive Insight

Health care organizations now draw on established models to guide communication after harm, moving away from the traditional "deny and defend" response toward openness and learning. Communication and Resolution Programs (CRPs) are one such approach, providing a systematic, transparent process for engaging patients and families after adverse events, facilitating early, honest conversations, timely investigation and explanation, support for affected individuals, and collaborative resolution of harm and its causes (Mello et al., 2014).

Within this broader category, the CANDOR model: *Communication and Optimal Resolution* offers a more prescriptive framework supported by toolkits developed by the Agency for Healthcare Research and Quality. The CANDOR Toolkit was designed to help health care organizations implement a structured approach to unexpected patient harm, emphasizing transparent communication with patients and families, systematic investigation and analysis of events, and resolution practices that support learning while maintaining respectful partnerships with those affected. The toolkit includes guidance on disclosure conversations, caregiver support, investigation processes, and organizational learning, reinforcing transparency as both a relational and a safety practice (Agency for Healthcare Research and Quality [AHRQ], 2016).

Together, CRPs and CANDOR illustrate that there is no single path to effective disclosure. Organizations adapt or blend approaches to support timely communication, accountability, and learning grounded in the voices of patients and families. As these models took hold, a broader realization followed. Transparency is not only a practice; it is a source of information. Disclosure created space for families to share what they noticed, questioned, or sensed during care. Those observations began to reveal patterns traditional reporting systems rarely captured. What felt confusing, what felt reassuring, and what felt unsafe became early indicators of system reliability. Communication patterns and emotional cues, once dismissed as subjective, started to function as predictive signals, setting the stage for experience to inform prevention.

## When Transparency Become Data

In one home care program, we compared HHCAHPS communication scores with medication error reports. The pattern was hard to ignore. Where patients said, "Staff explained things clearly," near misses declined. Where they said, "No one explained," incident reports rose. At first glance it looked like coincidence. It was not. Neuroscience helps explain why. Under stress, comprehension narrows; clear, compassionate explanation can reopen it (Van der Kolk, 2014). A discharge conversation, then, is not simply education. It is harm prevention.

## Listening as the First Act of Safety

The most powerful safety tools I have used were not forms or frameworks, but conversations. Early in my career, I asked patients, "Were you satisfied with your care?" It was a polite question, and it often produced polite answers. Later, I learned to ask something else: "Is there anything we could have done to make you feel safer today?"

The difference was immediate. The answers were specific and unvarnished: "The hallway was too dark." "You spoke too fast." "I didn't understand what to do if my pain returned." Those comments were not about comfort. They were about control. Patients were telling us what made them feel unsafe, not unsatisfied. Once we began asking, we could not pretend we hadn't heard what followed. Empathy became a form of surveillance. Listening became data (Wolf et al., 2021).

## A Voice That Changed How I Listen: Jamal's Story

One encounter involved Jamal during a home infusion visit years ago. He was seventeen, living with sickle cell disease, bright, skeptical, and tired of being misunderstood. His mother greeted me with the steady weariness of someone who had spent too many nights under hospital light.

As I reviewed the chart, Jamal said quietly, "You all write about my pain like it's a number. But it's my life. Why don't you ever ask what makes it worse?" That question stopped me. He wasn't being difficult. He was naming the gap. We had reduced suffering to a scale without asking for the story. Together, we mapped what triggered his crises: dehydration, stress, skipped meals. We adjusted his plan around his reality, not ours. Months later, his readmissions declined, not because we found a miracle medication, but because we changed the conversation. That encounter reshaped how I think about safety. Patients are not data points. They are partners in sense-making. When we listen carefully, they show us where our blind spots live.

## From Story to System: Embedding the Patient Voice

Jamal's story did not stay personal for long. It became a spark. Soon after, we began holding patient voice rounds, brief debriefs where staff shared one comment or story that had altered their understanding of safety. At first, the stories were small: a confusing label, a missed callback, a vague instruction. But over time, they accumulated into something larger: a shared language of empathy that no policy could replicate.

Those informal sessions eventually grew into structure, our first Patient and Family Advisory Council (PFAC). The early meetings were tentative, a circle of caregivers and clinicians waiting for someone to speak. Then one mother said softly, "We just want to know that when we speak, someone is really listening." That sentence shifted the room. Listening became an operational strategy rather than a symbolic value. As engagement deepened, PFAC members began reviewing educational materials, joining safety walk rounds, and participating in policy discussions. Their perspectives became part of decision-making, and teams began asking, "What did our advisors say?" before finalizing initiatives. The shift was cultural as much as procedural: feedback became relationship, not transaction, consistent with national guidance emphasizing partnership with patients and families in safety work (Agency for Healthcare Research and Quality [AHRQ], 2024).

## Why Patient Voices Matter in Safety

Patient and family voices matter because they reveal risks that routine clinical practice can miss. When patients are excluded from safety work, we lose some of our most reliable observers. They notice what clinicians may have learned to tolerate: the confusing label, the hurried explanation, the alarm no one seems to hear. Patients live inside the system continuously. Clinicians move through it episodically. That continuity holds its own wisdom.

Research supports this experiential insight. Organizations that engage patients and families in safety planning report fewer adverse events and stronger team engagement (Agency for Healthcare Research and Quality Patient Safety Network [AHRQ PSNet], 2024). Similarly, in one home health initiative, non English speaking patients rarely returned surveys until bilingual staff began follow up calls. Participation doubled, not because the questions changed, but because belonging did. This aligns with evidence that CMS approved HHCAHPS vendors use multilingual telephone follow up to increase response rates among non English speaking patients (Centers for Medicare & Medicaid Services, 2024). These patterns also underscore the importance of cultural humility, defined as curiosity, respect, and willingness to be changed by what we hear (Tervalon & Murray García, 1998). Equity begins with a question that is both simple and unsettling: *Whose story are we not hearing?* The answer often reveals gaps in communication and gaps in understanding how patients navigate care.

Most safety breakdowns do not begin with negligence. They begin with misunderstanding. A patient misinterprets instructions. A clinician assumes comprehension. A quiet gap widens into harm. One example still stays with me. A woman recovering from a diabetic foot ulcer nodded through discharge instructions she did not fully understand. Later, she admitted she hadn't changed her dressing, not from neglect, but because she physically could not reach it. Once home health support and an assistive tool were arranged, healing accelerated. The lesson was blunt: engagement is not persuasion. It is partnership. Shared decision making aligns clinical recommendations with patients lived realities, closing the gap between what we teach and what patients can do (Institute for Healthcare Improvement [IHI], 2022).

## Transparency as Trust, Not Risk

For years, some leaders feared disclosure would invite blame. In practice, silence does more damage. After a medication error that fortunately caused no injury, a physician apologized openly and described corrective steps underway. The mother's eyes filled not with anger, but relief. "You told us the truth," she said. "That means you'll tell us again if something else happens." That is trust in its most practical form. It also shaped how disclosure was approached: early communication, clear explanation, personal follow up. Within months, complaints decreased and gratitude letters increased (National Patient Safety Foundation, 2015).

In this light, transparency is more than a legal requirement. It is an act of respect. It is also the first step in turning harm into learning, shifting safety from a reporting system to a relational practice. This shift was illustrated powerfully at a recent national conference where Dr. Alisa Khan presented her research on family reported safety events. Her findings highlighted a persistent gap: much of our infrastructure still centers staff observation rather than family perception. In a 2017 JAMA Pediatrics study conducted across four U.S. children's hospitals, her team surveyed 746 parents or caregivers of 989 hospitalized children about safety related incidents. Families reported 255 events in total, including 22 preventable adverse events and 17 non harmful errors.

The implication was clear: families often detect harm earlier, more accurately, and in greater volume than traditional reporting systems. Their reports surface patterns clinical teams may miss and show why meaningful safety improvement requires systems built to listen, not only systems built to record.

## Why This Resonated

Hearing Khan's research presented made me think about a quiet gap in many safety programs, a gap not of data, but of voice. Our dashboards track falls, infections, readmissions. They rarely track what families notice: tone, delay, intuition. I have not yet implemented this particular model of structured family reporting in my own organization. But listening to Dr. Khan's work left me with urgency and hope in equal measure. It reminded me that sustainable improvement does not depend on one person's position. It depends on people who believe in the work enough to carry it forward. My role now is to create space, trust, and tools for others to make this real. The framework that follows offers a starting point, one I hope future leaders and teams will adapt, test, and strengthen.

Dr. Khan's study also named what I have witnessed repeatedly: families notice risk before it becomes harm. A caregiver sees a medication label that looks different. A beeping machine sits unattended. A child's pain cues don't match the chart. These are not anecdotes. They are early warnings. When systems invite family input, warnings can become prevention. Safety does not live only in protocols. It lives in perception. Families reveal friction points that clinical data alone may never capture.

## From Evidence to Action

Dr. Khan's work offers a practical model for embedding family participation into real time learning. The approach rests on four elements that reinforce each other:

- **Accessible reporting tools:** Simple bedside prompts and brief "family safety cards" invite caregivers to answer two questions: What happened? and What worried you most?
- **Integrated systems:** Family reports enter the same event tracking pathways used for staff findings, eliminating silos that keep patient input less visible.
- **Transparent follow up:** Families receive acknowledgment and timely updates on what was learned and what actions were taken, showing their voice leads to change.
- **Leadership framing:** Leaders consistently present family engagement as partnership and organizational strength, not scrutiny.

Together, these elements align with what psychological safety research has shown for decades: people speak up when they believe concerns will be met with appreciation rather than consequence (Edmondson, 2018). Applied to families, this turns them from silent observers into co analysts of care. It also reframes reporting from compliance into shared learning and trust building.

## Embedding the Family Voice in Systems

Reflecting on Dr. Khan's work, it became clear that the greatest opportunity is not creating more programs. It is rewiring the ones we already have to include the patient's voice. Family input should flow through the same quality channels that track events, reviews, and outcomes, not exist in a parallel track labeled feedback. The Patient and Family Centered I PASS intervention brought a structured approach to communication during inpatient rounds. Its purpose was simple: make conversations clearer, ensure shared understanding, and invite families into the dialogue in a way that mattered (Khan et al., 2018; Starmer et al., 2014).

The I PASS framework organizes rounds around five core elements: Illness Severity, Patient Summary, Action List, Situation Awareness and Contingency Planning, and Synthesis by Receiver. Clinicians explain the condition in plain language, outline the day's priorities, and discuss risks. Families restate the plan in their own words, confirming understanding and surfacing concerns. What was once a one way report becomes shared conversation that strengthens clarity and trust.

In practice, rounds followed a predictable sequence: illness severity, summary, action list, risks and contingencies, then family synthesis. Nurses contributed early so perspectives were complete. Health literacy and engagement were built in: families were invited to speak, clinicians used non technical language, and the exchange moved both ways. Interprofessional teamwork strengthened through consistent nurse physician huddles.

To reinforce verbal communication, teams provided short written summaries in the I PASS format (Figure 1) using whiteboards or paper completed in real time. Implementation relied on brief training, simulations, role playing, and accessible materials that introduced families to the process. Sustaining the work required observation, feedback, and visible reminders woven into daily workflow. Figure 6.1 illustrates; I PASS actions that structure family centered rounds. Adapted from the I PASS communication framework, originally developed to standardize clinician to clinician communication and later applied to family centered inpatient rounds (Starmer et al., 2014; Khan et al., 2018).

*Figure 1. This figure depicts the I-PASS structured handoff model*

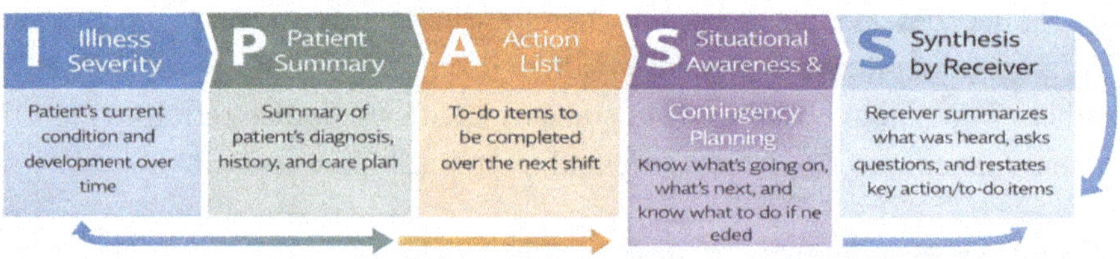


## Practice Impact

Embedding patient and family voices into everyday safety practice can measurably strengthen harm prevention, reliability, and trust by converting "feedback" into actionable clinical intelligence. Units that actively elicit concerns at key touchpoints (admission, rounds, discharge) and route reports into the same event tracking systems used for staff findings increase detection and accelerate corrective action (Khan et al., 2017; [AHRQ], 2024).

Psychological safety matters here, too. When teams are taught to respond with curiosity rather than correction, speaking up becomes more likely, learning becomes faster, and outcomes improve (Edmondson, 2018; Wolf, Niederhauser, Marshburn, & LaVela, 2021). Pairing transparent follow up ("You said, we did") with shared decision making operationalizes trust: families see their observations produce visible change, while clinicians gain context that reduces misunderstanding driven events across transitions of care (Institute for Healthcare Improvement [IHI], 2022; [NPSF], 2015).

Finally, measurement can reinforce the shift. Tracking family reported events per 1,000 patient days, documented follow up, and actions linked to family input turns empathy into a leading indicator of safety performance and equity, especially when paired with bilingual, accessible communication strategies that increase participation (Centers for Medicare & Medicaid Services, 2023; AHRQ PSNet, 2024).

## CONCLUSION

This chapter advances the idea that patient voice is not an adjunct to clinical quality but a driving force in safety itself. Speaking up is not simply a consumer behavior. It is an expression of psychological security. Patients and families share essential insights only when they feel protected, respected, and invited into the conversation. The narratives and practices explored here, from Jamal's experience to family inclusive safety rounds, show how listening reshapes clinical interactions, shifting care from a sequence of tasks to shared effort grounded in dignity and partnership. Evidence linking communication to outcomes reinforces what practice makes plain: when clinicians engage patients with clarity, compassion, and curiosity, errors decline and reliability strengthens.

Tools such as family initiated reporting pathways, integrated PFAC participation, and transparent follow up processes demonstrate how empathy becomes actionable and relational behaviors mature into measurable safety interventions. Drawing on the work of Dr. Alisa Khan and others, the chapter closes with a clear claim: embedding patient and family voices within governance, learning systems, and event analysis is not symbolic. It is a prerequisite for a resilient safety culture. When organizations operationalize this partnership, they accelerate learning, reduce preventable harm, and build the trust needed for high quality, equitable care across the continuum.

## REFERENCES


Agency for Healthcare Research and Quality. (2024). *Guide to patient and family engagement in hospital quality and safety*. U.S. Department of Health and Human Services.

Agency for Healthcare Research and Quality Patient Safety Network. (2024). *Patient- and family-centered I-PASS: Family-centered communication program to reduce medical errors*. https://psnet.ahrq.gov

AHRQ Communication and Optimal Resolution (CANDOR) Toolkit. Rockville, MD: Agency for Healthcare Research and Quality; May 2016.

Centers for Medicare & Medicaid Services. (2023). *CAHPS® Hospital Survey (HCAHPS)*. https://www.cms.gov

Centers for Medicare & Medicaid Services. (2024). *Home Health CAHPS Survey (HHCAHPS): Quality reporting and participation requirements*. https://www.cms.gov

Edmondson, A. C. (2018). *The fearless organization: Creating psychological safety in the workplace for learning, innovation, and growth*. Wiley.

Institute for Healthcare Improvement. (2022). *Partnering with patients and families to design a better health care system*. Institute for Healthcare Improvement.

Khan, A., Furtak, S. L., Melvin, P., Rogers, J. E., Schuster, M. A., & Landrigan, C. P. (2017). Parent-reported errors and adverse events in hospitalized children. *JAMA Pediatrics, 171*(4), 372–381. DOI: 10.1001/jamapediatrics.2016.4812 PMID: 28241211

Khan, A., Spector, N. D., Baird, J. D., Starmer, A. J., Rosenbluth, G., Simon, J. L., O'Toole, J. K., Yu, C. E., & Landrigan, C. P. (2018). Patient-centered I-PASS: Family-centered rounds to improve communication and safety. *Pediatrics, 142*(1), e20171873.

Mello, M. M., Boothman, R. C., McDonald, T., Driver, J., Lembitz, A., Bouwmeester, D., Dunlap, B., & Gallagher, T. (2014). Communication-and-resolution programs: The challenges and lessons learned from six early adopters. *Health Affairs, 33*(1), 20–29. DOI: 10.1377/hlthaff.2013.0828 PMID: 24395931

National Patient Safety Foundation. (2015). *Free from harm: Accelerating patient safety improvement fifteen years after To Err Is Human*. National Patient Safety Foundation.

Patient Safety Learning. (2024). *The missed bilirubin test: Cal Sheridan's story.* https://www.pslhub.org/learn/patient-safety-in-health-and-care/diagnosis/diagnostic-error/the-missed-bilirubin-test-cal-sheridans-story-r11885/

Starmer, A. J., Spector, N. D., Srivastava, R., West, D. C., Rosenbluth, G., Allen, A. D., Noble, E. L., Tse, L. L., Dalal, A. K., Keohane, C., Lipsitz, S. R., Rothschild, J. M., Wien, M. F., Yoon, C. S., Zigmont, K., Wilson, K. M., O'Toole, J. K., Wayne, D. B., & Landrigan, C. P. (2014). Changes in medical errors after implementation of a handoff program. *The New England Journal of Medicine, 371*(19), 1803–1812. DOI: 10.1056/NEJMsa1405556 PMID: 25372088

Tervalon, M., & Murray-García, J. (1998). Cultural humility versus cultural competence: A critical distinction in defining physician training outcomes in multicultural education. *Journal of Health Care for the Poor and Underserved, 9*(2), 117–125. DOI: 10.1353/hpu.2010.0233 PMID: 10073197

Van der Kolk, B. (2014). *The body keeps the score: Brain, mind, and body in the healing of trauma.* Viking.

Wolf, J. A., Niederhauser, V., Marshburn, D., & LaVela, S. L. (2021). Defining patient experience. *Patient Experience Journal, 8*(1), 10–14. DOI: 10.35680/2372-0247.159

## KEY TERMS AND DEFINITIONS

**Bridge Metrics:** Measures that connect data across inpatient, outpatient, and home settings to create a continuous, patient-centered safety narrative.

**Cultural Humility:** A practice of ongoing self-reflection and openness that helps clinicians understand and honor patients' diverse lived experiences.

**Emotional Safety:** A sense of psychological calm and respect that enables patients and families to speak up without fear of judgment or consequences.

**Family Reporting:** The structured inclusion of patients and caregivers in identifying, escalating, and interpreting potential or actual safety events.

**I-PASS:** A concise handoff framework, Illness severity, Patient summary, Action list, Situation awareness, and Synthesis, that promotes clarity and reduces communication errors.

**Patient Experience:** The totality of interactions shaped by organizational culture that influence how patients perceive the quality and humanity of their care.

**PFAC (Patient and Family Advisory Council):** A formal structure where patients and families partner with leaders to co-design policies, practices, and system improvements.

**Psychological Safety:** The belief that sharing concerns, questions, or mistakes is safe and will be met with respect rather than retaliation.

**Shared Decision-Making:** A collaborative process that aligns clinical evidence with patient values, goals, and preferences to guide care choices.

**Trust Loop:** A visible cycle in which patient feedback triggers system action, and the organization closes the loop by demonstrating what changed and why.

## APPENDIX

### Practice Vignette: I-PASS as a Tool for Family Engagement

During pediatric inpatient rounds, the attending physician invites the child's mother to speak first, asking if she has noticed any changes overnight. She reports increased fatigue and more difficulty breathing. Using the I-PASS framework, the team reviews illness severity with input from both the nurse and family, summarizes the patient's status, and outlines the day's action plan. When discussing situation awareness, the team explains warning signs to monitor and who to contact if concerns arise. The mother is then asked to restate the plan in her own words, confirming shared understanding with support from the bedside nurse. A written I-PASS summary is updated at the bedside for reference. Later that day, the family's concern is revisited during a nurse-physician huddle, prompting earlier reassessment and care plan adjustment. The structured I-PASS approach enables timely communication and reinforces the family's role as an active partner in patient safety.

### Applying I-PASS in Practice: Scenario Example

I, Illness Severity

The child's condition is slightly worse overnight. The family reports increased fatigue and more noticeable difficulty breathing, confirmed by nursing assessment.

P, Patient Summary

The patient is a 6-year-old admitted with pneumonia. Overnight, oxygen needs increased, and coughing caused visible discomfort. Current treatment includes antibiotics and supportive respiratory care.

A, Action List

- Reassess respiratory status this morning
- Adjust oxygen therapy as needed
- Obtain follow-up imaging
- Encourage mobility and monitor response to treatment

S, Situation Awareness & Contingency Planning

The team explains warning signs, including increased work of breathing or fever. The family is instructed to notify the nurse immediately if these symptoms occur.

S, Synthesis by Receiver

The mother summarizes the plan: the team will monitor breathing closely, adjust oxygen if needed, watch for fever or increased distress, and reassess later in the day. The nurse confirms understanding and updates the written bedside summary. Figure 6. 2. Application of the I-PASS framework in a clinical scenario, illustrating how the five structured elements, Illness severity, Patient summary, Action list, Situation awareness, and Synthesis, guide clear, consistent communication between clinicians and families.

*Figure 2. Scenario based representation demonstrates how the original I-PASS model, adapted from Starmer et al. (2014), supports safety, shared understanding, and family-centered decision making.*

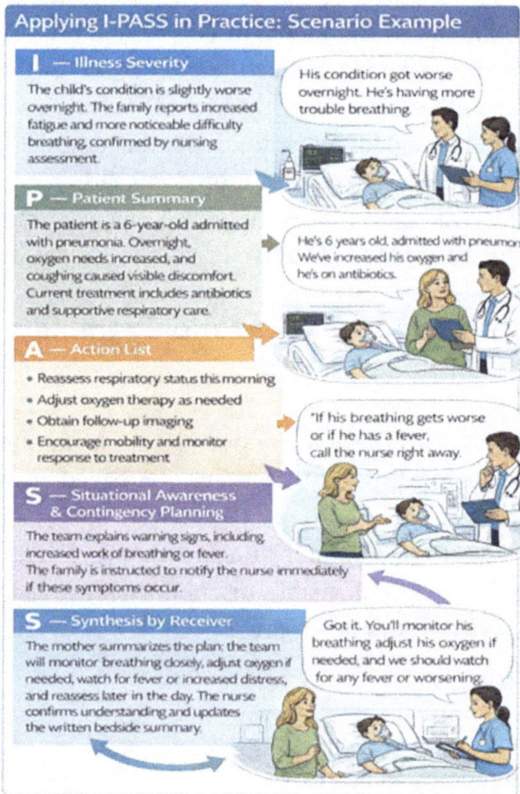

# Chapter 7
# Workplace Violence Prevention:
## Protecting Those Who Care


## ABSTRACT

*Safety in healthcare is often discussed as a patient outcome. Less often is it named for what it also is: a basic human right for those who deliver care. This chapter reframes workforce safety not as a compliance exercise, but as a foundational domain of quality itself. It explores how the very compassion that draws clinicians into service can, over time, expose them to fatigue, moral strain, and workplace violence. Through real world examples, the chapter shows how culture, environment, and leadership response determine whether harm is interrupted or quietly repeated. When psychological safety, shared accountability, and system design are treated as inseparable, organizations can move toward cultures of protection in which people feel not only physically safe, but genuinely valued.*


## INTRODUCTION

Across improvement efforts, one lesson surfaces again and again: patients cannot be protected in systems that fail to protect the people who care for them. Workforce safety is not an initiative layered onto clinical work; it is the infrastructure beneath it. Evidence consistently links unsafe working conditions, burnout, and exposure to aggression with poorer patient outcomes and diminished quality of care (Kim, Kitzmiller, Baernholdt, Lynn, & Jones, 2022; Lanctôt & Guay, 2014). Clinicians, whether in hospitals, clinics, or homes, routinely describe encounters with verbal hostility, physical threats, or emotional exhaustion. Many brush these experiences aside. *It comes with the job*, they say. But when harm becomes routine, something

DOI: 10.4018/979-8-3373-6496-4.ch007

deeper has failed. Culture has quietly absorbed risk and labeled it resilience (Chosewood, Nigam, & Cunningham, 2024).

Patient harm is tracked with precision. Staff harm is not. It often hides behind slogans about grit and endurance, particularly in home and community-based care where incidents unfold out of public view and reporting feels optional or futile (Felice et al., 2021; Occupational Safety and Health Administration, 2015). Over time, repeated exposure to threat or disrespect dulls empathy, the very capacity that safe, compassionate care depends on. As Berwick (1989) reminded the field decades ago, improvement is not only technical. It is moral. Systems that protect caregivers protect patients by design. Seen this way, workforce safety is not about self-preservation. It is about stewardship: protecting the human capacity to care. In healthy organizations, safety moves in both directions, creating conditions where compassion can persist without exacting a personal cost.

## Objectives of This Chapter

- **Reframe Workforce Safety as a Quality Imperative**

Position workforce safety as a core dimension of healthcare quality and patient protection, rather than a regulatory or compliance activity.

- **Provide an Evidence-Based Violence Prevention Framework**

Describe key components of effective workplace violence prevention, including leadership commitment, threat assessment structures, reporting pathways, training, and system-level safeguards.

- **Advance a Culture of Psychological Safety and Belonging**

Illustrate how organizations can move from reactive incident response toward proactive culture-building that supports speaking up, shared accountability, and inclusion.

## A Moment That Changed the Lens

My understanding of workforce safety shifted during a quiet conversation with a nurse after a difficult home visit. A family member had become verbally aggressive, the tension escalating enough to leave her shaken. She had not reported the incident. When I asked why, she paused before answering, almost apologetically: *"I didn't want to seem difficult. We're taught to manage."* That sentence lingered.

It captured what the literature has long suggested: silence in the face of risk is not resilience; it is resignation (Lanctôt & Guay, 2014).

Healthcare has historically rewarded endurance. Workers are trained to adapt, absorb, and continue, even when conditions are unsafe. This normalization of harm reflects a deeply embedded belief that caring for others requires personal sacrifice (Chosewood, Nigam, & Cunningham, 2024). Yet the evidence points in the opposite direction. Environments that tolerate violence and disrespect experience higher burnout, increased turnover, and worse patient outcomes (Kim, Kitzmiller, Baernholdt, Lynn, & Jones, 2022).

When staff are forced to choose between personal safety and professional duty, compassion itself is compromised. Occupational Safety and Health Administration (OSHA (2015) and NIOSH (2024) both emphasize that effective violence prevention depends less on equipment alone than on trust. When employees believe their concerns will be heard and acted upon, they report earlier, making prevention possible. That nurse's story became a catalyst. Protecting caregivers, I realized, is not adjacent to patient safety; it is where patient safety begins. Psychological safety rests on this foundation. As Edmondson (2018) notes, people must feel safe to learn. In healthcare, learning starts when endurance gives way to empathy, and courage is redefined; not as suffering silently, but as speaking honestly.

## Seeing Risk Through the Eyes of Staff

As conversations about safety deepened, risk began to look different. In many care environments, verbal threats, intimidation, and aggression are not rare disruptions; they are recurring features of systems that quietly normalize hazard as part of caregiving (Felice et al., 2021). Programs that rely only on retrospective reporting miss the opportunity to see harm forming in real time. Dashboards and incident logs told part of the story, but not enough. To understand risk as staff experienced it, we convened a focus group of clinicians, aides, and support personnel and asked a single question: *"Tell us about the violence you encounter in your daily work."*

What followed was unpolished and deeply revealing. Staff spoke of unpredictable behaviors in patient homes, escalating family dynamics, verbal threats, and the constant vigilance required when working alone. Many admitted they had never been asked these questions in a formal setting. Naming the harm aloud created a shared recognition: these were not isolated episodes, but patterns shaped by expectations, workflows, and culture. To honor those voices, the team created a short video using excerpts from the focus group. It was not refined. It was real. When the organization opened its annual Quality and Safety Forum with the video, the effect was immediate. The room fell quiet. Leaders later said it was the first time they had *felt* the problem, rather than reviewed it.

That moment mattered. The organization committed to building a comprehensive Employee Safety Program grounded in structure, training, and technology. The investment was framed not as regulatory compliance, but as a moral response to what staff had shared. Listening, as it turned out, was the first act of prevention.

## Bringing the Program to Life: A Case of Transformation

Sustaining that momentum required more than acknowledgment. It required architecture. Leadership recognized the need for dedicated expertise and recruited a Public Safety leader whose role was to translate urgency into operational discipline. This position became the anchor for turning intent into practice. The resulting Employee Safety Program was built around three reinforcing pillars: structure, training, and technology. The approach aligned with national guidance emphasizing workforce protection as integral to patient safety and system reliability (Occupational Safety and Health Administration, 2015; The Joint Commission, 2021).

1. Structure: Building Accountability

An interdisciplinary Employee Safety Committee was established, supported by a Threat Assessment and Management Team (TAMT). TAMTs are multidisciplinary, prevention-focused structures designed to identify and mitigate behavioral threats before harm occurs. These teams bring together clinical leadership, public safety, human resources, and partners from behavioral health, risk management, and operations as needed (Administration for Strategic Preparedness and Response [ASPR], 2024).

Rather than assigning blame, the TAMT evaluates patterns of concerning behavior and environmental contributors to escalation. Mitigation strategies are proportionate, coordinated, and centered on staff protection, service continuity, and psychological safety. Closed-loop communication, emotional support following incidents, and systematic capture of lessons learned are central features. Over time, findings are integrated into organizational dashboards, strengthening prevention and learning across settings (ASPR, 2024).

2. Training: Empowering Through Knowledge

Education became the bridge between awareness and action. Clinicians and support staff participated in hands-on training in crisis management, de-escalation, and situational awareness, reflecting evidence-based models that prioritize simulation and experiential learning (Somani et al., 2021).

Within six months, safety perception scores rose from 81% to 88%. Post-training surveys reflected increased confidence in recognizing early warning signs of aggression. Staff described a shift away from silent endurance toward shared preparedness, an indicator of psychological safety in practice (Edmondson, 2018).

3. Technology: Making Safety Tangible

Because many incidents occurred in isolated environments, the organization deployed a personal mobile safety device with GPS tracking and emergency alerts. Occupational safety literature consistently supports technological aids for lone workers (Felice et al., 2021). Yet the device's impact extended beyond function. It carried a message that mattered: *you are not alone*.

## Cultural and Measurable Impact

Improving reporting systems was necessary but insufficient. What changed behavior was the assurance that every report would lead somewhere. With the TAMT in place, reporting shifted from a bureaucratic exercise to a meaningful act. Evidence suggests that team-based violence prevention structures outperform individual escalation models by enabling shared accountability and timely action (Occupational Safety and Health Administration, 2015; Chosewood, Nigam, & Cunningham, 2024).

As review processes matured, staff noticed something unexpected. They felt less isolated. Reporting no longer meant shouting into a void. This shift mirrored Just Culture principles, where fairness and learning replace blame (Edmondson, 2018). One clinician put it simply: *"For the first time, I feel seen before something goes wrong."*

Metrics told part of the story. Incident reports grew richer in detail, reflecting trust. Workforce safety dashboards began appearing alongside patient safety metrics, signaling that the two were inseparable (Chosewood, Nigam, & Cunningham, 2024). Reporting volume increased by 27%, while follow up timeliness improved by 40%. These figures did not indicate more harm. They indicated more honesty (Agency for Healthcare Research and Quality, 2023). As psychological safety strengthened, staff began identifying risks earlier, often before incidents occurred. Departments that once operated in silos aligned their efforts. Safety officers joined patient safety committees. Workforce metrics entered leadership discussions. Frontline voices became part of executive rounds, echoing Joint Commission guidance on cross-functional visibility (The Joint Commission, 2021).

Over time, the organization moved from reacting to incidents toward anticipating vulnerability. Monthly debriefs included near misses and emotional strain, not just completed events. Leaders checked in after difficult visits. Peers offered debriefs without judgment. New employees were oriented to a simple expectation: *speak safety first.* The shift revealed a central truth. Safety endures where empathy and accountability meet. Protecting the workforce became less a project milestone than a moral stance embedded in daily work. Or, as one clinician summarized it, *"We finally measure what matters, the safety of the people who make care possible."*

## Designing Systems That Protect the Workforce

A truly safe organization is not one that reacts well after harm occurs, but one that anticipates risk before it surfaces. In healthcare, safety cannot rest on individual vigilance alone. It has to be designed, into environments, workflows, and everyday expectations. As Berwick (1989) observed, improvement is rarely about heroic individuals; it depends on systems that make the right actions easier and the wrong ones harder. The organization's safety redesign began with a simple but telling question: *Where do staff feel most vulnerable?* The answers were consistent. Home visits after dark. Working alone in unfamiliar environments. Encounters charged with emotional intensity. These local insights mirrored national findings showing that home health and community-based providers face disproportionate exposure to intimidation and violence (Felice et al., 2021; Occupational Safety and Health Administration, 2015).

Leaders responded with a combination of environmental and process changes. Secure parking, panic buttons, and clearer field safety protocols addressed physical exposure. Communication practices, daily check-ins, shared visit logs, and brief "safe arrival" texts created a sense of connection for staff who often worked in isolation. Together, these interventions reflected OSHA's (2015) guidance that effective prevention blends environmental design with behavioral response. Yet the most consequential redesign was not physical. It was cultural.

The team introduced a *Safety Pause* protocol, granting every staff member explicit authority to stop work if something felt unsafe, without penalty, explanation, or hesitation. This approach aligned with Just Culture principles by affirming professional judgment and discretion rather than rigid compliance (Edmondson, 2018). The first time the protocol was used, a nurse paused a home visit after noticing escalating agitation from a family member. The team regrouped, revisited the care plan, and returned the following day under safer conditions. The patient received uninterrupted care. The clinician was not harmed. The pause worked not because of policy language, but because permission was real.

Each Safety Pause was followed by a structured debrief focused on learning, not fault. Teams examined what conditions made risk possible and what supports were missing. These conversations echoed AHRQ's (2023) continuous learning model, treating near misses as sources of knowledge rather than failures. As one supervisor reflected, *"We stopped asking why the nurse didn't follow the process and started asking why the process didn't protect the nurse."*

To sustain engagement, leaders carried these lessons into daily safety huddles and leadership walk rounds. Executives attended debriefs not to investigate, but to listen. Their physical presence reinforced that safety was not delegated, it was shared (The Joint Commission, 2021). Staff later reported that seeing leaders show up, rather than follow up by email, reduced fear and improved response timeliness.

System design expanded further to include emotional safety. After critical incidents, the organization implemented psychological first aid, offering immediate, structured support. Emerging evidence suggests that early recovery interventions reduce post-incident trauma and burnout (Chosewood, Nigam, & Cunningham, 2024; Lanctôt & Guay, 2014). Leaders were trained to recognize distress and respond with empathy rather than efficiency.

Over time, the effects became visible, not only in metrics, but in demeanor. Incident response times shortened. Absenteeism linked to workplace stress declined. Engagement scores rose. More telling, the language of safety changed. Conversations shifted from reporting events to anticipating needs. These patterns reflect what AHRQ (2023) and NIOSH (2024) describe as the hallmark of resilient systems: the ability to learn faster than conditions change. Menendez et al. (2024) explicitly centers workplace violence as both a safety and mental health threat to healthcare workers. Designing for safety, the organization learned, is not a one-time intervention. It is an ongoing commitment to shape systems around human experience.

## From Safety to Belonging

As the organization's understanding of safety matured, something less expected began to emerge: belonging. What had once been defined by incident counts and compliance checklists became a lived experience of being valued and protected. The question subtly shifted, from *what keeps people safe* to *what makes them stay*. That distinction marked the transition from program to purpose.

Belonging, in this context, went beyond physical security. It meant emotional inclusion and mutual respect. When clinicians spoke about feeling safe, they used words like *supported*, *heard*, and *trusted*. This language echoed national research linking psychological safety to engagement, retention, and quality outcomes (Kim, Kitzmiller, Baernholdt, Lynn, & Jones, 2022; Edmondson, 2018). Teams that felt connected reported fewer errors and demonstrated stronger collaboration under pressure. Leadership played a decisive role in making belonging visible. During executive rounds, leaders asked not only, *"What happened?"* but also, *"How are you doing?"* They acknowledged that workforce well-being is not separate from operational performance, it underpins it (The Joint Commission, 2021). These moments of presence built trust more effectively than any dashboard could.

Recognition practices shifted as well. Acts of protection began to carry the same weight as clinical excellence. A nurse who successfully de-escalated a volatile situation was honored alongside colleagues recognized for patient satisfaction. The signal was clear: safety was not reactive. It was relational. The outcomes followed. Workforce turnover declined. Engagement surveys included comments such as *"I feel part of something that values me."* These words mattered. They reflected an emotional truth supported by the evidence: people who feel they belong do their best work and stay longer (Agency for Healthcare Research and Quality, 2023).

In time, workforce safety came to reflect organizational character. It was defined less by protocols than by how people treated one another when pressure mounted and no one was watching. The culture had moved from compliance to compassion, from reaction to prevention, and ultimately, from safety to belonging.

### The Moral Architecture of Safety

Every culture of safety rests on a moral architecture. Policies and metrics form the scaffolding, but trust is the structure itself. When organizations protect their people, body, mind, and spirit, they protect the integrity of care. What began as a workforce safety program evolved into something more enduring: a declaration that compassion and protection are inseparable. The same systems that prevent patient harm must also shield the hands and hearts that deliver care. As Berwick (1989) and AHRQ (2023) remind us, improvement is not merely technical. It is ethical.

Leaders shape that moral landscape long before safety is measured. Their language, presence, and willingness to listen define what safety feels like. When blame gives way to curiosity and belonging is made visible, leaders build what Edmondson (2018) describes as fearless organizations, places where people can speak honestly and act with courage. The lesson from this journey is clear. Safety is not a static goal. It is a living relationship. It grows where people are seen, valued, and trusted. It thrives where vulnerability is met with care. In the end, the measure of a safe organization is not the absence of harm, but the presence of confidence, the quiet assurance that those who give care will be cared for in return.

## PRACTICE IMPACT

Implementing a comprehensive workplace violence prevention program carries meaningful implications for clinical practice. Reframing workforce safety as a core quality domain reduces burnout and turnover while strengthening patient outcomes

(Kim, Kitzmiller, Baernholdt, Lynn, & Jones, 2022). Evidence-based strategies, including Threat Assessment and Management Teams (TAMTs) and structured reporting pathways, foster psychological safety and enable staff to speak up without fear of retaliation (Edmondson, 2018; Occupational Safety and Health Administration, 2015). These approaches move organizations from reactive response toward proactive prevention (Chosewood, Nigam, & Cunningham, 2024). Integrating technology such as mobile safety devices further supports lone workers, reinforcing that caregiver protection is inseparable from patient care (Felice et al., 2021). Together, these measures transform safety from compliance into ethical commitment, positioning organizations as learning systems that value both physical and emotional well-being (Agency for Healthcare Research and Quality, 2023; Berwick, 1989).

## CONCLUSION

Workforce safety is not peripheral to quality; it underwrites it. This chapter reframed the protection of caregivers as both an ethical and operational imperative, recognizing that unsafe conditions erode compassion and compromise care. Through strategies such as Threat Assessment and Management Teams (TAMTs), structured reporting, environmental design, and supportive technology, organizations can move beyond reaction toward anticipation. At the center of this shift is psychological safety, the belief that speaking up will lead to learning rather than blame. When that belief is present, organizations gain the capacity to see risk earlier and learn faster. Leadership engagement proved decisive, signaling that safety is a shared responsibility, not a delegated task.

Ultimately, protecting the protectors is about more than preventing harm. It is about creating conditions in which caregivers feel valued, connected, and empowered. In doing so, healthcare organizations affirm a simple but enduring truth: the path to high reliability begins with care for those who deliver it.

## REFERENCES


Administration for Strategic Preparedness and Response. (2024). *Workplace violence*. U.S. Department of Health and Human Services, Office of the Assistant Secretary for Preparedness and Response. https://asprtracie.hhs.gov/technical-resources/resource/2791/workplace-violence

Agency for Healthcare Research and Quality. (2023). *Patient safety culture surveys: User guide and resources*. U.S. Department of Health and Human Services. https://www.ahrq.gov/sops

Berwick, D. M. (1989). Continuous improvement as an ideal in health care. *The New England Journal of Medicine, 320*(1), 53–56. DOI: 10.1056/NEJM198901053200110 PMID: 2909878

Chosewood, L. C., Nigam, J. A. S., & Cunningham, T. R. (2024). Workplace violence prevention in healthcare: Integrating worker well-being and system safety. *Journal of Occupational and Environmental Medicine, 66*(3), 189–196. DOI: 10.1097/JOM.0000000000003098

Edmondson, A. C. (2018). *The fearless organization: Creating psychological safety in the workplace for learning, innovation, and growth*. Wiley.

Felice, S. T., Goodwin, S. G., Oliveri, A., Socias-Morales, C., Castillo, D., & Olawoyin, R. (2021). Home health care workers: A growing and diverse workforce at high risk for workplace violence. *Centers for Disease Control and Prevention: NIOSH Science Blog*. https://blogs.cdc.gov/niosh-science-blog/2021/09/02/hhc-violence

Kim, S., Kitzmiller, R., Baernholdt, M., Lynn, M. R., & Jones, C. B. (2022). Patient safety culture: The impact on workplace violence and health-worker burnout. *Workplace Health & Safety, 71*(2), 78–88. DOI: 10.1177/21650799221126364 PMID: 36476112

Lanctôt, N., & Guay, S. (2014). The aftermath of workplace violence among healthcare workers: A systematic literature review of consequences. *Aggression and Violent Behavior, 19*(5), 492–501. DOI: 10.1016/j.avb.2014.07.010

Menendez, C. C., Arespacochaga, E., Begley, R., Bhatnagar, M., Ross, P., Schaefer, M. E., Spring, C., & Tisdale-Pardi, J. (2024, May 29). *Prioritizing our healthcare workers: The importance of addressing the intersection of workplace violence and mental health and wellbeing*. †NIOSH Science Blog.‡ Centers for Disease Control and Prevention. https://blogs.cdc.gov/niosh-science-blog/2024/05/29/hcw_violence_mh/

Occupational Safety and Health Administration. (2015). *Guidelines for preventing workplace violence for health care and social service workers* (OSHA Publication 3148). U.S. Department of Labor. https://www.osha.gov/sites/default/files/publications/osha3148.pdf

Somani, R., Murnane, A., & Pinto, S. (2021). Effectiveness of interventions to decrease workplace violence toward emergency department nurses: A systematic review. *Journal of Emergency Nursing: JEN*, *47*(4), 620–632.

The Joint Commission. (2021, June 18). *Workplace violence prevention standards* ($R^3$ Report, Issue 30). https://www.jointcommission.org/standards/r3-report

## KEY TERMS AND DEFINITIONS

**Belonging in Healthcare Organizations:** A sense of being valued and supported that strengthens engagement, retention, and care quality.

**Just Culture:** An approach that promotes learning and fairness by separating human error from reckless behavior.

**National Institute for Occupational Safety and Health (NIOSH):** A CDC agency that conducts research and issues guidance to protect worker safety and health.

**Occupational Safety and Health Administration (OSHA):** A federal agency that sets and enforces workplace safety standards, including in healthcare.

**Organizational Resilience:** The ability of a healthcare system to anticipate, adapt to, and learn from risk and disruption.

**Psychological Safety:** A climate in which staff feel safe to speak up about concerns without fear of blame or retaliation.

**System Design for Safety:** The deliberate design of workflows and environments to make safe actions easier and more reliable.

**Threat Assessment and Management Teams (TAMTs):** Multidisciplinary teams that identify and address early warning signs of potential workplace violence.

**Workforce Safety:** The protection of healthcare workers from physical, emotional, and environmental harm as a core quality priority.

**Workplace Violence Prevention:** Proactive strategies used to reduce the risk of physical or psychological harm to healthcare workers.

# APPENDIX I

## How to Build a Robust Employee Safety Program

A strong Employee Safety Program is built on clear leadership commitment, frontline engagement, systematic risk assessment, and consistent follow through. Effective programs include:

1. Leadership Commitment

Set a zero-tolerance policy for violence, assign ownership to a designated safety leader and committee, allocate resources (training, alarms, security), and integrate safety metrics into organizational dashboards and walk rounds.

2. Frontline Participation

Include staff, security, and behavioral health experts in planning and the Threat Assessment and Management Team (TAMT). Promote reporting without retaliation, support anonymous options, and review near-misses during huddles.

3. Risk Identification

Conduct organization-wide violence-risk assessments, analyze incident and OSHA data, flag behavioral risks in the EHR, survey environmental vulnerabilities, and perform rapid post-incident debriefs.

4. Prevention and Control Measures

Implement a multidisciplinary TAMT to assess threats and coordinate response. Reinforce daily safety huddles, strengthen engineering and administrative controls (alarms, access control, screening), and provide structured recovery support after incidents, including psychological first aid and return-to-work checks.

5. Education and Training

Provide orientation on rights and reporting, annual de-escalation and self-protection training, supervisor instruction on investigation and response, and brief refreshers following emerging trends.

6. Ongoing Evaluation

Track key metrics (incident rates, DART, training completion, TAMT response time), conduct routine audits, and measure staff perceptions of safety through annual culture surveys.

7. Coordination and Communication

Facilitate consistent communication across HR, Public Safety, Security, Occupational Health, and Risk Management; maintain relationships with local emergency responders; and share lessons learned and success stories. Recognize teams demonstrating strong safety practices.

Figure 7.1 presents an integrated, cyclical model for employee safety grounded in leadership accountability and frontline engagement. The framework emphasizes continuous risk identification, targeted education and training, prevention and control strategies, effective coordination and communication, and ongoing evaluation. Together, these interdependent components support a learning system that strengthens workforce safety, reinforces organizational reliability, and sustains safe care delivery across complex healthcare environments.

*Figure 1. A simplified framework showing the core components of a robust employee safety program*

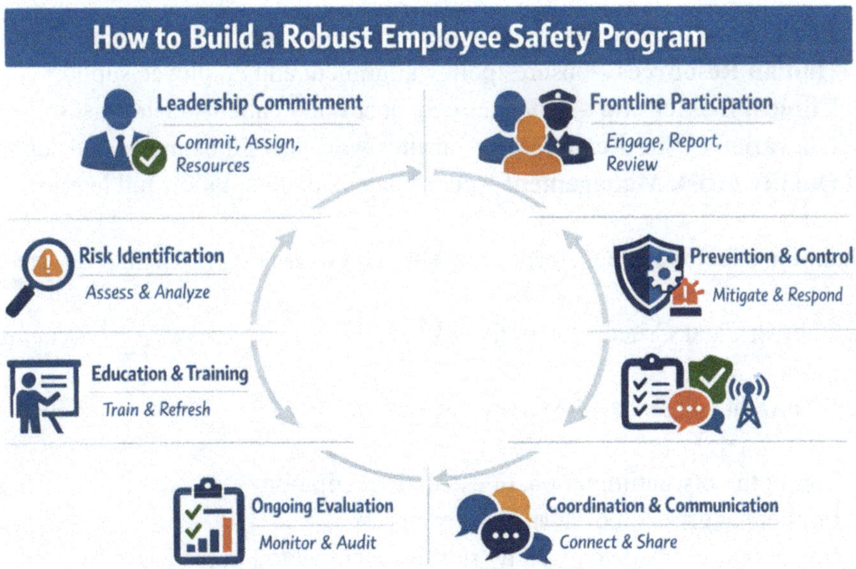
How to Build a Robust Employee Safety Program
Leadership Commitment
Commit, Assign, Resources
Frontline Participation
Engage, Report, Review
Risk Identification
Assess & Analyze
Prevention & Control
Mitigate & Respond
Education & Training
Train & Refresh
Ongoing Evaluation
Monitor & Audit
Coordination & Communication
Connect & Share

# APPENDIX II

## How to Establish a Threat Assessment and Management Team (TAMT)

A Threat Assessment and Management Team provides a structured, multidisciplinary approach for identifying, evaluating, and responding to behaviors that may pose a risk to staff or patients. Establishing a TAMT requires intentional design, clear governance, and reliable processes.

1. Define the Team's Purpose

Articulate the TAMT's role as the organization's central mechanism for evaluating concerning behaviors, coordinating interventions, and ensuring consistent follow up. The purpose statement should emphasize prevention, early action, and staff protection rather than punitive response.

2. Identify Core Membership

Build a multidisciplinary team with members who bring complementary perspectives. Core roles typically include:

- **Public Safety / Security Lead** – oversees risk evaluation and safety measures
- **Human Resources** – ensures policy alignment and employee support
- **Clinical Leadership** – evaluates care needs and patient-related risks
- **Operations / Site Leadership** – ensures workflow adjustments and support
- **Quality / Risk Management** – coordinates documentation and learning

Additional members (e.g., legal counsel, social work) may be engaged as needed.

3. Establish Clear Criteria for Activation

Define what triggers a TAMT review, such as:

- Verbal threats, intimidation, or escalating agitation
- Physical aggression or near-miss events
- Behavioral red flags flagged by staff or documented in the EHR
- Recurrent safety concerns involving the same patient, visitor, or employee

Clear criteria strengthen consistency and reduce hesitation in reporting.

4. Create a Standardized Referral Pathway

Develop simple, accessible methods for initiating a TAMT review:

- A dedicated reporting form or EHR trigger
- A direct email or hotline monitored by Public Safety
- Referral through leaders after huddles or incident reports

The process should require minimal burden on staff and guarantee timely review.

5. Build a Structured Assessment Process

Use a consistent framework for evaluating risk. A typical process includes:

1. **Gather information** from incident reports, staff interviews, EHR notes, and security logs.
2. **Assess risk level** using behavioral indicators and situational factors.
3. **Determine safe alternatives**, modified visit plans, paired visits, telehealth, or environmental controls.
4. **Develop an intervention plan** with clear roles, timelines, and follow-up.
5. **Document all actions** in a shared, secure system.
6. Define Response and Follow Up Expectations

Set expectations for:

- Initial review (e.g., within 24–48 hours for concerning behaviors)
- Documentation requirements
- Communication back to staff who submitted concerns
- Ongoing monitoring in subsequent huddles or leadership rounds

Reliable follow-through is what builds trust in the system.

7. Train Team Members and the Workforce

Provide TAMT members with training in threat assessment models, de-escalation strategies, trauma-informed communication, and decision-making under uncertainty.

Educate frontline staff on:

- When to notify the TAMT
- How the team works
- What to expect after submitting a concern

Transparency reduces fear and increases reporting.

8. Integrate TAMT Insights Into Organizational Learning

Incorporate trends and lessons learned into:

- Leadership dashboards
- Safety huddles
- Workflow redesign
- Policy updates
- Staff education

This signals that the TAMT is not an isolated function, but part of a broader culture of protection and prevention.

9. Evaluate and Refine the Program

Regularly assess:

- Volume and type of referrals
- Timeliness of response
- Staff perception of safety and reporting trust
- Effectiveness of intervention strategies
- Patterns that require system-level changes

Figure 2 outlines a structured, prevention-focused framework for establishing a Threat Assessment and Management Team. The model defines the purpose of TAMT, identifies core multidisciplinary membership, specifies criteria for activation, and delineates clear referral pathways and assessment and response processes. Together, these elements support early identification of behavioral risk, coordinated response, and proactive mitigation of threats to staff safety while reinforcing a non-punitive, learning-oriented safety culture.

*Figure 2. A streamlined framework outlining the essential components of a Threat Assessment and Management Team (TAMT)*

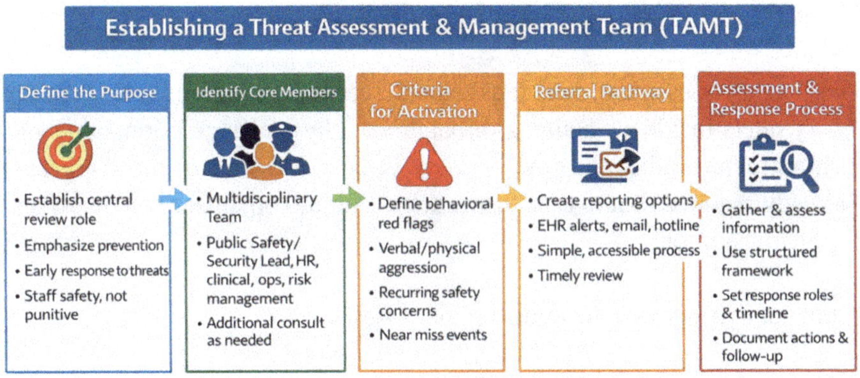

## APPENDIX III

### TAMT's Role in Post-Incident Review

The Threat Assessment and Management Team plays a central role in ensuring that every safety incident whether a verbal threat, physical aggression, or near miss, receives a structured, fair, and timely review. Its purpose is not to re-investigate what staff already reported, but to transform each event into organizational learning and actionable prevention.

1. Conduct a Structured, Multidisciplinary Review

After an incident is reported, the TAMT brings together perspectives from Public Safety, HR, clinical leadership, behavioral health, operations, and risk management to examine the event in context. This multidisciplinary lens helps determine what conditions contributed to the incident, rather than who is at fault.

2. Assess Ongoing or Escalating Risk

The team evaluates whether the behavior is likely to recur or intensify. This includes reviewing previous incidents, behavioral patterns, environmental factors, and staff concerns. TAMT's assessment ensures that risk is managed proactively, not reactively.

3. Develop a Coordinated Response Plan

Based on the review, TAMT outlines concrete actions such as:

- Adjusting visit plans or assigning paired visits
- Implementing telehealth alternatives when appropriate
- Modifying environmental or workflow controls
- Engaging behavioral health resources
- Establishing safety check-ins for affected teams

The goal is to provide practical, immediate protection for staff and continuity of safe care.

4. Communicate Back to Staff and Leaders

Timely communication builds credibility. TAMT informs involved staff and local leaders about:

- The actions taken
- What to expect next
- Who to contact for follow-up support

This closes the loop and reinforces that reporting leads to real action, not silence.

5. Support Emotional Recovery and Well-Being

TAMT ensures that staff affected by the incident receive appropriate support, such as psychological first aid, debriefing, or occupational health follow-up. Recognizing emotional impact is essential to restoring trust, confidence, and readiness to return to work.

6. Capture Lessons Learned and Update Protocols

TAMT converts post-incident insights into organizational learning by:

- Identifying system vulnerabilities
- Updating safety protocols or environmental controls
- Informing just-in-time training
- Sharing trends in huddles and leadership rounds

This reinforces a learning culture, where each event shapes safer future practice.

7. Track Trends and Integrate Findings Into Safety Dashboards

Patterns identified through TAMT reviews feed into broader safety analytics. By tracking repeated risks or high-risk settings, the team helps guide prevention strategies, resource allocation, and workforce support. Presenting TAMT insights alongside patient-safety metrics signals that caregiver safety is a core quality domain.

Figure 3 illustrates the Threat Assessment Management Team's (TAMT) structured role following an incident, moving from multidisciplinary review and risk assessment through coordinated response, communication, staff support, and organizational learning. The sequence emphasizes both immediate risk mitigation and long-term system improvement through trend tracking and integration into safety dashboards.

*Figure 3. TAMT's role in post-incident review*

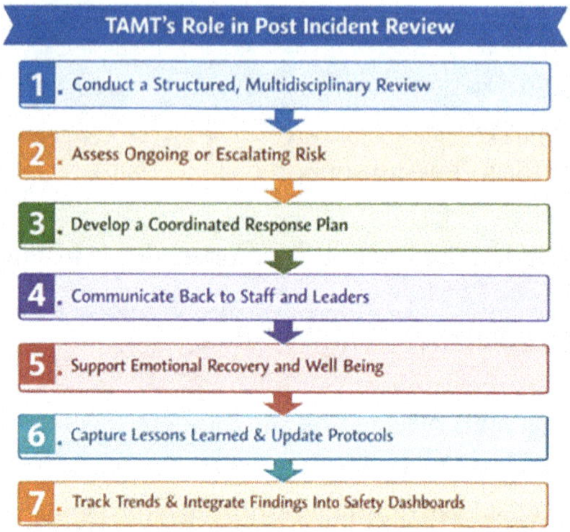


A streamlined process showing how TAMT conducts review, manages risk, supports staff, and feeds lessons learned into ongoing safety improvement.

# Chapter 8
# Seeing Risk Before It Sees You


## ABSTRACT

*Risk assessment in healthcare is shifting from a backwardlooking, compliancedriven exercise toward a more demanding focus on foresight. In this chapter, risk is treated not as a static checklist but as a living signal of system strain, human limits, and organizational resilience. Two complementary approaches are examined: Proactive Risk Assessment (PRA) and Proactive Latent Risk Assessment (PLRA, each contributing differently to safety and reliability. PRA focuses on protecting execution by identifying threats to scope, timelines, resources, and operational readiness, often within defined projects. PLRA broadens the lens to surface quieter risks introduced through structural decisions, workload assumptions, cultural norms, and environmental conditions that shape behavior long before harm occurs. Drawing on safety science and real world application, the chapter shows how PRA and PLRA reveal distinct yet interdependent forms of risk. Used together, they support early signal detection, reduce cognitive burden, strengthen psychological safety, and anticipate system strain under pressure.*


## INTRODUCTION

After decades of leading quality and safety initiatives, I've learned that the most consequential question is rarely *What failed?* More often, it is *What could fail next if we don't look closely enough?* Asked early, at the start of a project, before momentum takes over, that question has saved more time, trust, and credibility than any mitigation plan written after harm has already occurred. Early in my leadership career, risk assessment felt transactional. Identify the issue. Assign an owner. Update the spreadsheet. The work was tidy, bounded, and reassuring. Yet the deeper I moved into high reliability efforts, the more obvious its limits became. Risk, I learned, is

DOI: 10.4018/979-8-3373-6496-4.ch008

not a document. It is a conversation. And most failures are not the product of bad actors, but of unseen conditions.

Many risks originate not in individual actions but in what Reason (2008) termed *latent failures*: design weaknesses that lie quietly within systems until a particular alignment of circumstances exposes them. Proactive risk assessments helped keep initiatives on track, but many of the most painful surprises emerged outside the project boundary. They appeared in the handoffs between departments, in assumptions about readiness, or in the fatigue no dashboard ever captured. This is where latent risk assessment earns its relevance. Paine and Pronovost (2018) describe latent risk assessment as a leadership discipline, one that evaluates the risks embedded in organizational decisions *before* those decisions lead to harm. Rooted in Reason's framework, it asks leaders to examine how structure, staffing, and policy shape the conditions for reliability or failure. When this lens is integrated into everyday decision making, risk shifts from hindsight to foresight, a way of seeing the system before the system is tested.

## OBJECTIVE OF THIS CHAPTER

This chapter aims to:

- **Differentiate Proactive Risk Assessment (PRA) and Proactive Latent Risk Assessment (PLRA/LRA):** Clarify how each serves a distinct purpose, one focused on protecting project execution, the other on safeguarding system reliability and safety.
- **Guide leaders on when and how to apply each method:** Offer practical criteria for selecting PRA, PLRA, or both, depending on the nature of the initiative and the type of risk under consideration.
- **Describe the pitfalls of conflating the two:** Illustrate how misalignment can lead to overlooked vulnerabilities, erosion of safety culture, and preventable harm at both organizational and human levels.

## FROM REACTIVE TO PROACTIVE

Traditional risk assessment often begins once a hazard is already visible, an event report, a compliance gap, a near miss. Organizations operating in complex environments cannot afford to wait that long. Those that remain resilient treat risk not as a surprise, but as a signal. They pay attention to small frictions: the workaround that saves time, the quiet delay no one escalates, the phrase "that's just how we do it."

Safety science has long shown that some of the most valuable insights surface outside formal audits. They appear in off hand comments during a site visit, a pause during a huddle, or a hesitation before answering a routine question. These moments invite curiosity. Behind every "always" is often a latent risk, something that once solved a problem but now quietly conceals vulnerability. When leaders learn to notice these patterns before harm occurs, curiosity itself becomes a form of protection. As Pronovost and colleagues observe, high reliability systems depend on leaders who "anticipate and mitigate the risks their own decisions create" (Paine et al., 2018). That framing reshaped how I approached major initiatives. Instead of asking only whether something would succeed, I began asking what that success might quietly cost.

## PROACTIVE RISK VS. PROACTIVE LATENT RISK

### Understanding the Two Lenses

Every major initiative begins with a plan, and an implicit promise that the work will be done safely. Honoring that promise requires more than technical competence. It requires foresight. Two complementary forms of risk assessment support that work: Proactive Risk Assessment (PRA) and Proactive Latent Risk Assessment (LRA). Each operates with a different rhythm and focus. Together, they reveal how resilient an organization truly is.

1. Proactive Risk Assessment: Managing the Known

Proactive Risk Assessment is the structured, often spreadsheet based discipline that keeps implementation on track. Its role is to identify threats that could derail success, delays, budget constraints, technology failures, staffing gaps, and to manage those uncertainties within a clearly defined scope.

A typical PRA process includes:

- Identifying risks to scope, schedule, or quality
- Scoring probability and impact to prioritize threats
- Developing mitigation strategies, such as reallocating resources or adjusting timelines
- Tracking residual risk through routine reviews

PRA is essential for operational reliability. Its strength, however, is also its limitation. By design, its vigilance often ends when the project closes. A dashboard can turn green while the surrounding system quietly absorbs strain. I have seen implementations executed flawlessly on paper, only to unravel later as workarounds multiplied and fatigue accumulated. PRA protects execution. It does not always protect endurance.

2. Proactive Latent Risk Assessment: Managing the Invisible

Proactive Latent Risk Assessment (LRA), as described by Paine et al. (2018), widens the lens to examine organizational conditions that shape future risk. *Latent* refers to what exists beneath the surface, present, but not yet visible or acknowledged. In safety science, latent conditions are system level vulnerabilities introduced through design, policy, environment, or leadership decisions. They differ from active errors because they are embedded long before an event occurs, only becoming apparent when stress exposes them.

Rather than waiting for incidents, LRA seeks out these underlying conditions by examining structure, workflow, and decision making. Grounded in Reason's model of latent failure and high reliability theory, it emphasizes a difficult truth: leaders themselves create risk through the choices they make. In practice, LRA asks questions that rarely appear in project plans:

- What assumptions are we making about workload or capacity?
- How might this decision shift risk onto those doing the work?
- Which weak signals are we discounting because performance metrics look stable?

LRA is less about compliance and more about attentiveness. Silence, workarounds, and near misses are treated as early warnings, the quiet data that precede harm. When leaders map these signals, they gain the chance to redesign systems before failure occurs. In one organization I supported, a latent risk review conducted before launching a new scheduling platform revealed that night shift staff lacked reliable Wi-Fi access. That single finding prevented a cascade of downstream delays, frustration, and informal workarounds that would otherwise have been misread as individual resistance.

3. Comparing Both Approaches

These frameworks are not alternatives; they are companions. Proactive Risk Assessment secures outcomes. Proactive Latent Risk Assessment protects people and process integrity. Used together, they form a loop of anticipation and learning, one that supports a culture capable of seeing risk early, responding thoughtfully, and adapting before harm occurs.

Figure 1 contrasts proactive risk assessment, which focuses on identifying and managing known, visible, and documented hazards, with proactive latent risk assessment, which seeks to surface hidden, systemic, and emerging risks not yet apparent. Together, these approaches strengthen safety by addressing both what is known and what remains unseen in real world practice.

*Figure 1. Proactive risk assessment vs proactive latent risk assessment*

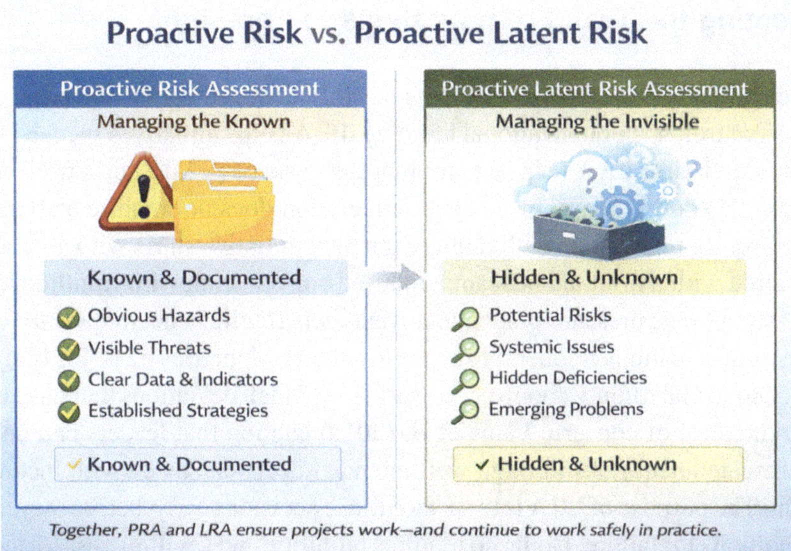


## Bringing Both Together

When Quality and Safety leadership aligns with project management disciplines, risk work can shift from a compliance obligation to a strategic practice. In reality, however, responsibility for risk assessment during large scale initiatives is often unclear. Quality and Safety leaders bring deep expertise in safety science, system reliability, and human factors. Yet many projects hinge on highly specific technical or operational details, details that only those embedded in the work can fully see.

In those moments, a project manager or process expert may be better positioned to notice where failures, disruptions, or unintended consequences are likely to emerge.

A more balanced approach pairs a traditional project risk log with a latent risk reflection. The first asks, *what could derail this plan?* The second asks, *what could this plan quietly disrupt?* Together, these questions integrate operational precision with safety awareness. They reduce tunnel vision and redefine success, not only as meeting deliverables, but as sustaining the people and processes that must live with the outcome. As Pronovost's high reliability framework reminds us, safety emerges when organizations "continually evaluate both active and latent risks across all layers of the system" (Paine et al., 2018).

## Connecting the Two: From Analysis to Foresight

When project and latent risk assessments are used together, the outcome is more than risk control, it is organizational learning. PRA helps initiatives succeed within defined boundaries; LRA helps ensure that those successes do not introduce new vulnerabilities downstream. In practice, integration does not require elaborate infrastructure. It often begins with habit. Each new initiative starts with a structured PRA, paired with a brief latent scan: a focused conversation with frontline leaders about assumptions, pressure points, and what feels fragile beneath the surface.

These conversations frequently surface what formal metrics miss. Early signs of fatigue. Quiet; uncertainty about a new workflow. Small deviations that have not yet risen to the level of concern. Paine et al. (2018) caution that leaders can unintentionally create latent risks through well intended decisions made with incomplete foresight. The purpose of LRA is to surface those decisions early, before they harden into conditions for failure. Doing so requires humility, and a willingness to question systems that appear to be performing well.

Figure 2 illustrates how Proactive Risk Assessment (PRA) concentrates on identifying and controlling known, project based risks within defined timelines, while Proactive Latent Risk Assessment emphasizes uncovering hidden system vulnerabilities through continuous, organization wide oversight. Together, these approaches demonstrate how addressing both visible risks and latent conditions strengthens reliability, safety, and long term performance.

Figure 2 illustrates how Proactive Risk Assessment (PRA) focuses on identifying and controlling known, project based risks within defined timelines, while Proactive Latent Risk Assessment emphasizes uncovering hidden system vulnerabilities through continuous, organization wide oversight. Together, these approaches demonstrate how managing both visible risks and latent conditions strengthens reliability, safety, and long term performance.

*Figure 2. Comparison of proactive risk assessment and proactive latent risk assessment. Consequences of confusion between PRA and PLRA*

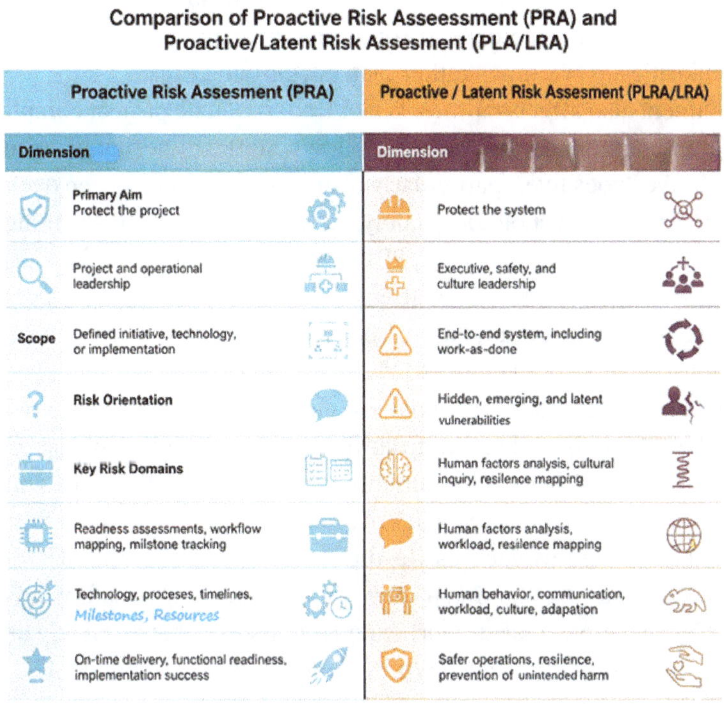


## Consequences of Confusion Between PRA and PLRA

Confusion between Project Risk Assessment (PRA) and Proactive Latent Risk Assessment (PLRA/LRA) is common in healthcare organizations, particularly during large scale operational or technology initiatives. Although both use the language of "risk," they serve fundamentally different purposes. PRA protects project deliverables, scope, schedule, budget, and resources, while PLRA protects the system itself, focusing on hidden vulnerabilities, human factor dynamics, and organizational conditions that shape future harm (Paine et al., 2018). When these approaches are conflated, leaders tend to narrow their attention to what is visible on a project plan, overlooking system forces that evolve quietly beneath the surface.

The consequences are substantial. When organizations rely solely on PRA, latent conditions often go unnoticed: communication gaps, workload strain, brittle design assumptions, cultural fatigue, and informal workarounds that gradually redefine how work is done. Evidence consistently shows that these latent factors, not frontline actions, are the primary contributors to adverse events (Reason, 2008). Without PLRA, even well executed projects can introduce downstream hazards, erode reliability, or increase cognitive burden. As Weick and Sutcliffe (2015) emphasize, high reliability performance depends on noticing weak signals early and treating small irregularities as warnings rather than background noise.

Misalignment also affects culture. When leaders equate project completion with system safety, a compliance mindset often follows. Staff may hesitate to raise concerns once an initiative "goes live," particularly if success has already been declared. This dynamic undermines psychological safety, a critical predictor of speaking up, early reporting, and learning (Edmondson, 2018). Over time, organizations drift toward reactivity, responding to harm only after it occurs. Empirical studies demonstrate that when latent risks remain unaddressed, patient safety culture deteriorates and adverse events increase (Cui et al., 2025).

The human consequences are equally real. When new workflows or technologies introduce unanticipated strain, frontline teams absorb the impact. Over time, this contributes to frustration, burnout, moral residue, and self blame when system flaws lead to near misses or errors, patterns well documented in the safety literature (Dekker, 2011). Programs such as Resilience in Stressful Events (RISE) underscore that acknowledging emotional impact is not ancillary to safety but central to resilience. Organizations that support caregivers recover more quickly and sustain engagement after stressful events (Wu & Connors, 2017). When PLRA is absent, these protective structures are often underdeveloped, leaving clinicians exposed during periods of heightened stress.

When PRA and PLRA are intentionally integrated, risk management becomes a strategic capability rather than a project artifact. PRA helps ensure the initiative succeeds; PLRA ensures that success does not conceal emerging vulnerability. Together, they support anticipation, early detection, and adaptive learning, the conditions required for a resilient, psychologically safe, high reliability organization (Pronovost & Paine, 2019; Paine et al., 2018).

## PRACTICE IMPACT

Safety science consistently demonstrates that latent conditions, not frontline behaviors, are the primary drivers of adverse events, and that early identification of these conditions measurably strengthens resilience and safety culture (Reason, 2008; Weick & Sutcliffe, 2015). When PRA and PLRA operate together, leaders detect risks that traditional project tools overlook: workload mismatches, usability burdens, communication drift, and growing reliance on informal workarounds. These weak signals typically surface through frontline insight, psychological safety, and attention to small operational frictions that dashboards rarely capture (Dekker, 2011; Edmondson, 2018).

This dual lens approach also reinforces the cultural foundations of safety. Research shows that when leaders reduce blame, encourage open reporting, and address latent risks directly, safety culture improves and adverse events decline (Cui et al., 2025; Edmondson, 2018). PLRA further supports resilience by explicitly integrating emotional realities into system design. Programs such as RISE demonstrate that structured caregiver support reduces moral distress, improves well being, and strengthens organizational recovery after stressful clinical events, linking emotional resilience to operational performance (Wu & Connors, 2017).

Figure 3 illustrates how Proactive Risk Assessment (PRA) and Latent Risk Assessment (LRA) serve complementary roles across the project and system life cycle. PRA focuses on managing scope, budget, timelines, and technical risks to ensure project delivery, while LRA examines safety, reliability, human factors, and hazard analysis to ensure systems work safely in practice. Their overlap highlights a shared goal: achieving both project success and sustained operational safety through coordinated mitigation and safety controls.

*Figure 3. Integrating proactive and latent risk assessment for project success and operational safety*

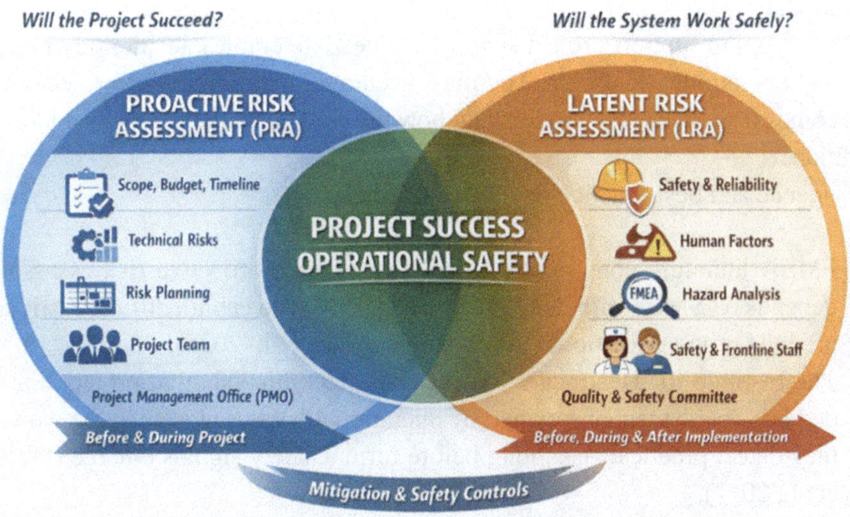

## WHO SHOULD CONDUCT PROACTIVE RISK ASSESSMENT VS. PLRA: ROLES, RATIONALE, AND EVIDENCE

Effective risk assessment depends not only on the tools used, but on who leads the analysis. In healthcare, confusion often arises about whether subject matter experts, project teams, or safety leaders should conduct proactive risk reviews. The distinction becomes clearer when separating Proactive Risk Assessment (PRA), which addresses project specific vulnerabilities, from Proactive Latent Risk Assessment (PLRA/LRA), which examines system wide conditions and human factor implications.

Both processes are essential, but they require different vantage points, expertise, and governance.

1. Who Should Conduct Proactive Risk Assessment (PRA)

Primary owners:

- Project managers and operational SMEs
- Technical leads with detailed process knowledge
- Frontline representatives who perform the work being redesigned
- IT, finance, workflow SMEs, or vendor partners (depending on the initiative)

Rationale:

PRA exists to support project success, scope, deliverables, technology integration, and operational readiness. The most accurate identification of project based risks comes from those who understand how the work actually functions under real conditions.

Evidence and best practice recommendations:

- FMEA literature consistently shows that reliable proactive risk assessment depends on SMEs with deep process expertise who can identify realistic failure modes and operational dependencies (Cui et al., 2025).
- The Institute for Healthcare Improvement recommends that project embedded risk assessments be owned by operational leaders closest to the work, as they detect practical risks long before formal safety signals emerge (Frankel et al., 2017).
- In digital health initiatives, PRA relies heavily on technical experts and workflow owners to surface integration failures, data sync risks, and usability challenges that are often invisible at higher governance levels (Waseem et al., 2025).

2. Who Should Conduct Proactive Latent Risk Assessment (PLRA/LRA)

Primary owners:

- Quality and Safety leaders
- Human factors specialists
- Leaders trained in high reliability science
- Interdisciplinary safety committees (often including psychology, risk management, and operations)
- Frontline staff as contributors, but not primary analytical owners

Rationale:

PLRA examines system reliability, workload strain, policy design, leadership decisions, coordination gaps, and cultural signals. These are organization level risks, not project specific issues, and require a panoramic view of the system.

Evidence and best practice recommendations:

- Paine and Pronovost emphasize that LRA must be led by leaders trained in safety science and organizational behavior, as the aim is to identify vulnerabilities created by leadership decisions, not frontline tasks (Paine et al., 2018).
- Reason's model locates latent risks in management decisions, resource allocation, supervision, and policy, underscoring the need for system level authority in their assessment (Reason, 2008).
- Weick and Sutcliffe note that recognizing weak signals and organizational drift is a leadership skill set typically held by safety leaders and human factors experts rather than project teams (Weick & Sutcliffe, 2015).
- LRA is most effective when facilitated by neutral governance bodies, such as quality and safety committees, reducing bias introduced by project delivery pressures (Pronovost & Paine, 2019).

## CONCLUSION

This chapter reframes risk assessment in healthcare as a discipline of foresight rather than a checklist driven compliance activity. It distinguishes two complementary approaches: Project Risk Assessment (PRA), which protects project deliverables within defined timelines and constraints, and Proactive Latent Risk Assessment (LRA), which surfaces hidden system vulnerabilities that shape safety long before harm occurs. PRA supports execution; LRA strengthens the system by examining human factors, capacity assumptions, and organizational conditions that influence reliability.

Across both approaches, the central insight is that risk is not a static inventory. It is an evolving conversation. Effective leaders learn to notice subtle signals of strain, workarounds, fatigue, communication drift, and silence where questions should be. These signals offer the clearest window into emerging vulnerability. When integrated into everyday decision making, they allow leaders to move from reacting to failure toward anticipating the conditions that make failure possible.

Together, PRA and LRA form a more complete safety architecture, one that delivers projects successfully while preserving the resilience of the people and processes required to sustain them. This integration shifts risk management from after the fact mitigation to proactive insight, enabling organizations to learn earlier, adapt faster, and absorb stress without losing integrity.

## REFERENCES


Cui, Y., Wang, Y., Liu, H., Xu, S., & Zhang, X. (2025). Exploring the correlation between patient safety culture and adverse medical events using failure mode and effect analysis (FMEA). *Risk Management and Healthcare Policy, 17*, 163–176. DOI: 10.2147/RMHP.S502725 PMID: 40264504

Dekker, S. (2011). *Drift into failure: From hunting broken components to understanding complex systems*. Ashgate.

Edmondson, A. C. (2018). *The fearless organization: Creating psychological safety in the workplace for learning, innovation, and growth*. Wiley.

Frankel, A., Haraden, C., Federico, F., & Lenoci-Edwards, J. (2017). *A framework for safe, reliable, and effective care*. Institute for Healthcare Improvement. https://www.ihi.org/resources/Pages/IHIWhitePapers/AFrameworkforSafeReliableandEffectiveCare.aspx

Paine, L. A., Holzmueller, C. G., Elliott, R., Kasda, E., Pronovost, P. J., Weaver, S. J., Sutcliffe, K. M., & Mathews, S. C. (2018). Latent risk assessment tool for health care leaders. *Journal of Healthcare Risk Management, 38*(2), 36–46. DOI: 10.1002/jhrm.21316 PMID: 29631323

Pronovost, P. J., & Paine, L. (2019). Creating learning health systems to improve patient care and safety. *BMJ Quality & Safety, 28*(5), 389–392. DOI: 10.1136/bmjqs-2018-008726 PMID: 30337498

Reason, J. (2008). *The human contribution: Unsafe acts, accidents and heroic recoveries*. Ashgate.

Waseem, H. M., Ul Islam, S., Harrison, S., Epiphaniou, G., Matragkas, N., Arvanitis, T. N., & Maple, C. (2025). Data driven FMEA approach for hazard identification and risk evaluation in digital health. *Scientific Reports, 15*(1), 11929. DOI: 10.1038/s41598-025-11929-4 PMID: 40702036

Weick, K. E., & Sutcliffe, K. M. (2015). *Managing the unexpected: Sustained performance in a complex world* (3rd ed.). Wiley. DOI: 10.1002/9781119175834


## KEY TERMS AND DEFINITIONS

**Cognitive Load:** The mental effort required to perform tasks or make decisions, which increases the likelihood of error when excessive.

**Failure Mode and Effects Analysis (FMEA):** A proactive tool used to identify potential failure modes in a process and prioritize them based on severity, occurrence, and detectability.

**Human Factor Vulnerabilities:** Risks arising from the interaction between people, tasks, technology, and environment that influence safety and performance.

**Latent Conditions:** Underlying system weaknesses created by design, policy, culture, or environment that remain undetected until triggered by stress.

**Organizational Drift:** The gradual normalization of deviations from intended practice that increases exposure to latent risks.

**Proactive Latent Risk Assessment (PLRA/LRA):** A system level evaluation that identifies hidden organizational vulnerabilities before they contribute to harm.

**Project Risk Assessment (PRA):** A structured method used to identify and mitigate risks that may affect a project's scope, timeline, resources, or implementation readiness.

**Psychological Safety:** A team's shared belief that speaking up about concerns or risks is expected and will not result in negative consequences.

**System Resilience:** An organization's capacity to anticipate, absorb, and adapt to disruption while maintaining safe, reliable operations.

**Weak Signals:** Early, subtle indicators of system strain such as workarounds or silence that precede more obvious failures.

# APPENDIX I

## Vignette: Using PRA and PLRA During a Major EHR Transition

A large healthcare organization prepared to transition from a legacy electronic health record (EHR) to a new enterprise wide system. The project was well resourced, governance was clear, and early testing showed the system was technically sound. Leadership expected the go live to be complex but manageable. Based on prior experience, leadership chose to run two parallel assessments: a traditional Proactive Risk Assessment (PRA) to protect the project, and a Proactive Latent Risk Assessment (PLRA) to protect the system once it entered daily clinical use.

## Proactive Risk Assessment (PRA): Protecting the Project

The PRA was led by the project management office with participation from IT leaders, clinical informatics, operational subject matter experts, and frontline representatives. The focus was on risks that could disrupt delivery, adoption, or technical performance.

The PRA identified several foreseeable risks:

- Delays in interface mapping between the legacy system and external applications
- Uneven training completion, especially among night and weekend staff
- Risk of downtime during data migration
- Limited vendor staff availability to support all clinical areas at once

Mitigation plans were put in place. Training schedules were adjusted, vendor coverage was expanded during go live week, interface testing was staged earlier, and downtime procedures were rehearsed. From a project standpoint, the organization was prepared. Milestones were met, risks were documented, and leadership confidence was high. What the PRA did not address was how the new system would behave once embedded in real work, under real conditions, with real staffing constraints.

## Proactive Latent Risk Assessment (PLRA): Protecting the System

At the same time, the Quality and Safety Office led a PLRA with support from human factors specialists. The focus was not the project plan, but the environment the system would enter. Through unit walk rounds, staff interviews, observation of clinical workflows, and review of policies, the PLRA surfaced risks that were not visible in the project risk log:

- The new EHR generated a significantly higher volume of alerts, particularly during medication reconciliation, increasing cognitive load for clinicians
- Several older inpatient units had unreliable Wi-Fi coverage, especially overnight, increasing the likelihood of delayed documentation and workarounds
- Staffing assumptions did not reflect reality; vacancy rates in float pools meant unfamiliar staff would often be managing new workflows
- Residents and nurses were unclear about escalation pathways during system downtime
- Staff in multiple units expressed reluctance to raise concerns, believing the implementation was "too far along to change," signaling reduced psychological safety

These issues were not technical defects. They were system conditions: environmental, human, and cultural that could compromise safety after go live.

## Actions Taken Before Go Live

Based on the PLRA findings, leadership made several targeted adjustments:

- Wi-Fi infrastructure was reinforced in high risk areas
- Alert thresholds were modified to reduce unnecessary interruptions
- Safety coaches were deployed to high acuity units during the first 72 hours of go live
- Downtime escalation pathways were clarified and reinforced during huddles
- Leaders explicitly invited staff to report concerns during go live, reinforcing that adjustments were still possible

These changes did not alter the project timeline, but they materially changed how the system would function under pressure.

Figure 4 illustrates how successful EHR implementation requires attention to both project delivery and clinical use. Project Risk Assessment (PRA) supports timely, in scope deployment, while Patient Logistics Risk Assessment (PLRA) addresses workflow, safety, and human factors once the system is live. When applied together, these approaches reduce workarounds, support the workforce, and promote safe, reliable care.

## What the Dual Approach Achieved

The PRA ensured the EHR implementation was launched on time, within scope, and with appropriate technical controls. The PLRA ensured that once the system went live, it could be used safely, reliably, and without overwhelming the workforce. Had the organization relied only on PRA, the project would still have succeeded but clinicians would have faced avoidable strain, workarounds would likely have emerged, and safety risks would have surfaced only after harm or burnout occurred. By using PRA and PLRA together, leadership addressed both sides of risk: the risks that threaten delivery and the risks that threaten care.

*Figure 4. Dual approach to EHR implementation*

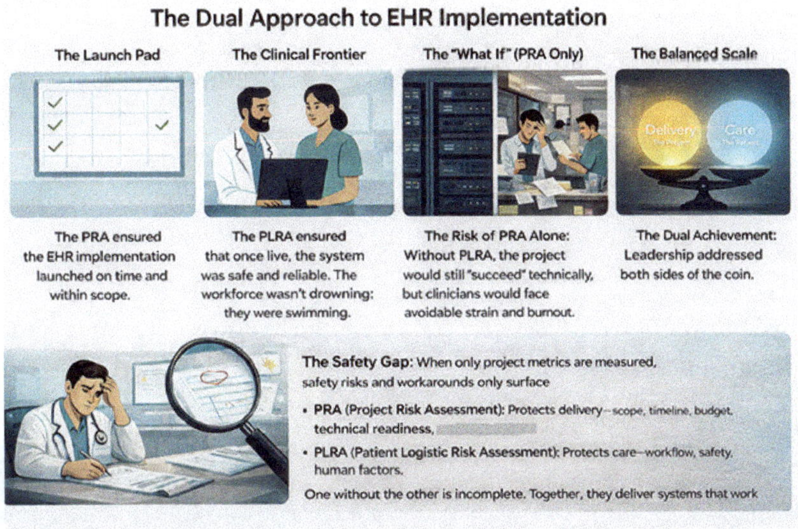

# Chapter 9
# Building Bridges:
## Transitions of Care and Safety at the Edges


## ABSTRACT

*Every transition in healthcare carries a story, one that rarely fits neatly into a discharge summary or an electronic note. This chapter looks closely at what happens at the fragile edges where systems meet and, at times, fail to connect. Drawing on real cases and evidence based frameworks, it explores how communication, accountability, and empathy shape whether a transition strengthens safety or quietly undermines it. By reframing continuity of care as both a technical process and a human relationship, the chapter argues that improvement does not begin with more checklists, but with presence, verification, and connection at the moment responsibility changes hands. What emerges is a call to build bridges that honor both process and person, turning each transition into an act of shared responsibility rather than a procedural endpoint.*


## INTRODUCTION

Safety during transitions of care sits at the center of patient safety, even though it often unfolds quietly. When a patient moves from one setting to another, hospital to home, and inpatient unit to clinic, there is a moment when responsibility shifts. That moment can determine whether recovery continues or begins to unravel. Most preventable errors during transitions trace back to a familiar source: breakdowns in communication during the handoff.

A handoff is not simply the transfer of information. It is the transfer of understanding. It requires that the next clinician knows not only what happened, but why it matters and what remains uncertain. When handoffs are rushed, incomplete, or


DOI: 10.4018/979-8-3373-6496-4.ch009

treated as transactional, patients move forward without a shared plan. Small gaps, an unclear medication change, an unspoken concern, an assumption that someone else will follow up, can quickly become safety risks. A strong handoff, even when brief, does something different. It creates a shared mental model, invites questions, and confirms that the patient's story has been heard and carried forward. Safe care does not end at the doorway of a unit; it depends on how deliberately we guide patients into the next setting.

The most fragile moments in healthcare are rarely the emergencies. They are the quiet transitions between them. As patients leave one place of care for another, carrying instructions, medications, and expectations, every discipline is tested at once. Research continues to show that nearly half of preventable readmissions stem from communication failures during discharge or transfer (Ghosh et al., 2021). Patients do not experience departments; they experience a single, continuous story and assume that professionals are walking alongside them throughout. Early in my career, I believed better forms could fix these gaps. Over time, it became clear that what was missing was not information alone, but relationships, empathy, accountability, and confidence that someone would catch the baton when it left my hand.

## Objectives of the Chapter

- Identify and mitigate risks during transitions of care by addressing communication failures, system gaps, and social determinants that affect patient safety.
- Strengthen relational continuity through structured, empathetic handoff communication that supports accountability, trust, and clarity between providers.
- Integrate evidence-based frameworks and contextual awareness, such as medication reconciliation, teach-back, and warm handoffs, into sustainable programs that align clinical precision with patient-centered care.

## Ms. Patel's Story: What a Safe Discharge Requires

By traditional measures, Ms. Patel's discharge was successful. Her hospitalization ended on schedule. The paperwork was complete. Medication changes and follow up recommendations were documented. From the system's perspective, the boxes were checked. From the patient's perspective, the transition was fragile.

When Ms. Patel arrived home, she sat at her kitchen table with a stack of discharge papers spread in front of her. The instructions were accurate, but dense. Medication names were unfamiliar. Dosing schedules had changed. Follow up plans were described but not scheduled. Her daughter, usually the person who helped interpret medical information, was unavailable. Home health services had been ordered, but no one had told Ms. Patel when to expect the nurse. The oxygen delivery company arrived hours earlier than planned, leaving equipment she did not fully understand. Nothing had gone "wrong" in a technical sense. No policy was violated. Yet the system assumed coordination that did not exist, and capacity Ms. Patel did not have. The discharge process emphasized completion rather than comprehension. This is where many transitions fail, not through error, but through misalignment.

A safer discharge would have looked different. The discharge summary would have reached Ms. Patel's primary care clinician before she left the hospital. Medication changes would have been reviewed with both Ms. Patel and her daughter, using plain language and clear distinctions between new, changed, and discontinued medications. Home health services would have been scheduled, not merely ordered. Oxygen delivery would have been coordinated around Ms. Patel's availability, with instructions provided at the time of setup. Follow up appointments would have been made before discharge, not deferred as future tasks.

In the days that followed, the gap widened. Without early follow up, small concerns, fatigue, dizziness, uncertainty about medications, went unaddressed. By the time Ms. Patel saw her ambulatory clinician, information was incomplete and recovery had already begun to fray. I saw the same pattern during a home visit with a nurse caring for another recently discharged patient. The nurse found a petite woman struggling with a standard adult walker that met ordering criteria but did not fit her body or her home. The nurse adjusted the walker, retaught the gait sequence, and said quietly, "Now let's make it fit you." That moment captured the difference between process and safety.

Transitions succeed when systems are designed for real people, real homes, and real work. Hospital, ambulatory, and home care must function as a connected pathway rather than a series of discrete handoffs. When discharge is measured by documentation alone, risk shifts quietly to patients and caregivers. When it is measured by understanding, coordination, and early follow-up, safety improves. Ms. Patel's story reminds us that discharge is not a single event, but a series of aligned actions across settings. The goal is not faster discharge or cleaner paperwork. The goal is continuity, care that makes sense at home and remains connected in ambulatory follow up.

## Discharge Planning at the Core of Safety

Discharge planning has its greatest impact in the in-between spaces, where patients feel fragmentation most acutely. At the point of discharge, hospital teams, ambulatory clinicians, and home environments converge around the same patient, yet often operate as separate worlds. Effective discharge planning closes this gap by deliberately linking these settings and extending care beyond hospital walls.

At transitions, discharge planning is not about adding tasks; it is about alignment. It brings nurses, physicians, pharmacists, social workers, care managers, home health partners, and ambulatory teams into a shared view of the patient's journey. Seen from the patient's perspective, gaps become visible: medication changes that are unclear, follow-up appointments recommended but not scheduled, social needs left unaddressed, assumptions about caregiver support that do not match reality. These gaps are rarely intentional. They arise because each discipline sees only its portion of the transition. Strong discharge planning creates the structure that ties these pieces together. It ensures medication lists are accurate and understood, teaching is confirmed rather than assumed, and communication is closed loop across settings. It also allows care to be tailored, adjusting equipment to fit the patient, accounting for the home environment, and recognizing the family's capacity to support recovery. Equally important, effective discharge planning includes those receiving the handoff. Ambulatory clinicians, home health teams, and pharmacists are engaged early, not positioned as downstream recipients of a plan they did not help shape.

Most importantly, discharge planning makes transitions visible. It shifts the definition of "complete" from a signed document to a successful handoff. It asks whether information reached the next provider, whether the patient understood the plan, whether follow-up occurred in time, and whether the transition held once the patient was home. When discharge planning is treated as a coordinated, cross disciplinary process, safety no longer depends on individual heroics or last-minute fixes. Instead, the system accompanies patients across settings with clarity and support, bridging care rather than handing it off across a gap.

## The Role of Handoff

Before technology can fully transform coordination, healthcare must preserve one of its most enduring instruments of continuity: the handoff. No digital interface can replace the deliberate transfer of accountability that occurs when one clinician ensures another is prepared, not just informed, but ready, to assume care. Effective handoffs turn empathy into practice through structure, translating conversation into reliability. Evidence from high-reliability systems consistently shows that these intentional exchanges remain among the strongest predictors of patient safety during transitions (Starmer et al., 2014; Shahid & Thomas, 2018; The Joint Commission, 2017). In an era increasingly shaped by automation, the handoff stands as both a relational and ethical act, a reminder that safety advances not only through smarter systems, but through shared human presence at moments of transfer.

## Handoff Communication: Where Continuity Becomes Conversation

Handoff communication is the bridge on which continuity travels. It is the point where safety is either carried forward or quietly lost. The Joint Commission defines a handoff as "a real time process of passing patient specific information from one caregiver to another to ensure continuity and safety of care" (The Joint Commission, 2017). Despite its apparent simplicity, failures in handoff communication remain one of the most common root causes of sentinel events (Paine et al., 2018a).

An effective handoff is not a checklist; it is a conversation anchored in accountability. Structure matters, but structure alone is insufficient. What distinguishes safe handoffs is the combination of clarity and connection, ensuring that information is not merely transmitted, but understood. Rushed or inconsistent handoffs create knowledge gaps that lead to delayed follow-up, duplication, and error (Starmer et al., 2014). In contrast, structured exchanges that invite questions and encourage read-back reduce communication failures and strengthen mutual trust (Shahid & Thomas, 2018; Paine et al., 2018b) High-reliability organizations treat handoffs as team behaviors rather than administrative tasks. They rely on standardization, but with room for professional judgment when complexity demands it (Pronovost et al., 2016). These exchanges are safest when psychological safety is present, when team members feel able to surface uncertainty without fear of judgment (Edmondson, 2018). Technology can support these moments, but it cannot replace them. Electronic records capture events; conversation carries context. Whether in a hallway or over telehealth, the quality of the exchange shapes the care that follows.

A reliable handoff accomplishes three essential transfers:

- **Information:** a shared understanding of the patient's current status, recent changes, and ongoing needs.
- **Accountability:** clarity about who assumes care next and what actions are required.
- **Trust:** confidence that care will continue seamlessly because both parties share responsibility for the patient's safety.

In this sense, every handoff is both clinical and ethical, a moment where the promise of safety is either realized or deferred.

## Handoff Communication Template (SBAR + Contextual Continuity)

The Handoff Communication Template (SBAR + Contextual Continuity) builds on the traditional SBAR framework, Situation, Background, Assessment, Recommendation, by integrating relational and anticipatory elements drawn from the Institute for Healthcare Improvement and The Joint Commission. The intent is not to lengthen handoffs, but to deepen them, preserving both informational accuracy and human connection across settings.

- **Identification and Setting:** Clearly establish who is speaking and the context of the transition.

*"This is [Name], [Role], calling from [Unit or Agency]. I'm handing off [Patient Name, Age, Diagnosis] transitioning from [Setting A] to [Setting B]."*

- **Situation:** State the immediate reason for the transition and current priorities.

*"The patient was admitted for [Condition] and is now stable for discharge. Key current issues include..."*

- **Background:** Provide concise medical and psychosocial context relevant to the transition.

*"Significant history includes..., current medications..., no complications in the past 24 hours."*

- **Assessment:** Summarize the patient's current condition and practical considerations.

*"Patient ambulates with assistance, pain controlled with oral medications, incision healing well. Home has one step at entrance; PT follow-up scheduled."*

- **Recommendations / Next Steps:** Clarify required actions and ownership.

*"Please reinforce wound-care teaching and monitor for swelling. First follow-up visit is scheduled for [Date]."*

- **Patient and Family Understanding (Teach-Back):** Confirm comprehension.

*"The patient and caregiver demonstrated understanding of medication timing using teach-back."*

- **Verification and Contact:** Close the loop.

*"Do you have any questions? You can reach me at [Contact]. Please confirm receipt of this handoff."*

This expanded SBAR approach reframes routine handoffs as purposeful exchanges that emphasize clarity, accountability, and relational continuity.

Implementation Notes:

- Conduct handoffs verbally whenever possible, supported by written or electronic summaries.
- Encourage two-way communication, with confirmation or read-back by the receiver.
- Integrate safety cross-checks such as medication reconciliation and goals of care.
- Document participants, timing, and confirmation of understanding (The Joint Commission, 2017).

This figure extends the SBAR framework to support continuity, verification, and patient understanding during care transitions, informed by guidance from the Institute for Healthcare Improvement (IHI) and The Joint Commission (IHI, n.d.; The Joint Commission, 2017).

*Figure 1. Handoff communication template (SBAR + contextual continuity)*

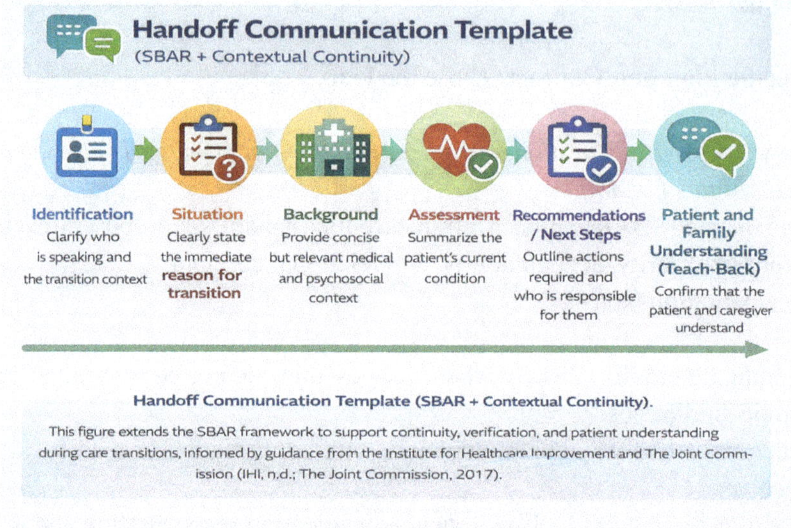


## PRACTICE IMPACT

At one hospital, leadership noted that unplanned 30-day readmissions remained high despite standardized discharge paperwork and checklists. Performance data suggested that the transition from hospital to home was not holding. In response, the organization implemented a structured, in-person discharge planning model, assigning a dedicated discharge planner to meet with high-risk patients before they left the hospital.

The role extended well beyond document review. The discharge planner met face-to-face with patients and families to review medication changes, confirm understanding, and clarify what had changed since admission. Prescriptions were filled or had a clear pickup plan. Transportation and equipment needs were verified. Outpatient follow-up appointments were scheduled before discharge, rather than deferred. Coordination with home health agencies and ambulatory clinics occurred in real time. This approach aligns with evidence showing that completed outpatient follow-up is associated with lower 30-day readmission rates, with reductions of approximately 20–30% depending on population and condition (Balasubramanian et al., 2025; Bilicki & Reeves, 2024). Discharge planning models that emphasize personalized coordination and scheduled follow-up are also associated with improved continuity, particularly among older adults and patients with chronic illness (McMartin, 2013).

Within a year, the hospital saw measurable improvements. Readmissions declined, especially among patients with complex medical and social needs. Follow up completion rates increased, ensuring that patients were seen during the high risk period after discharge. What changed was not treatment, but coordination. The discharge planner became a consistent point of connection across inpatient, outpatient, home health, and patient domains, reducing avoidable returns by replacing confusion with clarity.

## Key Takeaways

- Transitions of care are high-risk moments where communication failures often lead to preventable harm.
- Safety depends on both technical precision and human connection.
- Structured handoffs, warm handoffs, and teach-back reduce errors and improve comprehension.
- Medication reconciliation and attention to social determinants are essential for continuity.
- Psychological safety among teams strengthens accountability.
- Technology supports coordination but cannot replace human presence.
- Embedding these practices transforms vulnerable gaps into resilient bridges of care.

## CONCLUSION

Transitions of care represent some of the most vulnerable points in the healthcare continuum. This chapter reframes those moments as both technical and relational processes, arguing that continuity depends as much on trust and shared accountability as on accurate information. Evidence based strategies, structured handoffs, medication reconciliation, teach back, and warm handoffs, emerge as essential tools for reducing harm and supporting patient understanding. Real-world examples underscore that safety at the edges requires adaptability and humility, along with attention to contextual realities such as transportation and food security. Technology can assist coordination, but human connection remains the cornerstone of reliable transitions. When these principles are embedded into daily work and supported by psychological safety, handoffs become more than exchanges, they become bridges that carry care forward across settings.

## REFERENCES

Balasubramanian, I., Andres, E. B., & Malhotra, C. (2025). Outpatient follow-up and 30-day readmissions: A systematic review and meta-analysis. *JAMA Network Open, 8*(11), e2541272. DOI: 10.1001/jamanetworkopen.2025.41272 PMID: 41186947

Bilicki, D. J., & Reeves, M. J. (2024). Outpatient follow-up visits to reduce 30-day all-cause readmissions. *Preventing Chronic Disease, 21*, 240138. https://www.cdc.gov/pcd/issues/2024/24_0138.htm. DOI: 10.5888/pcd21.240138 PMID: 39325638

Edmondson, A. C. (2018). *The fearless organization: Creating psychological safety in the workplace for learning, innovation, and growth.* Wiley.

Ghosh, S., Chawla, N., & Sinha, S. (2021). Communication failures and patient safety: A systematic review. *Journal of Patient Safety, 17*(3), 157–165. DOI: 10.1097/PTS.0000000000000798 PMID: 29994818

Institute for Healthcare Improvement. (n.d.). *Care transitions: Key strategies from evidence to implementation.* https://www.ihi.org/resources/Pages/ImprovementStories/Care-Transitions.aspx

McMartin, K. (2013). Discharge planning in chronic conditions: Effects on readmissions and length of stay. *Canadian Journal of Respiratory Therapy.* https://pmc.ncbi.nlm.nih.gov/articles/PMC3804053/

Paine, L. A., Rosenstein, A. H., & Sexton, J. B. (2018a). Safety culture and handoff communication: Implications for patient safety. *Journal of Nursing Care Quality, 33*(3), 213–220. DOI: 10.1097/NCQ.0000000000000333 PMID: 29035906

Paine, L. A., Rosenstein, B. J., Pronovost, P. J., & Bagian, J. P. (2018b). Safety as a system property: Lessons from high-reliability organizations. *Joint Commission Journal on Quality and Patient Safety, 44*(7), 377–384. DOI: 10.1016/j.jcjq.2018.02.006 PMID: 30008350

Pronovost, P. J., Berenholtz, S. M., & Needham, D. M. (2016). Translating evidence into practice: A model for large-scale knowledge translation. *BMJ (Clinical Research Ed.), 333*(7565), 1210–1212. DOI: 10.1136/bmj.333.7565.1210 PMID: 18838424

Shahid, S., & Thomas, S. (2018). Situation, background, assessment, recommendation (SBAR) communication tool for handoff in health care: A narrative review. *Safety in Health, 4*(1), 7. DOI: 10.1186/s40886-018-0073-1

Starmer, A. J., Spector, N. D., Srivastava, R., West, D. C., Rosenbluth, G., Allen, A. D., Noble, E. L., Tse, L. L., Dalal, A. K., & Landrigan, C. P. (2014). Changes in medical errors after implementation of a handoff program. *The New England Journal of Medicine, 371*(19), 1803–1812. DOI: 10.1056/NEJMsa1405556 PMID: 25372088

The Joint Commission. (2017). *Improving handoff communications: Meeting National Patient Safety Goal 02.05.01.* https://www.jointcommission.org

## KEY TERMS AND DEFINITIONS

**Care Transition:** A shift of a patient from one care setting to another, where responsibility moves to a new team.

**Continuity of Care:** Consistent, coordinated care that follows the patient across settings.

**Handoff Communication:** A structured exchange of essential patient information between clinicians during a transition.

**Medication Reconciliation:** Comparing medication lists to correct discrepancies during transitions.

**Readmission:** An unplanned return to the hospital.

**Teach Back:** A method where patients repeat instructions in their own words to confirm understanding.

**Warm Handoff:** Direct person-to-person communication to ensure the receiving clinician understands the patient's needs.

# APPENDIX I

## Vignette: SBAR in a Hospital-to–Home Health Handoff for Heart Failure

Mr. Lewis is a 68-year-old man hospitalized for worsening heart failure after several days of increasing shortness of breath and weight gain. Following treatment with intravenous diuretics and medication adjustments, his breathing improves and his weight decreases. He is medically stable and scheduled to discharge home with home health services.

On the morning of discharge, the hospital nurse calls the home health agency to hand off care using SBAR.

Situation:

"This is Maria, the nurse on 5 East. I'm calling about Mr. Lewis, a 68-year-old patient with heart failure who is being discharged home today with home health services."

Background:

"He was admitted three days ago for fluid overload and responded well to IV diuretics. His discharge weight is five pounds lower than admission. His medication regimen has changed, his diuretic dose was increased, and a new beta-blocker was started."

Assessment:

"At discharge, he's breathing comfortably at rest but becomes short of breath with exertion. His blood pressure has been running low-normal since the medication changes, and he has reported occasional dizziness. He lives alone, but his daughter visits daily."

Recommendation:

"He needs close monitoring of weight, blood pressure, and symptoms during the first week at home. Please reinforce daily weights and symptom reporting. If he gains more than two pounds in a day, feels dizzy, or becomes more short of breath, we recommend contacting the cardiology clinic immediately. Labs are ordered to be drawn before his follow-up appointment."

The home health nurse confirms the first visit for the next day and reviews the medication changes and monitoring plan. Questions about equipment, medication timing, and emergency contact numbers are clarified during the call.

The day after discharge, the home health nurse visits Mr. Lewis and notices mild dizziness when he stands. Because expectations were clearly communicated, the nurse contacts the cardiology clinic right away. The diuretic dose is adjusted, symptoms improve, and Mr. Lewis avoids an emergency department visit.

In this case, SBAR created continuity across settings. The handoff focused on risks that often emerge after discharge and gave the home health team clear guidance on what to watch for and when to escalate concerns. By aligning hospital and home health teams around the same priorities, SBAR supported a smoother transition and safer recovery at home.

## APPENDIX II

### Vignette: Extended SBAR + Contextual Continuity

Mr. Ramirez, a 72-year-old man with COPD and diabetes, was preparing for discharge after stabilizing from an exacerbation. He lived alone with no nearby family or caregiver support. During discharge planning, the team realized that the clinical plan would not hold unless his social needs were addressed directly. The inpatient nurse used the extended SBAR + Contextual Continuity handoff template to create a reliable connection between the hospital and community partners.

### Identification and Setting

"This is Jordan, RN from 4 West. I'm handing off Mr. Juan Ramirez, 72, admitted for a COPD exacerbation. He is transitioning from inpatient care to home with home-health services."

### S, Situation

"He is clinically stable for discharge today. Key current issues include limited endurance, difficulty managing medications, and no social support at home."

### B, Background

"He was admitted with shortness of breath related to missed inhaler doses. He has COPD, diabetes, limited health literacy, and does not drive. He recently lost the informal neighbor support he relied on for groceries and transportation."

### A, Assessment

"His breathing is stable at rest but worsens with activity. He becomes fatigued easily and required multiple attempts during teach-back to correctly identify his inhalers. Home safety risks include food insecurity, medication non-adherence, lack of transportation, and no one at home to monitor symptoms."

### R, Recommendations / Next Steps

"He will need daily home-health nursing this week for inhaler review, symptom monitoring, and reinforcement of COPD action steps. Please arrange:

- prescription delivery
- meals-on-wheels enrollment
- transportation assistance for his follow-up appointment in five days

He also needs coaching on when to call for help, especially if breathing worsens or he gains weight rapidly."

## Patient and Family Understanding (Teach-Back)

"Mr. Ramirez was able to repeat inhaler timing and the early warning signs of a flare after several rounds of teach back. He expressed worry about managing alone, which makes early home-health contact essential."

## Verification and Contact

"Do you have any questions before we close? Please confirm receipt of this handoff. You can reach me directly if anything needs clarification."

The home health nurse confirmed the first visit for the next morning and immediately coordinated food, transportation, and medication delivery services.

## Outcome

On day two after discharge, the home-health nurse noticed mild shortness of breath and early weight gain both early signs of a COPD flare. Because escalation pathways were clearly established in the handoff, she contacted the clinic promptly. His medications were adjusted, preventing a return to the emergency department. The extended SBAR (figure 2) approach ensured not only clinical accuracy, but also continuity, verification, and acknowledgment of the social realities shaping his safety at home.

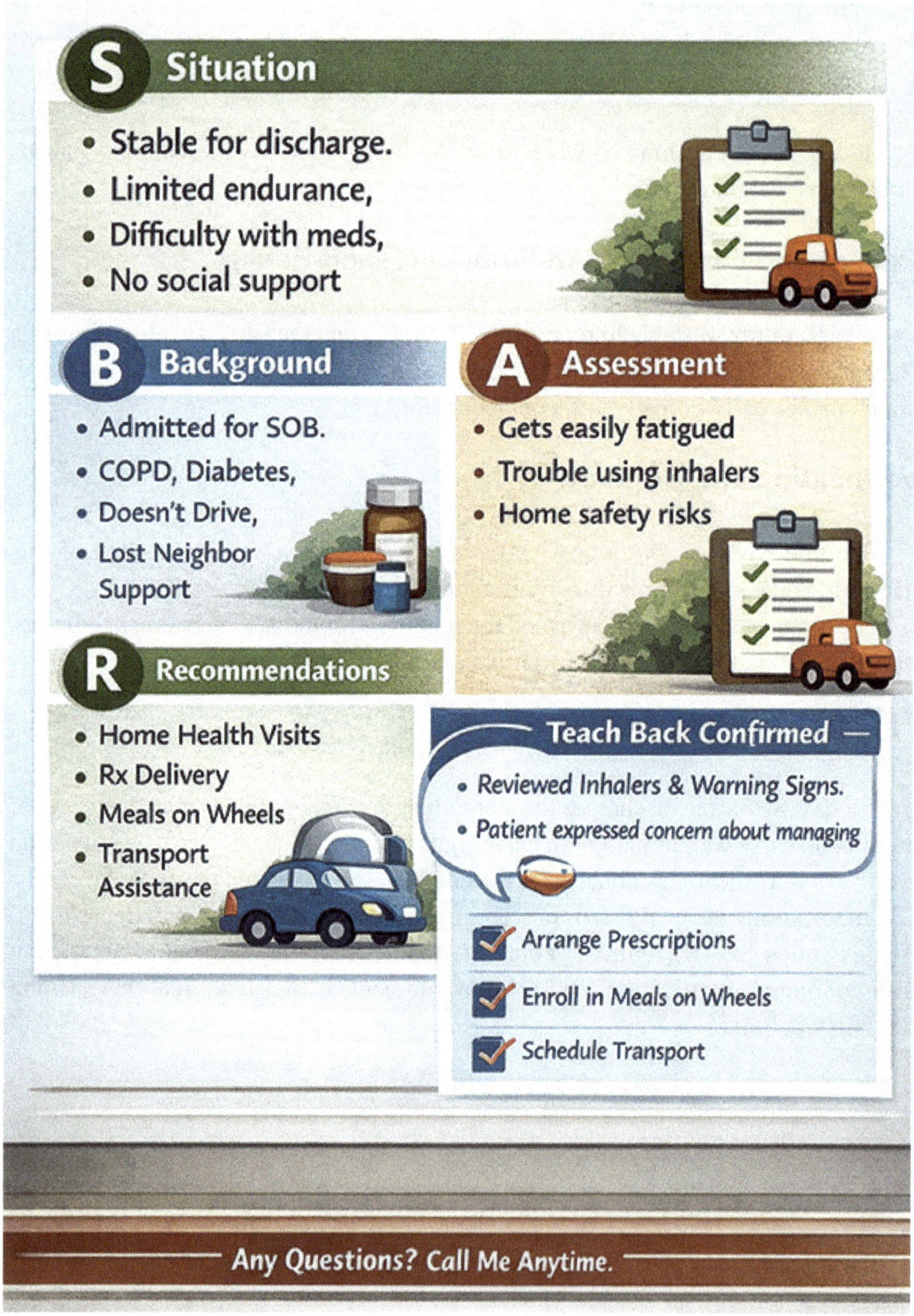
S Situation
• Stable for discharge.
• Limited endurance,
• Difficulty with meds,
• No social support
B Background
• Admitted for SOB.
• COPD, Diabetes,
• Doesn't Drive,
• Lost Neighbor Support
A Assessment
• Gets easily fatigued
• Trouble using inhalers
• Home safety risks
R Recommendations
• Home Health Visits
• Rx Delivery
• Meals on Wheels
• Transport Assistance
Teach Back Confirmed
• Reviewed Inhalers & Warning Signs.
• Patient expressed concern about managing
Arrange Prescriptions
Enroll in Meals on Wheels
Schedule Transport
Any Questions? Call Me Anytime.

# Chapter 10
# Real Tools, Real Impact:
## Templates, Scripts, and Checklists


## ABSTRACT

*The real test of improvement is not how polished a framework looks in a slide deck, but how it holds up when the day becomes unpredictable. This chapter brings together practical tools that steady teams in those moments: scripts that make it easier to speak up, checklists that prevent quiet drift, and reflection prompts that turn experience into learning. Each tool emerged from lived settings, a hospital corridor, a clinic hallway, a patient's home, and evolved through necessity rather than theory. What connects them is purpose. These are not static templates to replicate, but living guides shaped by real voices and grounded in trust. At its core, improvement is not an abstract ideal; it is the daily discipline of noticing, asking, and following through.*


## INTRODUCTION

I've learned that culture change begins with what we repeatedly do. Language sets direction, but structure sustains it. Without structure, even the most compelling ideas fade into good intentions. A well designed checklist or form may seem ordinary, yet it acts as a quiet anchor. It signals that the work matters enough to be done the same way again, that safety is a habit, not a project (Health Quality & Safety Commission New Zealand, 2016).

Early in my quality journey, I assumed the best ideas would emerge from data reviews or planning retreats. In practice, the most durable improvements almost always began somewhere smaller: a nurse asking, "Can we make this step easier?" or a technician wondering why the same mistake kept repeating. Those questions were not complaints. They were design prompts. When we give teams practical tools, we do more than offer direction, we offer permission. Permission to notice,

DOI: 10.4018/979-8-3373-6496-4.ch010

to act, and to take ownership of the system they inhabit. Every checklist, debrief, or reflection form carries the same message: safety belongs to everyone (World Health Organization [WHO], n.d.). Over time, I've come to think of tools as language made visible. They translate values into verbs. They make accountability tangible.

## Objectives of This Chapter

- **Provide practical, adaptable tools:** Equip teams with field tested checklists, briefs, huddles, and reflection prompts that translate safety principles into reliable daily habits across hospitals, clinics, and home care.
- **Foster psychological safety and shared accountability:** Use structured communication to encourage speaking up, learning from experience, and co-creating solutions.
- **Demonstrate real-world impact:** Show how simple tools, born from front-line challenges, reduce errors, improve clarity, and turn improvement into a lived practice.

## Mr. Alvarez's Notes: The Power of Observation

Mr. Alvarez, a retired bus driver recovering from cardiac surgery, was one of my earliest teachers. During his home infusion therapy, I noticed a small spiral notebook resting beside his medication pump. Its pages were filled with careful notes, when the nurse arrived, which supplies were running low, what felt better that day. When I asked why he started writing things down, he smiled. "Because I don't want to forget what to thank her for, or what to remind her about next time."

That small habit captured what many checklists aspire to do: honor what works while noticing what doesn't. Later, we added a single line to our post-visit debrief template: *"Patient Voice: What They Noticed."* That change altered the tone of our reviews. Instead of opening with "What went wrong?" we began with "What did the patient see that we didn't?" Documentation became dialogue, reflecting the principles behind reflective practice models that convert tacit observation into shared learning (Chance et al., 2024).

## Tools That Emerge from Real Life

The most effective tools are rarely imported wholesale. They grow out of friction, out of moments when something didn't quite work. A discharge checklist may trace back to one missed follow-up call. A communication script may emerge after a tense huddle. Each tool in this chapter was shaped through those small, necessary lessons (Treadwell et al., 2013). What I've seen repeatedly is that consistency builds confidence. When teams encounter the same questions, framed the same way, they begin to trust the process, and one another. That trust becomes invisible infrastructure, holding safety in place when pressure rises (Edmondson, 2019).

## Reflection: From Templates to Trust

If years of applying these tools taught me anything, it's this: the form is never the goal. The relationship is. A checklist will never replace empathy, but it can prompt a pause, to ask, to listen, to notice. Mr. Alvarez's notebook reminded me that observation itself is an act of care. His handwritten notes became part of a larger conversation about how patients participate in safety, echoing the philosophy behind the WHO Safe Surgery Checklist, which uses structured dialogue to promote shared vigilance (WHO, n.d.). These tools don't replace judgment; they refine it. They bring discipline to compassion. Used well, they turn improvement from something we discuss into something we practice.

## Hospitals: The Discipline of Clarity

Hospitals move fast. That speed is both strength and risk. I've watched how small communication shortcuts, taken in the name of efficiency, quietly open the door to error. Over time, I've come to see tools not as restrictions, but as breathing space for clarity (American Hospital Association/Health Research & Educational Trust, 2013).

One example was a shift-to-shift handoff checklist co-designed with bedside nurses. It contained just five prompts:

1. Identify the patient's biggest risk.
2. Confirm medication changes.
3. Highlight one success from the shift.
4. Name what still feels uncertain.
5. Ask: *What does the next nurse need to succeed?*

Within weeks, reports of missed medication updates dropped by nearly 30%, consistent with evidence that checklists reduce communication errors and near misses (Treadwell et al., 2013). What changed wasn't workload, but rhythm. In healthcare, clarity is kindness. Every checklist that promotes clear language is compassion disguised as process (Joint Commission Resources, 2025).

## Ambulatory Settings: When Every Minute Counts

Ambulatory care runs on momentum. One clinic struggled with handoffs between nurses and physicians. Together, we introduced a "Red Dot Board", a low-tech visibility tool inspired by human factors principles that emphasize shared situational awareness (HQSCNZ, 2016). Nurses placed small red magnets beside patient names when safety concerns surfaced, from abnormal vitals to medication hesitation.

At first, it seemed too simple to matter. Within weeks, missed follow-ups fell sharply. As one nurse said, "It feels like we finally work in the same story." The board didn't just track tasks; it created a shared mental model, a hallmark of reliable teams (Edmondson, 2019).

## Home Care: Home Observation Visit (HOV)

The Home Observation Visit (HOV) is a structured, field-based assessment designed to reveal how care is actually lived at home. (Despite the shared acronym, it has nothing to do with the traffic lane.) Unlike routine home visits focused on task completion, the HOV centers on observation, environmental conditions, routines, and caregiver practices that shape success or risk. The HOV follows a simple three-part flow, *Before Entry, During the Visit, and Before Leaving.* By watching what patients do rather than what documentation assumes, clinicians uncover issues often missed: unsafe equipment placement, inaccessible supplies, dosing confusion, or caregiver strain masked by politeness. The tool shifts the clinician's role from task execution to pattern recognition, enabling earlier, more realistic adjustments to care plans.

## Briefs, Debriefs, and the Leadership Habit

Before major procedures or meetings, I pause for what I think of as a purposeful moment. In aviation, it's a brief. In healthcare, it's the breath before motion, when teams align around what matters (WHO, n.d.). Our brief template evolved from small failures, missing supplies, misunderstood timing, unspoken concerns, until it settled into five questions:

1. What are we trying to accomplish today?
2. Who owns each step?
3. What could go wrong, and how will we catch it early?
4. Who else needs to know?
5. What will success look like by day's end?

Briefs like these are now recognized globally as core to safety culture and communication reliability (Treadwell et al., 2013).

## Debriefs: Turning Action into Insight

If the brief prepares the team, the debrief keeps learning alive. It's often skipped when days run long, yet it's where improvement takes shape (Joint Commission Resources, 2025). We began closing projects with two questions:

- What went well, and why?
- What do we never want to repeat?

This simple structure reflects reflective practice models shown to strengthen team learning and resilience (Edmondson, 2019). The power of the debrief isn't the data, it's honesty. Once invited, honesty becomes habit.

## Huddles: The Rhythm of Real Time Safety

Huddles are among the most underestimated safety tools. Unlike meetings that analyze the past, huddles look forward. They are short, structured pauses to anticipate risk and align priorities before the day unfolds (Health Quality & Safety Commission New Zealand, 2016). Typically lasting less than ten minutes, they value proximity over presentation.

Where meetings review performance, huddles scan for vulnerability:

- What could put a patient, staff member, or process at risk today?
- Who needs help or extra resources?
- What did we learn yesterday that applies now?

Many organizations use a three-question format:

1. What's working well today?
2. What concerns us right now?
3. What help or escalation do we need?

Five ten-minute huddles often do more for safety than a single long meeting (Joint Commission Resources, 2025). Over time, patterns surface, equipment issues, workload surges, handoff gaps, allowing leaders to respond in real time. A respiratory therapist once told me, "The huddle makes it feel like we start the day as a team, not a task list." That captures their value: restoring connection and foresight.

## Quick Comparison: Huddle vs. Meeting

- **Duration:** Huddles (5–10 minutes) vs. meetings (30–90 minutes)
- **Focus:** Immediate operations vs. review and planning
- **Tone:** Collaborative and action-oriented vs. informational
- **Participants:** Frontline staff and supervisors vs. broader teams
- **Output:** Rapid fixes and escalation vs. reports and plans
- **Cadence:** Daily or per shift vs. weekly or monthly
- **Goal:** Keep the system safe today vs. improve it for tomorrow

Huddles are the heartbeat of reliability, small, predictable pulses that keep complex systems alert. Figure 1 contrasts huddles and meetings by duration, focus, participants, cadence, and purpose, highlighting how huddles support real time safety while meetings drive longer term improvement.

*Figure 1. Comparison of huddles and meetings*

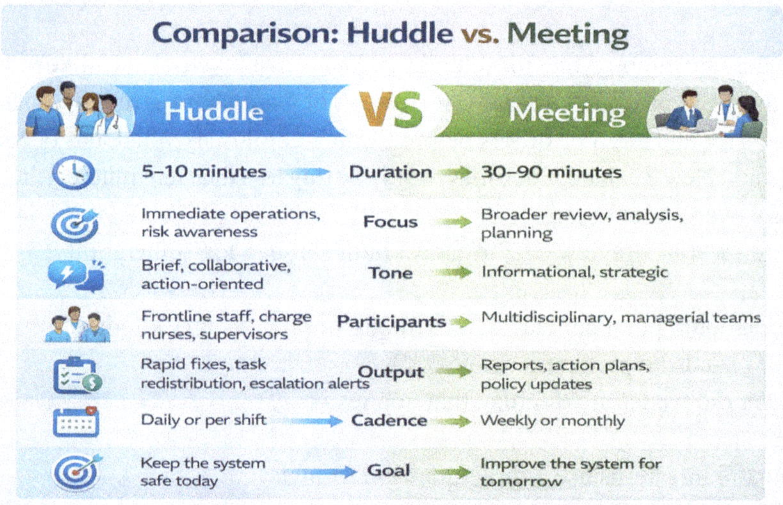


## Real Tools, Real Impact

From Mr. Alvarez's notebook to a nurse's field card, a single thread runs through these stories: structure in the service of humanity. We don't create tools to control behavior; we create them to make insight visible. We don't rely on checklists to catch people doing something wrong; we use them to notice what's going right, consistently (American Hospital Association/Health Research & Educational

Trust, 2013). The most powerful effect of any tool isn't the data it collects; it's the confidence it builds. Confidence that learning happens in real time, across shifts, conversations, and encounters. When that confidence takes hold, safety stops feeling like a departmental responsibility and becomes a shared habit.

That is what *real tools* truly means.

## Tool-to-Outcome Map: Turning Structure into Safety and Culture

Every improvement journey eventually reaches the same realization: tools matter, but only when trust and consistency give them life. The Tool-to-Outcome Map: Turning Structure into Safety and Culture brings together the most frequently used tools from this chapter into a single view. It links each tool to its purpose, everyday application, and observable impact, offering teams a practical reference for daily reliability. These are not abstract frameworks. They are lived practices; checklists that slow the rush toward error, huddles that turn awareness into foresight, briefs and debriefs that convert experience into learning, and reflection prompts that make empathy actionable. While the Tool-to-Outcome Map and Reliability Chain Concept are drawn from this chapter's applied work, they reflect broader safety science insights that reliability emerges through reinforcing practices rather than isolated tools (Weick & Sutcliffe, 2015).

This is also where the Reliability Chain Concept becomes visible. Reliability rarely emerges from one tool used perfectly. It develops when simple structures reinforce one another; briefs informing clean handoffs, huddles surfacing risks those handoffs miss, debriefs shaping tomorrow's brief, and reflective prompts keeping the patient's voice present. Each tool forms a link; consistency provides the tensile strength. Whether in a hospital ward, clinic hallway, or patient's living room, these practices serve the same purpose: turning intention into action and culture into safety. Figure 2 illustrates the Reliability Chain Concept, showing how interconnected practices function together as a continuous, self-correcting safety system.

*Figure 2. Reliability chain concept*

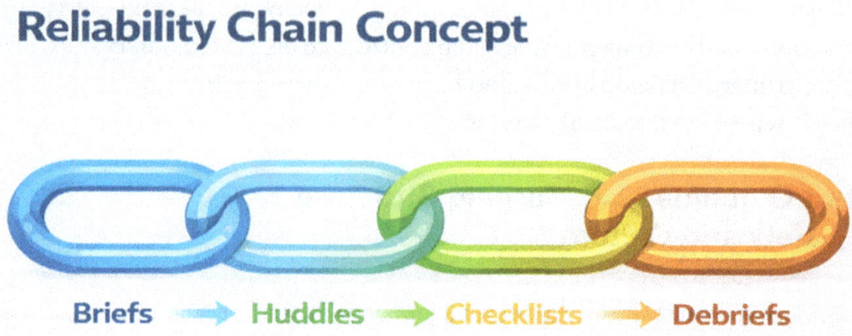


## REAL-WORLD TOOLS AND THEIR EVERYDAY FUNCTION

Here are the most used and field-tested tools and how they function in practice (Table 1).

- **Shift-to-Shift Handoff Checklist:** Standardizes transfer of critical information using a five-point bedside format covering risks, medication changes, successes, uncertainties, and needs. *Outcome:* 30% fewer missed medication updates and improved team reliability.
- **Red Dot Board:** A visual management tool for ambulatory flow that flags real-time safety concerns, red for unresolved, green for resolved before discharge. *Outcome:* Enhanced situational awareness and reduced post-visit safety calls.
- **Home Observation Visit:** A structured, field-based assessment that strengthens safety, reliability, and patient capability by examining how care is actually delivered and lived in the home
- **Team Brief:** A five-question micro-brief conducted before procedures or outreach rounds to clarify purpose, roles, and anticipated risks. *Outcome:* Increased readiness and improved teamwork satisfaction.
- **Debrief:** A short reflection after events using "What went well?" and "What should never repeat?" to capture lessons and emotional tone. *Outcome:* Higher psychological safety and fewer repeat failures.
- **Reflective Form / Patient Voice Prompt:** Converts patient feedback into improvement data through prompts such as, "What did the patient see that we didn't?" *Outcome:* Strengthened trust and empathy-based learning.

- **Quarterly Tool Review Dialogue:** Encourages teams to ask, "Which tools still help, and which need redesign?" to prevent checklist fatigue. *Outcome:* Sustained adoption and shared ownership of improvement.
- **Just Culture Script (Leadership Cue Card):** Helps leaders respond constructively after errors using three questions, "What happened?", "What was reasonable?", and "What supports are needed?" *Outcome:* Fairer responses and higher event reporting.
- **Daily Safety Huddle:** A 10-minute stand-up each morning asking "What's working?", "What's risky?", and "What help is needed?" *Outcome:* Greater situational awareness, fewer unplanned escalations, and a stronger teamwork climate.

Figure 3 depicts. Simple, high-reliability tools that support everyday safety and quality work from handoffs and huddles to observation, reflection, and Just Culture leadership designed to strengthen situational awareness, teamwork, learning, and sustained improvement across care settings.

*Figure 3. Practical safety and quality tools that build reliability, learning, and teamwork in daily care*

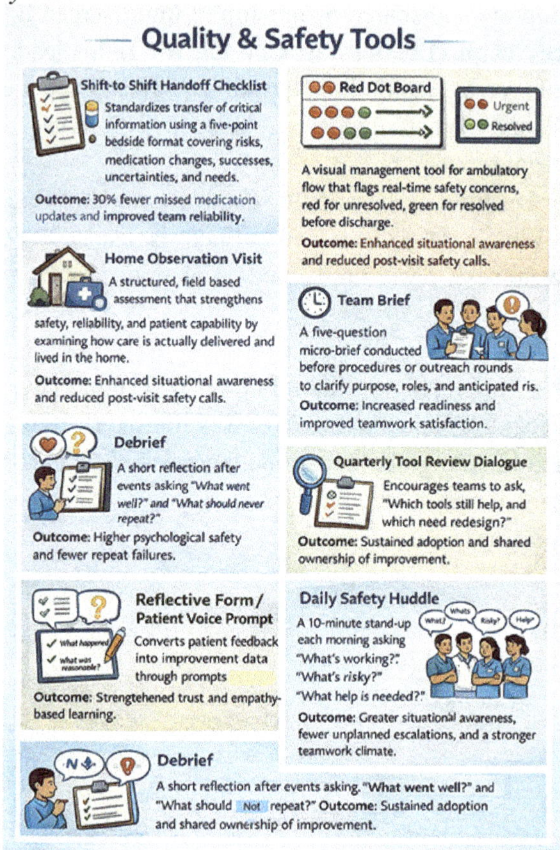


## PRACTICE IMPACT

In day-to-day practice, the effect of simple, well-designed tools is visible and measurable. Checklists, briefs, huddles, and debriefs reduce communication failures, near misses, and process variation by creating shared situational awareness and dependable rhythms of care (Treadwell, Lucas, & Tsou, 2013; Chance, Shah, & Ali, 2024). Their value lies not in standardization alone, but in how they make it easier for people to speak, clarify roles, and learn in real time. In this way, structure becomes the mechanism through which psychological safety is expressed and sustained, strengthening team reliability and resilience at the point of care (Edmondson, 2019).

Daily safety huddles offer a clear example. Rather than reacting to problems as they surface, teams learn to anticipate risk, align resources early, and reduce unplanned escalations (Health Quality & Safety Commission New Zealand, 2016; Joint Commission Resources, 2025). Similarly, concise handoff checklists and pre-procedure briefs help teams surface "what matters most," cutting through cognitive overload during busy shifts (American Hospital Association/Health Research & Educational Trust, 2013; World Health Organization, n.d.). Importantly, these tools travel well. Whether used in hospitals, ambulatory clinics, or home care, portable field cards and reflection prompts carry vigilance and learning into varied environments, translating intention into reliable action that sustains both compassion and safety (Health Quality & Safety Commission New Zealand, 2016; Chance et al., 2024).

## Closing Call to Action: Making Tools Work for You

Tools should never feel like one more obligation layered onto an already full day. When designed well, they do the opposite. They make the right actions easier and the work lighter. The checklists, huddles, and debriefs in this chapter are not meant to slow care down; they are meant to remove friction, confusion, duplication, and second-guessing, that quietly drains energy.

A two-minute huddle can prevent an hour of rework. A clear checklist can spare a night spent worrying about what might have been missed. The invitation is intentionally modest: start small, start anywhere, but start. Let these tools support you rather than work against you. When structure carries the stress, people are free to carry the purpose. That is how safety strengthens, fatigue eases, and care becomes, almost imperceptibly, more humane.

## Key Takeaways

- **Structure sustains safety:** Checklists, briefs, huddles, and debriefs create predictable rhythms that reduce error and cognitive overload.
- **Tools translate values into action:** Practical templates and scripts operationalize psychological safety, shared accountability, and reliability in everyday work.
- **Adaptability matters:** The most effective tools evolve from frontline realities and flex across hospitals, clinics, and home care.
- **Culture grows through habit:** When teams consistently use and refine tools, they shift from interventions to habits, and eventually to culture.

- **Impact is observable:** Structured communication improves clarity, reduces missed handoffs, and turns reactive firefighting into proactive risk anticipation.
- **Small steps count:** Even brief pauses, a two-minute huddle or a simple checklist, can prevent harm and lighten workload.

## CONCLUSION

This chapter underscores that safety and reliability are sustained through practice, not theory. The tools described here, checklists, briefs, huddles, and reflection prompts, emerged from real healthcare settings and persist because they work. Rather than abstract frameworks, they offer structured habits that translate values into action. Through examples drawn from hospitals, clinics, and home care, the chapter illustrates how these tools reduce error, clarify responsibility, and strengthen psychological safety by inviting voice and shared accountability. Their power lies in their evolution from frontline challenges and their ability to build trust, consistency, and resilience under pressure. Ultimately, these tools are not ends in themselves. They are vehicles for culture change, turning intention into reliable action and protecting both patients and caregivers through structure that supports compassion.

## REFERENCES

American Hospital Association / Health Research & Educational Trust. (2013). *Checklists to improve patient safety*. Health Research & Educational Trust.

Chance, E. A., Shah, N., & Ali, R. (2024). The effectiveness of checklists and error reporting systems on enhancing patient safety and reducing medical errors in hospital settings. *Journal of Patient Safety*, *20*(3), 145–153. https://pmc.ncbi.nlm.nih.gov/articles/PMC11329062/ PMID: 39156684

Edmondson, A. C. (2019). *The fearless organization: Creating psychological safety in the workplace for learning, innovation, and growth*. Wiley.

Health Quality & Safety Commission New Zealand. (2016). *Checklists, briefings, debriefings, and huddles: Evidence summary*. https://www.hqsc.govt.nz

Joint Commission Resources. (2025). *Health care worker safety checklists: Protecting those who serve* (2nd ed.). Joint Commission Store.

Treadwell, J. R., Lucas, S., & Tsou, A. Y. (2013). Surgical checklists: A systematic review of impacts and compliance. *BMJ Quality & Safety*, *22*(4), 299–314. DOI: 10.1136/bmjqs-2012-001797 PMID: 23322751

Weick, K. E., & Sutcliffe, K. M. (2015). *Managing the unexpected: Sustained performance in a complex world*. John Wiley & Sons. DOI: 10.1002/9781119175834

World Health Organization. (n.d.). *Safe surgery: Tools and resources (WHO surgical safety checklist and adaptations)*. https://www.who.int/teams/integrated-health-services/patient-safety/research/safe-surgery

## KEY TERMS AND DEFINITIONS

**Daily Safety Huddle:** A 5–10 minute forward looking check in focused on what's working, what's risky, and what help is needed today.

**Debrief:** A two question reflection after work ("What went well?" "What should never repeat?") that turns experience into learning.

**Home Observation Visit (HOV):** A field based home care assessment that surfaces environmental and routine based risks that are invisible in traditional visits.

**Just Culture Script:** A leader's three question cue card ("What happened? What was reasonable? What supports are needed?") that ensures fairness after errors.

**Patient Voice Prompt / Reflective Form:** A structured tool capturing what the patient noticed to integrate lived experience into improvement.

**Purposeful Moment / Pre Action Pause:** A brief pause before action to align expectations and identify risks, reducing cognitive overload.

**Red Dot Board:** A visual clinic tool that flags real time safety concerns with simple red to green indicators to align team awareness.

**Reliability Chain Concept:** A model showing how briefs, huddles, checklists, and debriefs work together as interconnected habits that strengthen safety culture.

**Shift to Shift Handoff Checklist:** A structured five point bedside prompt that standardizes critical information transfer and reduces missed updates.

**Team Brief (Micro Brief):** A short, pre action conversation that clarifies purpose, roles, risks, and what success looks like for the day.

# APPENDIX I

## Simulation Toolkit for Reliability in Practice

This appendix presents a set of **short, practical simulations** designed to help interprofessional teams practice everyday reliability tools in real care settings. The simulations are intentionally brief, repeatable, and embedded in routine work so that teams can practice safety behaviors without disrupting operations. Table 1 below serves as a navigation map. Each scenario aligns a specific reliability tool to a care setting, a focused simulation objective, and a clear reliability outcome. Together, these scenarios reinforce how small, consistent practices: briefs, huddles, checklists, pauses, and debriefs function as a connected system to prevent drift, surface risk, and support psychological safety.

*Table 1. Simulation scenarios and reliability outcomes*

| Scenario | Primary Tool | Care Setting | Simulation Focus | Key Reliability Outcome |
|---|---|---|---|---|
| Shift-to-Shift Handoff | Handoff Checklist | Inpatient unit | Conduct a complete, unhurried handoff under distraction | Risks surfaced; clarity for next clinician |
| Red Dot Board | Visual Risk Board | Ambulatory clinic | Align team on real-time risk | Rapid reprioritization and resolution |
| Home Observation Visit (HOV) | Environmental Scan + Teach-Back | Patient home | Observe routines before advising | Environmental and behavioral risks reduced |
| Team Brief (Micro Brief) | Five-Question Brief | Pre-rounds huddle | Define success and dependencies | Early risk identification |
| End-of-Shift Debrief | Two-Question Debrief | Nursing station | Reflect on work just completed | One actionable improvement identified |
| Daily Safety Huddle | Three-Question Huddle | Unit hallway | Reallocate resources in real time | Escalation prevented |
| Huddle vs. Meeting | Decision Script | Supervisor office | Choose correct coordination structure | Time protected; action prioritized |
| Tool-to-Outcome Map | Tool Matching Guide | Leader huddle | Match tool to failure mode | Targeted intervention selected |
| Reliability Chain | Reliability Chain Concept | Mini-workshop | Map how tools connect | Weak link identified and strengthened |

## How to Use the Simulation Toolkit

Each scenario is designed to run in **15–30 minutes**, followed by a **10–15 minute debrief**. Facilitators may select individual scenarios based on local risks or run several over time to reinforce a shared reliability culture.

Simulations follow a consistent structure:

1. **Brief:** Set the context and tool intent.
2. **Action:** Run the tool as designed in a realistic scenario.
3. **Observation:** Track whether risks were surfaced and communication remained clear.
4. **Debrief:** Identify one success, one vulnerability, and one small improvement to carry forward.

The emphasis is not on performance perfection, but on learning how the tool behaves under real conditions, including interruptions, time pressure, and uncertainty.

## Implementation Notes for Facilitators

Psychological Safety

- Use neutral, curiosity-based language.
- Invite multiple voices before acting.
- Separate learning from blame.

Timing Discipline

- Simulations are intentionally short.
- Extending time reduces fidelity and impact.
- Protect the cadence to preserve the tool's purpose.

Optional Quick Scoring (0–2 scale)

- Prompts used as intended
- Risk named and next step identified
- Right roles engaged
- Communication loop closed
- Dignity and clarity preserved

Learning Data to Collect (Optional)

Organizations may track:

- Percentage of simulations where a key risk was surfaced
- Number of micro-fixes identified per session
- Time to complete brief, huddle, or handoff
- Use of teach-back during home observation visits

These data support learning and adaptation without converting simulations into audits.

## Simulation Script

Scenario 1. Shift-to-Shift Handoff Checklist

*Figure 4. Scenario 1. Shift-to-shift handoff checklist*

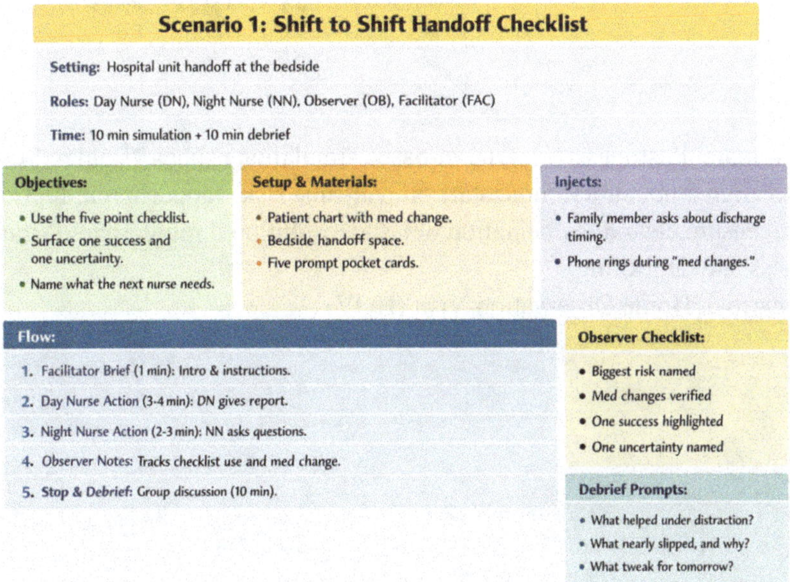


This figure depicts a brief, simulation-based bedside handoff designed to strengthen communication, surface risk, and support reliable transfer of care between nursing shifts through structured prompts and focused debriefing.

Scenario 2. Red Dot Board

*Figure 5. Scenario 2: Red dot board*

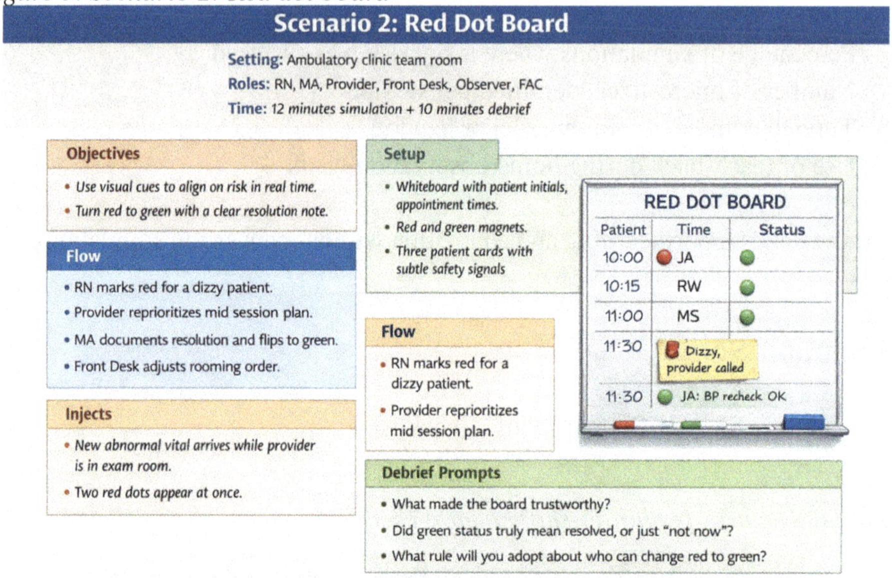


This figure illustrates a brief, team-based simulation using a visual red-to-green board to align ambulatory clinic staff on real-time risk, support rapid reprioritization, and ensure clear documentation of issue resolution through shared situational awareness and debriefing.

Scenario 3. Home Observation Visit (HOV)

*Figure 6. Scenario 3: Home Observation Visit (HOV)*

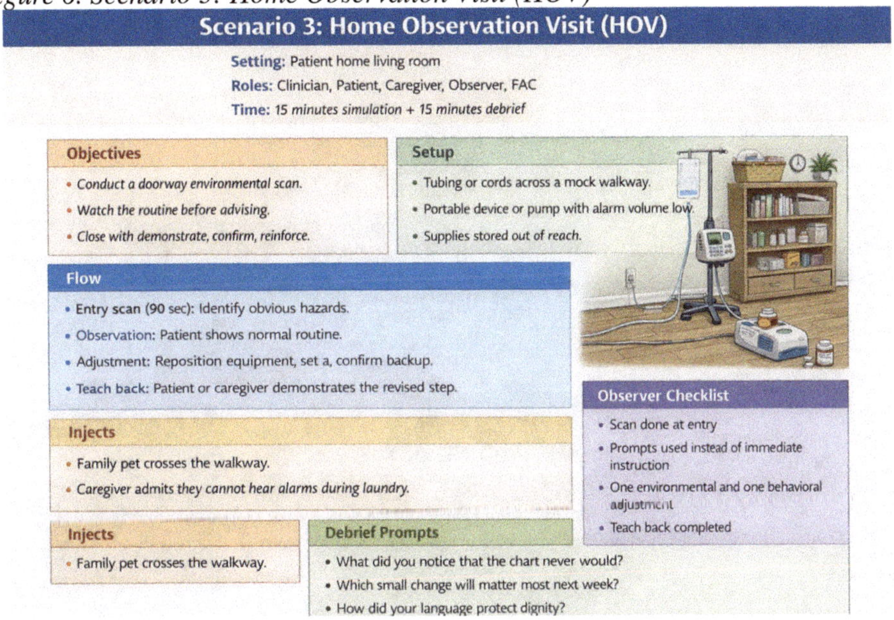


This figure depicts a structured home based simulation that emphasizes environmental scanning, observation of real routines, and teach back to identify safety risks and reinforce reliable care practices in the patient's home.

Scenario 4. Team Brief (Micro-Brief)

*Figure 7. Scenario 4: Team brief (micro brief)*

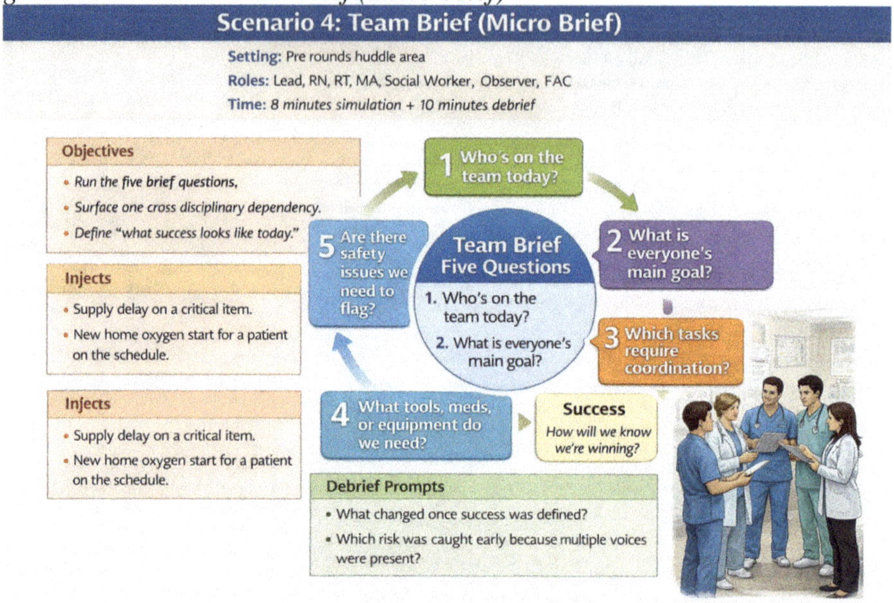


This figure illustrates a brief, pre-rounds team huddle using five focused questions to align roles, surface cross-disciplinary dependencies, define daily success, and identify risks early through shared team awareness and debriefing.

Scenario. Daily Safety Huddle

*Figure 8. Scenario: Daily safety huddle*

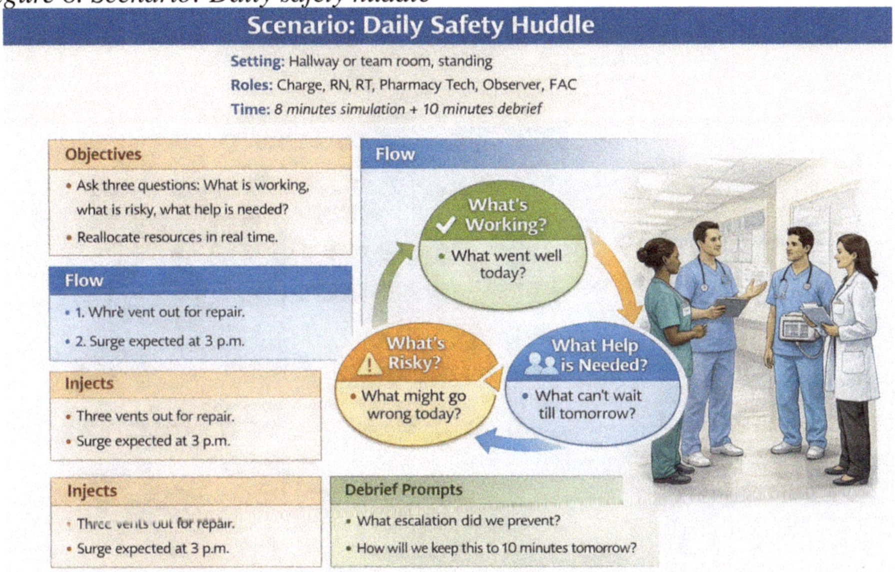


This figure illustrates a brief, standing safety huddle that uses three focused questions to surface real-time risks, reallocate resources, and prevent escalation through rapid team coordination and structured debriefing.

Scenario. Tool-to-Outcome Map

*Figure 9. Scenario: Tool-to-outcome map*

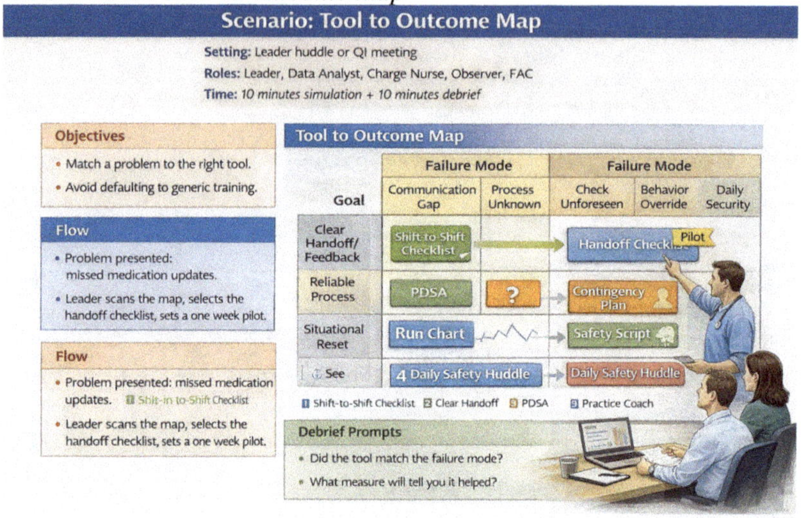


This figure illustrates a leader-led simulation in which teams match a specific failure mode to the most appropriate improvement tool, reinforcing purposeful tool selection and measurable outcomes rather than defaulting to generic training.

Scenario. Reliability Chain Concept

*Figure 10. Scenario: Reliability chain concept*

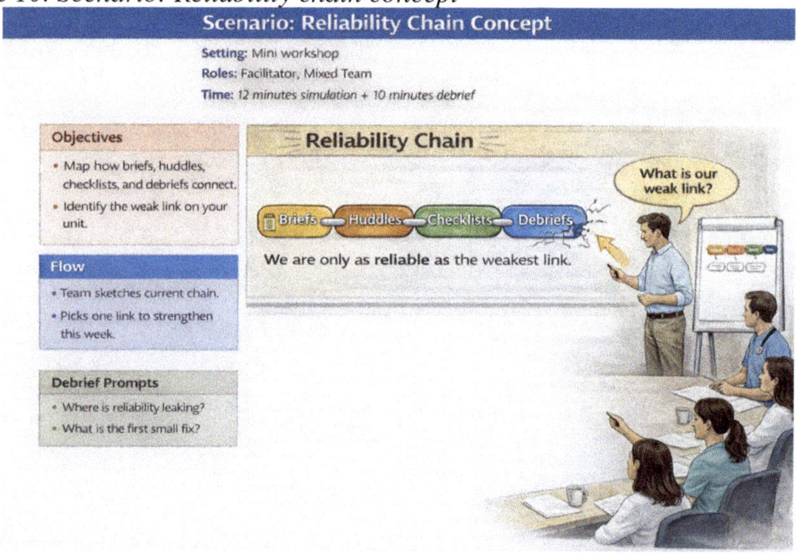

This figure shows a brief workshop exercise where teams map how briefs, huddles, checklists, and debriefs connect as a reliability chain, identify the weakest link in their system, and select one focused improvement to strengthen reliability.

# Chapter 11
# Assessing Organizational Readiness Through Awareness, Desire, Knowledge, Ability, and Reinforcement


## ABSTRACT

*This chapter reframes change management as a human sequence rather than a technical rollout, using the Awareness–Desire–Knowledge–Ability–Reinforcement (ADKAR) model as its guide. Instead of treating change as something organizations deploy, it positions adoption as a progression of mindsets, motivations, skills, and behaviors that must be supported over time. The chapter introduces practical tools for assessing readiness, identifying barriers, and strengthening adoption at each stage of the model. Through applied examples and leaders facing guidance, it illustrates how ADKAR can be used across diverse organizational initiatives to improve engagement, reduce resistance, and sustain new practices. Readers are provided with readiness diagnostics, targeted interventions, common pitfalls, and reinforcement strategies designed to move organizations beyond surface compliance and toward durable cultural change.*


## INTRODUCTION

Organizations often invest heavily in planning and launching new projects, systems, or initiatives, yet overlook one of the strongest predictors of success: understanding how ready people are to take on the change. Timelines, training plans, and technical

DOI: 10.4018/979-8-3373-6496-4.ch011

requirements tend to dominate early conversations, while the human experience of change receives far less attention. As a result, many initiatives struggle not because the design is flawed, but because readiness was assumed rather than examined.

Although numerous change management models exist to help leaders navigate this complexity, this chapter centers on the Awareness–Desire–Knowledge–Ability–Reinforcement (ADKAR) model as a practical, people centered framework for supporting individual adoption. ADKAR offers a way to slow the work just enough to notice where people are and where they are not before behaviors begin to fracture.

The ADKAR model was developed by Prosci, Inc., a change management research organization founded by Jeff Hiatt in the 1990s to study why large organizational initiatives succeed or fail (Hiatt, 2006). Through extensive cross industry benchmarking, Prosci identified consistent patterns in how individuals experience change and distilled those findings into the ADKAR sequence: Awareness, Desire, Knowledge, Ability, and Reinforcement. Their research underscored a simple but often overlooked truth: adoption depends less on technical execution and more on individual motivation, capability, and support. By framing change as a human process rather than an organizational mandate, ADKAR gives leaders a practical way to assess readiness, anticipate resistance, and intervene before breakdowns occur. Its strength lies in its clarity. Each stage functions as both a diagnostic checkpoint and an opportunity for support.

When I first encountered the ADKAR model during a leadership development session, it struck me as deceptively simple. Over time, its depth became evident. It gave structure to what I had long practiced intuitively in quality and safety work, guiding people through uncertainty while still holding systems, outcomes, and reliability in view. For years, I led initiatives with detailed plans and dashboards yet rarely paused to measure readiness from the perspective of those living the change: nurses adapting to new workflows, technicians learning unfamiliar technology, or leaders adjusting long held habits. We tracked compliance, not comprehension, rollout, not readiness.

## Objectives of the Chapter

- **Explain the ADKAR Model as a Framework for Change Readiness**

Describe how the five stages—Awareness, Desire, Knowledge, Ability, and Reinforcement—guide leaders in assessing and supporting organizational change.

- **Demonstrate Practical Application of ADKAR in Healthcare Initiatives**

Show how the model can be applied to real-world efforts such as Gemba Walks, EHR implementations, and safety culture initiatives to identify readiness gaps and strengthen engagement.

- **Provide Tools and Strategies for Measuring and Sustaining Change**

Introduce readiness self-assessment tools, implementation approaches, and reinforcement practices that help leaders move from planning to sustained cultural transformation.

## ADKAR: WHERE CHANGE REALLY BEGINS

ADKAR (Figure 11.1) reshaped how I understood improvement. Each element: Awareness, Desire, Knowledge, Ability, and Reinforcement became a mirror, reflecting how well we were supporting people rather than simply managing processes. For the first time, I began to see improvement not as implementation, but as accompaniment: walking alongside people through uncertainty instead of pushing them toward completion.

Understanding ADKAR conceptually is only the starting point. Its real value emerges when each element is explored in depth. These stages are not abstract categories; they are practical checkpoints that determine whether change will take hold or quietly stall. Figure 11.1 illustrates the ADKAR framework—Awareness, Desire, Knowledge, Ability, and Reinforcement (Adapted from the ADKAR change management model developed by Prosci).

*Figure 1. ADKAR model for change adoption (Adapted with change from the ADKAR change management model developed by Prosci)*

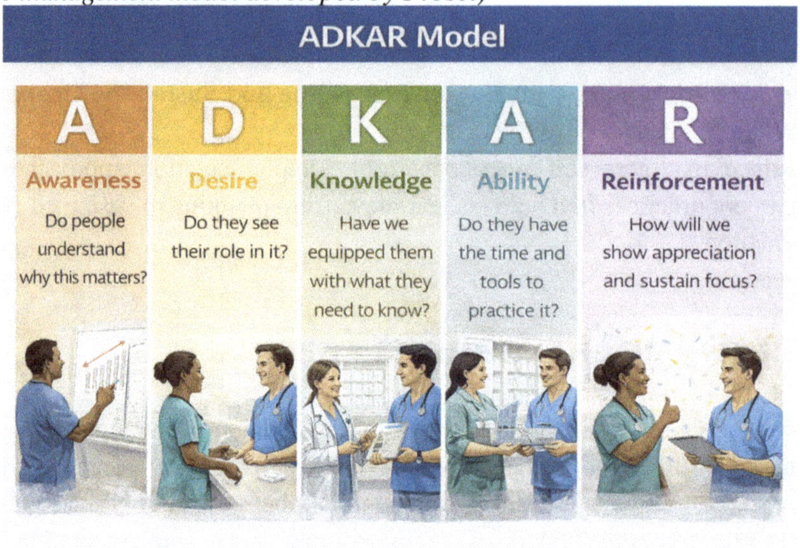
ADKAR Model
A
Awareness
Do people understand why this matters?
D
Desire
Do they see their role in it?
K
Knowledge
Have we equipped them with what they need to know?
A
Ability
Do they have the time and tools to practice it?
R
Reinforcement
How will we show appreciation and sustain focus?

## Awareness

Beginning with Awareness, the foundation of readiness, we move through Desire, Knowledge, Ability, and Reinforcement, examining how each stage shapes behavior and culture. Let's start with the first and most critical step: building awareness.

Awareness is more than an email or a memo. It is the moment when people connect change to something that matters to them. I've learned that awareness built on logic alone rarely holds; it must also reach emotion. During one organization wide safety initiative, I chose not to open with data. Instead, I shared a single story about a missed fall risk assessment that led to a preventable injury. I told it during leadership rounds, in huddles, and in small staff meetings. Each time, I watched the same shift occur, people leaned forward. The story grounded the "why" in lived experience. Awareness grows when people recognize themselves in the narrative. I often ask teams a simple question: *"What does this change mean for you and for the patients you care for?"* The responses reveal more than any readiness survey. Awareness is built in those exchanges, one conversation at a time.

That said, awareness fades quickly if it is not revisited. Competing priorities, new mandates, and daily pressure can blur the original purpose. To sustain it, I've learned to return to the "why" repeatedly, sometimes through brief reminders during huddles, other times through recognition stories that reconnect improvement to real outcomes. Change begins to root itself when people start articulating the "why" in their own words. That is the moment awareness shifts from compliance to conviction.

## Desire: When Change Becomes Personal

If awareness answers *why*, desire answers something more intimate: *why now, and why me?* Desire is the most fragile and most powerful stage of the ADKAR model. It cannot be mandated. It grows in spaces where people feel capable, respected, and included.

I've learned that desire often appears quietly, not in declarations but in moments of recognition. I think of a home care nurse who openly resisted a new digital documentation platform. Her concern wasn't philosophical; it was practical. She worried it would slow her down during already compressed home visits. Rather than pushing compliance, I asked her to walk me through a typical visit using the old process. As she described each step, I timed them. We noted the delays introduced by handwritten notes, later transcription, and double entry. When we compared totals, she paused. The new system could save nearly 20 minutes per visit. Her willingness to adopt the platform didn't come from my explanation. It came from her own realization.

Building desire means helping people locate personal meaning inside organizational goals. It is not about persuading; it is about connecting change to what already matters; efficiency, safety, pride in work, or patient trust. I often remind leadership teams, *"People don't resist change; they resist loss."* Loss of autonomy. Loss of confidence. Loss of predictability. When leaders take time to understand what feels at risk, their responses shift from frustration to empathy. Desire also strengthens through visibility. When progress is seen and named through peer recognition, patient thank you notes, or shared improvements effort gains emotional weight. These moments may seem small, but they become fuel. Over time, they sustain momentum long after the initial launch energy fades.

## Knowledge: Turning Understanding into Skill

Once awareness and desire take root, knowledge provides direction. But knowledge does not begin with slides or checklists. It begins with clarity. People cannot practice what they do not understand, and they cannot understand what has not been explained in the context of their daily work. Early in my career, I equated education with learning. If staff completed the training, I assumed readiness followed. Shadowing them afterward proved otherwise. In home care, nurses could recite a new infusion policy word for word yet struggled when something unexpected appeared;

a missing supply, a malfunctioning device, a home environment that didn't match assumptions.

That gap between knowing and doing reshaped how I approach education. Now, when introducing any new process, I start with a single question: *"What does this look like in your world?"* The question invites context. It allows theory to meet reality. Learning accelerates when people can see themselves in the change where it fits, where it helps, and where it still needs refinement. I've also learned that knowledge spreads faster in circles than in rows. Formal training has its place, but peer learning carries a different credibility. When a nurse explains a new process to another nurse, or a technician shares a safe shortcut discovered in practice, the knowledge sticks. It becomes social, not transactional. Within ADKAR, knowledge is not just information transfer; it is the bridge that equips people with confidence to act. Every successful change I've witnessed shared one trait: people didn't just know *what* to do, they understood *why* it worked.

## Ability: Where Change Meets Reality

Ability is where intention encounters the pressure of real work. This is the point where plans either hold or quietly unravel. Even motivated teams struggle when systems fail to support them. I recall a pilot project introducing a new home oxygen safety protocol. The policy was solid. Training was thorough. Yet within weeks, reports showed inconsistent completion. Rather than enforcing compliance, I joined staff in the field. The problem surfaced quickly: the required form depended on internet access, and many rural homes had none. The barrier wasn't motivation or skill, it was infrastructure. Once we created an offline version, compliance climbed above 95%. That experience reinforced a hard truth: ability depends as much on system design as on individual performance. Leaders must ask whether people have the time, tools, and conditions to succeed. When the answer is no, motivation alone cannot close the gap.

Ability also grows through coaching. In complex environments, skills are reinforced through guided practice, feedback, and modeling. During one clinic rollout, we paired staff with "change buddies" for their first week using a new scheduling system. Hesitation gave way to confidence. By week two, requests for help dropped by half. Change becomes real when people experience success. The goal is not perfection; it is momentum.

## Reinforcement: Making Change Stick

Reinforcement is the quiet force that determines whether change becomes culture or fades from memory. It is not celebration alone, but consistency, feedback, acknowledgment, and visible presence. I once heard it said, *"Change doesn't fail at launch; it fails at sustainment."* I've seen that play out repeatedly. Early enthusiasm gives way to new priorities, and without reinforcement, progress thins.

In my teams, reinforcement thrives on transparency. Sharing results especially when they slip, keeps engagement honest. When performance dips, I frame it as information rather than failure: *"This is what the system is telling us. What needs to adjust?"* That framing invites ownership instead of defensiveness. Recognition matters too. A brief note of thanks or a mention during huddles often carries more weight than formal awards. Reinforcement is emotional; it signals that effort mattered and was noticed.

At an organizational level, reinforcement shows up as alignment. Expectations embedded into orientation, performance reviews, dashboards, and policies make change durable. In one large scale culture initiative, we incorporated ADKAR milestones into quarterly leadership evaluations. The message was unmistakable: change was not optional, it was how we worked. Reinforcement closes the ADKAR loop by anchoring new behaviors in daily practice rather than letting them drift after launch.

## Real World Application: Using ADKAR to Strengthen Gemba Walk Implementation

When preparing to launch our Gemba Walk initiative, I chose to slow down before moving forward. Instead of focusing solely on logistics, I wanted to understand how ready people actually felt. Readiness, I've learned, is not created by announcements; it is revealed through attention. Using the ADKAR model, we conducted a pre-launch readiness assessment across departments. Some questioned the need. *"Do we really need a survey before we even start walking?"* one manager asked. That question answered itself. What we were measuring wasn't compliance, it was the organization's emotional temperature.

We gathered both numeric scores and narrative comments. The picture that emerged was nuanced. People were interested, even hopeful, but unsure. Many understood what a Gemba Walk was, but not yet why it mattered. That insight reshaped the launch. We set aside checklists and expectations and began with conversation. Why presence mattered, what listening looked like, and how this work connected to daily frustrations staff already carried. To move from stories to patterns, we complemented these qualitative insights with a structured assessment using the ADKAR scale.

## The ADKAR Scale

The ADKAR scale translates each stage: Awareness, Desire, Knowledge, Ability, and Reinforcement into measurable indicators using a 1–5 Likert rating. Scores within each domain are averaged to reflect the relative strength of readiness, capability, or sustainability. Leaders review these domain averages to identify the primary constraint; the lowest scoring element most likely to impede adoption.

Used over time, the ADKAR scale becomes more than a snapshot. It functions as a practical learning tool, tracking progress, surfacing barriers early, and guiding targeted support throughout a change initiative.

## Readiness Thresholds

Organizations often rely on thresholds to make readiness visible and actionable. Table 1 translates average ADKAR scores into graduated levels of organizational readiness, using visual cues to signal when performance is likely to hold, when reinforcement is needed, and when targeted or immediate intervention is warranted. The goal is not categorization for its own sake, but guidance: helping leaders decide where to slow down, where to coach, and where risk may be quietly accumulating.

*Table 1. Readiness thresholds using ADKAR*

**Readiness Score Interpretation**

| Average Score | Readiness Level | Action Guidance |
|---|---|---|
| 4.2 - 5.0 | Strong readiness | Sustain and scale |
| 3.6 - 4.1 | Moderate readiness | Reinforce and support |
| 3.0 - 3.5 | Weak readiness | Targeted intervention |
| < 3.0 | High risk | Immediate action |

## Pre-Launch Assessment Findings

Our organization's pre-launch ADKAR survey revealed a mix of strong engagement and clear opportunities for growth.

- **Awareness (Avg. 4.35 | 78.6%)**

Staff demonstrated a solid understanding of program goals, reflecting consistent and effective communication.

- **Desire (Avg. 4.43 | 85.7%)**

Motivation to participate was high, with many expressing interest in observing leadership in action.

- **Knowledge (Avg. 4.26 | 67.9%)**

Baseline understanding was present, though participants asked for clearer guidance on what to observe and how to contribute insights.

- **Ability (Avg. 4.09 | 64.3%)**

This domain scored lowest, pointing to the need for hands-on demonstrations and clearer role expectations, particularly for non-leadership staff.

- **Reinforcement (Avg. 4.36 | 75.0%)**

Teams expressed confidence in leadership follow-through and emphasized the importance of celebrating small wins to maintain momentum.

Taken together, the results confirmed strong awareness and desire, while signaling that ability required more intentional support through experiential learning and timely feedback.

## Key Lessons from the Assessment

The findings were more than numbers; they were stories in disguise. Preparation shifted first. Rather than assuming shared understanding, we integrated readiness insights directly into the launch plan, using short, scenario based demonstrations during huddles to model what good observation and communication looked like in practice. Engagement followed. Teams were invited to choose their own focus areas, which changed the tone from obligation to ownership.

The launch itself became interactive. We opened with a brief activity designed to surface examples of teamwork and innovation during early Gemba rounds, setting expectations through participation rather than instruction. Transparency mattered. Results and narrative feedback were shared openly with both leaders and staff, reinforcing that their input actively shaped the process. Recognition closed the loop. Each week, one observation that led to measurable change was highlighted, turning insight into visible improvement.

Over time, the data became less about readiness and more about resilience. Staff began saying things like, *"These walks aren't inspections anymore; they're conversations."* That was the moment I knew the model had taken hold.

## What the Data Revealed and How We Responded

The numbers told a consistent story. People understood why the Gemba Walk mattered and wanted to participate, but many were unsure how to contribute meaningfully. That gap between intent and execution is where improvement efforts often stall. So before launch, we changed course. Instead of refining logistics, we focused on connection.

## Actions Taken Pre-Launch

- **Integrated readiness insights into training:** Short, scenario based simulations showed how to identify and communicate safety or workflow barriers in real time.
- **Encouraged local ownership:** Each team selected a focus metric such as patient flow time or equipment readiness building pride and accountability.
- **Used light gamification:** Recognition badges acknowledged actionable ideas and meaningful safety observations.
- **Closed the feedback loop:** Findings from each walk were shared within 48 hours, making follow through visible and timely.

Within weeks, participation shifted from compliance to curiosity. Staff began anticipating the walks rather than bracing for them, because they could see their observations translated into action.

## Mid-Implementation Adjustment

By week four, a pulse re-survey showed measurable progress:

- **Ability** scores increased to **4.31** following on-the-job coaching.
- **Reinforcement** rose to **4.55** as leaders consistently acknowledged contributions in public forums.
- **Participation** exceeded 90%, and feedback evolved from surface-level concerns ("We need more supplies") to systems-level insights ("Let's re-sequence setup to prevent delays").

Gemba had shifted from inspection to collaboration a living expression of ADKAR's intent: turning awareness into action, and action into ownership.

## Sustaining the Gains

To prevent drift, quarterly ADKAR reassessments were embedded into the improvement cycle. The model was no longer a pre-launch exercise; it became a standing way to check engagement and psychological safety.

Each reassessment prompted reflective dialogue:

- Where are we strong, and where are we slipping?
- Are we reinforcing outcomes or only celebrating them?
- What new skills do teams need to sustain curiosity and presence?

By the end of the first year, the Gemba Walk program had matured into a system wide rhythm of reflection. Staff reported greater confidence in speaking up, and leaders gained clearer visibility into frontline realities previously seen only through dashboards. Figure 11.2 illustrates how ADKAR supported the shift from readiness assessment to sustained cultural change highlighting leadership modeling, shared ownership, rapid feedback, and the evolution from inspection to conversation through reinforcement.

*Figure 2. From readiness to resilience using ADKAR framework*

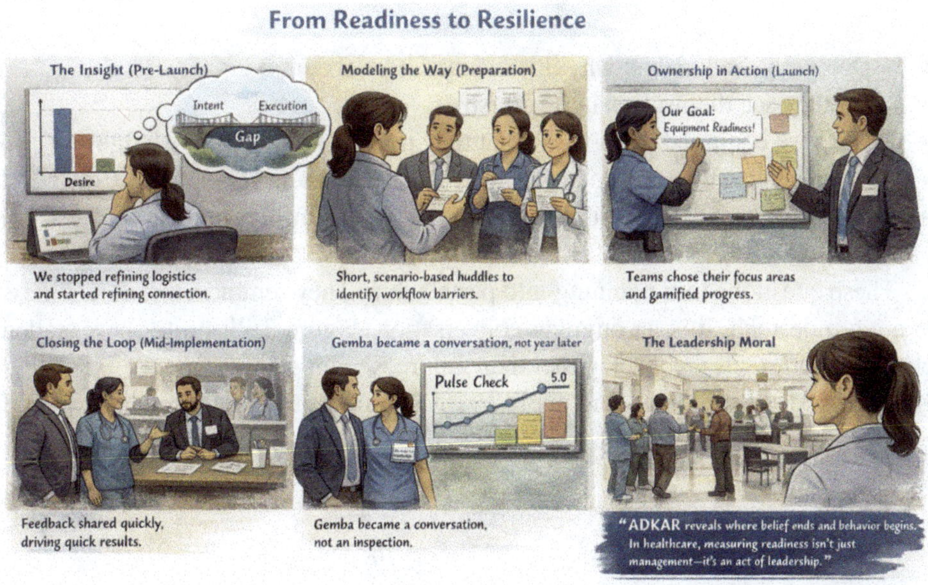
From Readiness to Resilience
The Insight (Pre-Launch)
Intent
Execution
Gap
Desire
We stopped refining logistics and started refining connection.
Modeling the Way (Preparation)
Short, scenario-based huddles to identify workflow barriers.
Ownership in Action (Launch)
Our Goal: Equipment Readiness!
Teams chose their focus areas and gamified progress.
Closing the Loop (Mid-Implementation)
Feedback shared quickly, driving quick results.
Gemba became a conversation, not year later
Pulse Check
5.0
Gemba became a conversation, not an inspection.
The Leadership Moral
"ADKAR reveals where belief ends and behavior begins. In healthcare, measuring readiness isn't just management—it's an act of leadership."

## When Change Feels Stuck

Even with thoughtful design, some change efforts lose momentum. When that happens, I no longer see failure; I see feedback.

When progress stalls, I ask which letter of ADKAR is missing.

- Lack of **Awareness** sounds like confusion: *"Why are we doing this again?"*
- Lack of **Desire** sounds like fatigue: *"We've tried this before."*
- Lack of **Knowledge** shows up as repeated mistakes.
- Lack of **Ability** appears as frustration.
- Lack of **Reinforcement** reveals itself as drift, quiet returns to old habits.

That lens has saved me from labeling resistance as defiance. Most people aren't resisting change; they're responding to not being heard. There are also moments when fatigue is real. During one particularly heavy year of concurrent rollouts, a nurse said to me, *"I'm tired of being resilient."* I wrote it down. It reminded me that resilience without recovery becomes burnout. As leaders, we must pace change, not just drive it. Improvement that ignores human bandwidth rarely lasts.

## From Framework to Habit

The strength of ADKAR lies in its simplicity. It is not a one time checklist, but a rhythm. I now use it informally, as a mental map. Before introducing any initiative, I pause to ask:

- Do people understand why this matters? (**Awareness**)
- Do they see themselves in it? (**Desire**)
- Have we equipped them with what they need to know? (**Knowledge**)
- Do they have the time and tools to practice it? (**Ability**)
- How will we notice effort and sustain focus? (**Reinforcement**)

These questions turn planning into partnership. They remind me that readiness is not a milestone, it is an ongoing conversation. Figure 3 illustrates how stalled change functions as feedback rather than failure, showing how leaders use the ADKAR lens to identify gaps and apply targeted support to restore momentum and re-engage teams.

*Figure 3. When change feels stuck*

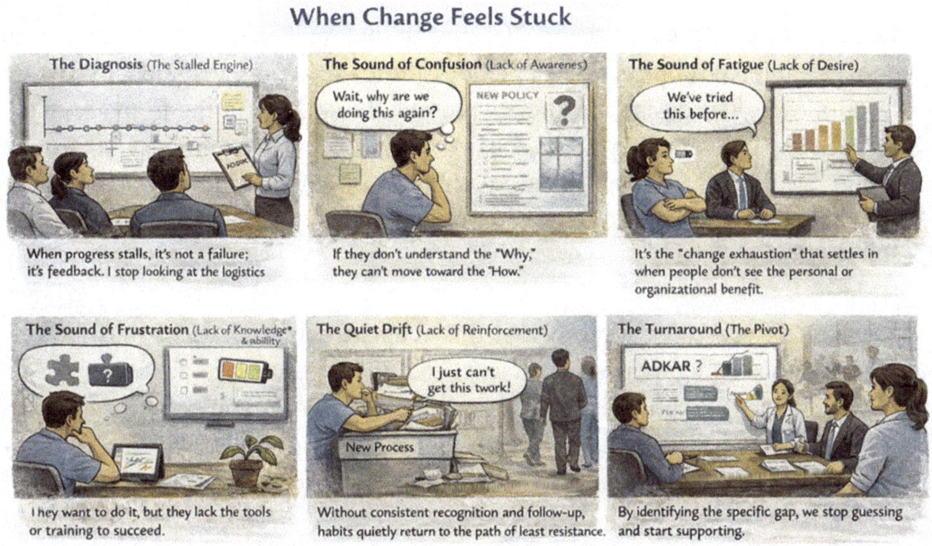


## A Note on Sustainability

Sustaining change requires rhythm, not heroics. It is built through follow-up huddles, visible dashboards, and everyday recognition. It also requires humility, the willingness to admit when something isn't working and adjust course. The organizations that thrive are not those that avoid missteps, but those that keep learning out loud. As I often tell my teams, *"Change doesn't have to be perfect; it just has to stay alive long enough to grow."* ADKAR reminds us that readiness is relational. It grows where leaders listen and accountability feels fair. Awareness and motivation matter but they are only the beginning.

## PRACTICE IMPACT

One of my clearest lessons came from a senior respiratory therapist after a ventilator management policy change. She told me, "Once I understood the why, the how took care of itself." That insight became even more evident when she worked with her team and our leadership group to draft a Respiratory Therapy Services program that clearly differentiated clinical from non-clinical respiratory regulatory requirements.

Once everyone understood *why* the distinctions mattered. How accreditation guidelines reinforced clinical safety practices; the team was able to build the program with confidence. The desire was already present, the ability was there, and once the knowledge gaps closed, the "how" became straightforward to implement. As she later said, "When we feel the drift, we go back to reinforcing the why.

## CONCLUSION

Figure 4 reflects the central idea of this chapter: that ADKAR is most powerful when it stops being treated as a formal change tool and starts functioning as a way of thinking. In practice, it becomes a quiet pause before action, a mental map leaders carry into everyday decisions. Rather than asking teams to "implement a framework," leaders return to a small set of human questions: *Do people understand why this matters? Do they see themselves in it? Have we given them what they need to succeed? Do they have the time and tools to practice? How will effort be noticed and sustained?*

When used this way, change shifts from compliance to habit (Figure 4). Awareness and desire ground the work in purpose. Knowledge and ability make the work doable in real conditions. Reinforcement ensures that progress does not fade once attention moves elsewhere. Over time, the framework recedes into the background, but its rhythm remains; shaping how initiatives are introduced, how resistance is interpreted, and how leaders stay anchored to meaning rather than checklists. This is how change endures: not through perfect execution of a model, but through repeated, human centered use in the flow of daily work.

*Figure 4. From framework to habit*

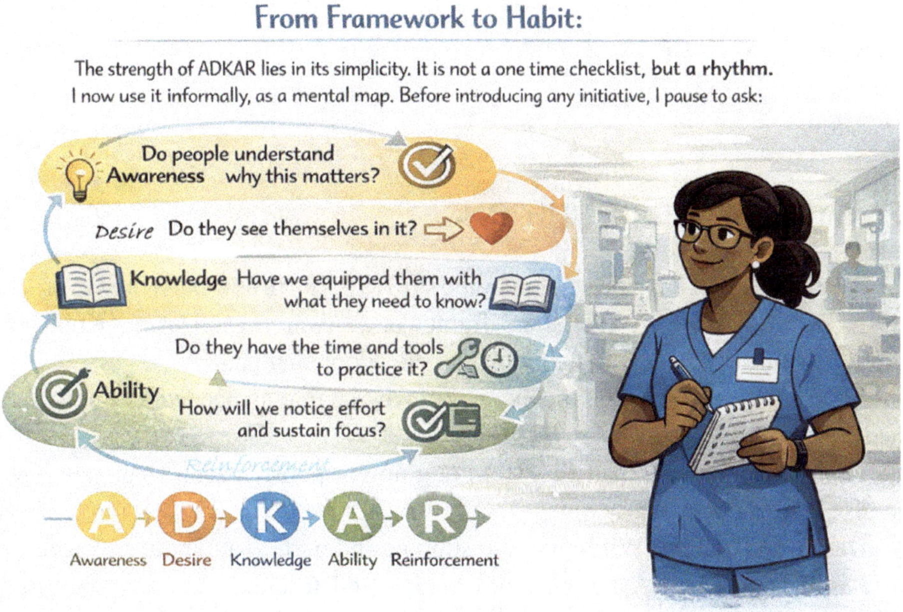
From Framework to Habit:
The strength of ADKAR lies in its simplicity. It is not a one time checklist, but a rhythm.
I now use it informally, as a mental map. Before introducing any initiative, I pause to ask:
Awareness
Do people understand why this matters?
Desire
Do they see themselves in it?
Knowledge
Have we equipped them with what they need to know?
Do they have the time and tools to practice it?
Ability
How will we notice effort and sustain focus?
Reinforcement
A D K A R
Awareness
Desire
Knowledge
Ability
Reinforcement

## REFERENCES

Hiatt, J. (2006). *ADKAR: A model for change in business, government, and our community*. Prosci.

## KEY TERMS AND DEFINITIONS

**Ability (ADKAR):** The demonstrated skill to perform new behaviors in practice.

**ADKAR Model:** A five-stage framework, Awareness, Desire, Knowledge, Ability, Reinforcement, showing how people adopt change.

**Awareness (ADKAR):** Understanding why change is needed and how it connects to goals.

**Change Fatigue:** Exhaustion from ongoing or poorly paced change that leads to disengagement.

**Desire (ADKAR):** Willingness to support and participate in the change.

**Knowledge (ADKAR):** The information and training required to carry out change effectively.

**Organizational Readiness:** The extent to which an organization and its people are prepared for change.

**Psychological Ownership:** A personal sense of responsibility and commitment to the change.

**Reinforcement (ADKAR):** Actions that sustain new behaviors and make change stick.

**Stakeholder Engagement:** Involving those affected by change to build ownership and reduce resistance.

# APPENDIX I

## ADKAR-Relevant Healthcare Initiatives

Across multiple improvement programs, the ADKAR model helps clarify where readiness thrives and where reinforcement is needed:

- **EHR Rollout:** Focused on *Knowledge Ability.* Common challenges included workflow fatigue and fear of technology errors. *Reinforcement strategies:* peer mentorship and live support stations.
- **Just Culture / Safety Reporting:** Focused on *Awareness Desire.* Barriers involved fear of blame and lack of trust. *Reinforcement strategies:* leadership storytelling and positive recognition of reporting behavior.
- **Gemba Walk / Lean Initiatives:** Focused on *Awareness Reinforcement.* Teams experienced role confusion and uneven engagement. *Reinforcement strategies:* visible leadership presence and gamified participation.
- **Workforce Safety / Violence Prevention:** Focused on *Desire Ability.* Main challenges were confidence gaps and underreporting. *Reinforcement strategies:* scenario-based practice and public recognition.
- **Health Equity / Patient Experience:** Focused on *Awareness Desire.* Seen by some as "extra work." *Reinforcement strategies:* values-based messaging and shared storytelling.
- **Telehealth Expansion:** Focused on *Knowledge Reinforcement.* Challenges included technology anxiety and patient skepticism. *Reinforcement strategies:* simulation training and ongoing peer coaching.

Together, these initiatives show how ADKAR domains interconnect, building awareness and desire sets the stage for ability, while reinforcement transforms short-term change into sustainable culture. The ADKAR Playbooks Matrix (Figure11.5) provides a practical view of how change adoption is intentionally supported across multiple initiatives by aligning each playbook with the five elements of the ADKAR model. Rather than treating change as a single training event, the matrix shows how awareness, desire, knowledge, ability, and reinforcement are addressed differently depending on the context; whether implementing a new EHR, strengthening Just Culture, advancing Gemba Walks, improving workforce safety, promoting health equity, or expanding telehealth. By making these connections explicit, the matrix helps leaders identify where adoption may stall and where targeted support is needed. It also reinforces that sustainable improvement depends not only on technical solutions, but on consistent attention to human factors, leadership behaviors, and reinforcement mechanisms that keep new practices embedded in daily work.

*Figure 5. ADKAR playbooks matrix*

**ADKAR Playbooks Matrix**

| Playbook | A Awareness | D Desire | K Knowledge | A Ability | R Reinforcement |
|---|---|---|---|---|---|
| EHR Implementation | Staff can explain the "why" (safety, interoperabil) | Clinicians see personal value time saved, fewer errors) | Role-specific clarity (ordering; documentation, inbox tasks) | Confident use under peak workload; contingency plans for common glitches. | Visible leader follow up, rapid fixes, recognition of adoption milestones. |
| Patient Safety & Just Culture | Staff understand Just Cultures purpose and link to safer care | Willingness to report near misses without fear; leaders model | Clear 'how to' for reporting and debriefing; role clarity in reviews | Teams conduct learning reviews and implement' corrective actiors porpply. | Routine storytelling on improvements from reporting; timely feedback to reporters |
| Quality Improvement & Gemba Walks | Staff articulate purpose (observe work, learn, remove barriers) | Teams anticipate walks as partnership, not audit | Clear roles, observation focus, and escalation pathways. | Real time identification: of barners, leader follow up within 48 hours | Recognition of actionable ideas and visible changes from walk insights. |
| Workplace Violence Prevention | Clear rationale linking policies to staff well-being and patient safety | Staff view safety behaviors as part of professional identity; leaders model | Role-specific steps for de-escalation and reporting; quick guides | Demonstrated responses in simulations, access to supports (e.g. alams) | Feedback after incidents, public acknowledgement; policy alignment. |
| Health Equity & Patient Experience | Staff link equity to outcomes and trust | Motivation grounded in compassion and fairness; reduced "extra work" sentiment | Concrete scripts, troubleshooting; patient friendly instructions | Protocols, scripts, troubleshooting; patient friendly instructions | Recognition, of equity behaviors, patient stories highlighting impact |
| Remote Monitoring & Telehealth | Staff and patients understand purpose (access, convenience, safety) | Clear personal value (time saved, reduced exposure, better follow up) | Protocols, scripts troubleshooting patient friendly instructions | Betcord vising despite connectivity gaps, back up plans (phone, offline tools) | Share metrics (no show reduction, satisfaction); recognize effective practices. |

# APPENDIX II

## How the ADKAR Scale Is Calculated

Many organizations operationalize the ADKAR model by using it as a quantitative readiness scale. Each element: Awareness, Desire, Knowledge, Ability, and Reinforcement is measured through brief survey items rated by participants. While Prosci does not prescribe a single scoring method, the approach below reflects common practice across healthcare settings.

### Step 1. Rate Each ADKAR Element

Each ADKAR domain is assessed using several survey questions (typically 3–8 per domain) rated on a 1–5 Likert scale, where higher scores indicate stronger readiness.

### Step 2. Calculate Domain Averages

For each ADKAR element, item scores are averaged to produce a single domain score (e.g., Awareness = 4.35). Decimals may be retained or rounded based on organizational preference.

### Step 3. Convert to Percent Readiness (Optional)

To support leader interpretation, some organizations convert average scores into percentages using the formula:

Average score $\div 5 \times 100$

This step is optional and does not change the underlying interpretation.

### Step 4. Identify the Constraint

The lowest scoring ADKAR domain is treated as the primary adoption constraint. Interventions are prioritized to address this specific gap rather than applying broad, non-targeted solutions.

## Step 5. Track Change Over Time

ADKAR scores are typically reviewed at multiple points (pre-launch, mid-implementation, post-launch, and sustainment) to assess progress and guide course correction.

## Step 6. Apply Readiness Thresholds

Organizations commonly interpret scores using predefined readiness thresholds to guide action (e.g., strong, moderate, weak, or high-risk readiness).

## ADKAR Calculation at a Glance

- Collect Likert-scale responses for each ADKAR domain
- Calculate average domain scores
- Identify the lowest-scoring domain
- Target interventions to that constraint

# Chapter 12
# From Continuous Improvement to Enduring Impact: Sustaining Change Through Safety Stories


## ABSTRACT

*Sustaining improvement in healthcare requires more than technical fixes or increasingly refined performance measures. While metrics remain essential for tracking outcomes, they often lose meaning when separated from the human experience of care. This chapter examines patient safety stories as a mechanism for sustaining improvement and shaping organizational culture over time. Drawing on published cases, national exemplars, and a real-world, multi-agency CLABSI collaborative, it illustrates how patient narratives influence leader attention, staff behavior, and system level priorities. Safety stories translate abstract measures into lived experience, reinforce escalation norms, and preserve the intent of improvement efforts across leadership transitions. When embedded ethically and consistently into routine practice, storytelling complements data by keeping attention anchored on people. Durable improvement emerges when organizations intentionally integrate structure and narrative to support learning, accountability, and cultural continuity.*


## INTRODUCTION: WHEN MEASURES IMPROVE BUT MEANING FADES

Sustaining improvement over time remains one of the most persistent challenges in healthcare quality and safety work (Institute for Healthcare Improvement [IHI],

DOI: 10.4018/979-8-3373-6496-4.ch012

n.d.; Deming, 1986). While performance metrics such as readmission rates, infection rates, and compliance scores are indispensable for monitoring outcomes, research consistently shows that gains often erode once focused initiatives conclude or leadership attention shifts (Cowie et al., 2020; *Lennox et al., 2023).*

Anyone who has worked in healthcare long enough recognizes the pattern. Performance improves with concentrated effort. Results are celebrated. Attention moves on. Gradually, outcomes drift. I have seen this cycle repeat across acute care, home health, and post acute settings, not because teams forget how to improve, but because organizations slowly lose connection to why the work mattered in the first place.

Early in my career, readmissions were framed as discrete improvement projects. Discharge instructions were refined, follow-up calls standardized, medication reconciliation strengthened. The gains were real, but they were often temporary. A home care nurse once reframed the problem for me with a single sentence: *"We talk about readmissions as a number, but for the patient, it's just another hospital stay."* That comment changed how I understood sustainment. Lasting improvement depends not only on technical reliability, but on whether teams remain connected to the lived experience behind the metric. Measures do not sustain themselves. Meaning has to be actively protected.

## KEEPING IMPROVEMENT CONNECTED TO PEOPLE

Improvement initiatives are often launched in response to a sentinel event, patient harm, or a compelling failure story, consistent with early patient safety literature emphasizing the catalytic role of narrative (Institute of Medicine, 2000). Over time, however, that origin story is frequently replaced by dashboards, thresholds, and reporting cadence, increasing the risk of what has been described as metric fatigue (Berwick, 1989; Tawfik et al., 2023).

Storytelling is one of the most effective ways to prevent this drift. Patient safety stories do not replace data; they give it context. They remind teams that every data point represents a person navigating illness, uncertainty, and transitions of care. Simple, repeatable practices such as opening meetings with a brief safety story or a "home care moment" help keep improvement grounded without adding operational burden.

In one home based care team, meetings began with short stories tied to safety or reliability in the home. These were rarely dramatic. More often, they described a missed cue caught early, a workaround that introduced risk, or a small adjustment that made care safer. New staff consistently reported that this practice helped performance data feel tangible rather than abstract. The stories did not compete with metrics; they made them legible.

## EXAMPLE IN PRACTICE: HARDWIRING SAFETY THROUGH STORY AND SYSTEM DESIGN

Central line associated bloodstream infections (CLABSIs) in home infusion present unique challenges. Hospital based definitions and surveillance systems do not fully capture the realities of home environments, caregiver involvement, and care transitions. To address these gaps, five regional home infusion agencies partnered in an AHRQ-funded, IRB approved collaborative to establish a shared definition and develop practical tools for real world use.

Guided by the Systems Engineering Initiative for Patient Safety (SEIPS) 2.0 framework which examines how people, tasks, tools, environments, organizational conditions interact to shape safety and the RE-AIM framework, which supports implementation, measurement, and sustainment, the collaborative created a standardized surveillance dashboard and a CLABSI prevention toolkit designed specifically for home infusion care. The Home Infusion CLABSI Collaborative, led by Dr. Sarah Keller and colleagues from agencies across the country, demonstrates how improvement becomes durable when system design and storytelling are intentionally paired. Building on a consensus definition developed through a modified Delphi process (Keller et al., 2020), the team consistently integrated patient and caregiver narratives alongside outcome data in governance and education forums. This pairing preserved meaning even as attention inevitably shifted over time. Infection prevention moved from being a metric to monitor toward a shared responsibility teams could explain, adapt, and sustain.

What ultimately sustained the work was not the dashboard alone, but how meaning was protected. Patient and caregiver experiences were embedded into training, educational materials, and leadership discussions. Literacy matched materials, QR-coded videos reflecting real home setups, and environmental safety checklists acknowledged variability rather than assuming ideal conditions. As implementation progressed, CLABSI rates declined year over year, caregivers reported increased confidence in line care, and teams could articulate why specific safeguards mattered. Pairing outcome data with brief narratives in leadership forums reduced normalization of risk and reinforced purpose. This example underscores a central lesson of sustainment: when improvement is framed through both system design and human story, reliability becomes part of organizational identity rather than a time limited initiative.

## ROUTINES AND LEADERSHIP PRACTICES THAT SUPPORT SUSTAINMENT

Sustainment research consistently highlights the importance of leadership behaviors, routines, and social reinforcement in maintaining improvement gains (Foster et al., 2023; Murray et al., 2024). Simple, repeatable practices, brief reflection pauses, recognition of safety catches, shared learning stories, reinforce culture without adding operational weight. Leadership transitions pose particular risk. Written documentation captures what was done, but stories preserve why it mattered. Structured handoffs that include key patient examples, lessons learned, and risks to protect often provide greater continuity than policies alone. When leaders routinely invite teams to explain decisions through patient examples, ownership deepens and judgment matures. Over time, teams adapt improvements independently because they understand both the process and the people it protects.

## INTEGRATING DATA, STORY, AND DAILY PRACTICE

Sustainment science emphasizes that improvement lasts when system design and evaluation are intentionally linked (Cowie et al., 2020; Lennox et al., 2023). SEIPS 2.0 provides a framework for understanding how system elements interact, while RE-AIM ensures redesigned processes are implemented, measured, and maintained rather than treated as one-time fixes (Holden et al., 2013; Glasgow et al., 1999). High reliability and learning organizations balance quantitative and qualitative understanding (Deming, 1986; Berwick, 1989). Dashboards offer visibility and consistency. Stories explain why trends exist and how they surface in real world care, particularly in complex environments such as the home (Vehviläinen et al., 2024). In the CLABSI collaborative, pairing data with brief patient or caregiver stories allowed teams to interpret variation without blame and detect early signs of drift. Improvement became enduring when teams stopped referring to "the new process" and began saying, *"This is how we do it here."*

## THE ART OF WRITING A PATIENT SAFETY STORY

Writing a patient safety story is not documentation; it is interpretation. At its best, it makes risk visible without assigning blame, translates lived experience into system insight, and creates emotional resonance while remaining analytically disciplined. Effective stories begin with context, not conclusions. They situate the reader in the care environment, describe conditions under which decisions were made, and resist hindsight bias. Events are described with restraint; what happened, where risk emerged, and why it mattered without dramatization or moral judgment. Details are chosen for what they reveal about system performance, not for effect.

The turning point lies in learning. Human factors, workflow design, cognitive load, and environmental constraints are named explicitly so readers can recognize similar vulnerabilities in their own settings. The story earns its place when it clearly articulates what changed: the safeguard introduced, where it lives in the workflow, and who owns it. Without this, storytelling risks becoming symbolic rather than practical.

Sustainment completes the narrative. Metrics, early warning signs, and leadership routines are named so that safety is framed as stewardship rather than correction. Ethical practice underpins every step; de-identification, consent awareness when needed, and a system focused, no blame stance. This ethical grounding is not a disclaimer; it is what allows stories to circulate and be used constructively. In this way, patient safety storytelling becomes both a leadership practice and a cultural signal. It communicates how an organization learns, how it treats its people, and how seriously it takes the responsibility to turn experience into safer care.

Figure 1 presents a structured, ethics centered framework for writing patient safety stories that move from context and event description to learning, system change, sustainment, and accountability. By explicitly linking what happened to what changed and how improvement is monitored, the framework supports system-focused learning, prevents blame, and ensures insights translate into durable practice through clear ownership and closed loop follow up.

*Figure 1. Writing a patient safety story*

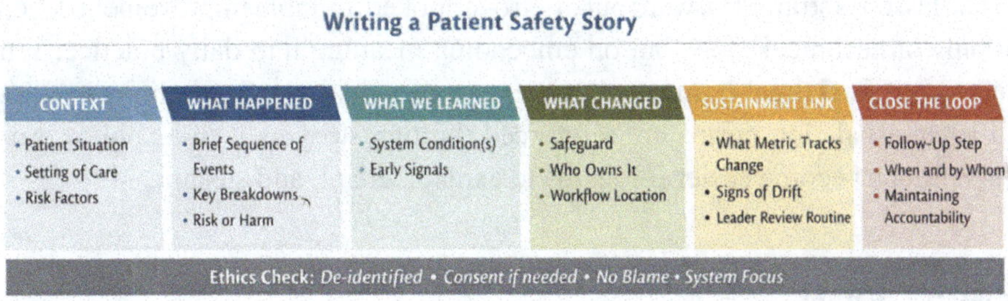

## PRACTICE IMPACT

Turning stories into sustained practice requires more than good intentions; it requires structure that keeps meaning close to the work. Safety stories are most effective when they are woven directly into the processes they are meant to influence, rather than shared as stand-alone reflections. When stories travel alongside metrics and decisions, they help teams connect numbers to lived experience and experience to action. In practice, this integration shows up in small, repeatable routines. Teams pair a brief safety story with the relevant measure in the same forum, reinforcing why the metric matters. Stories follow a short, familiar format so they remain consistent without becoming burdensome. Each narrative is anchored to action: what changed, what teams should do today, and what leaders will follow up on. Just as important, the loop is closed publicly. Staff see system response; not just discussion reinforcing that speaking up leads somewhere. Throughout, ethical discipline matters. De-identification, consent when appropriate, and non-blaming, system focused language create the psychological safety that allows stories to circulate and be used constructively.

The practical implications of this approach are clear in home infusion safety work. By pairing SEIPS informed system design with the RE-AIM framework, teams can design interventions that improve performance initially and are intentionally structured to be sustained and adapted over time. The Home Infusion CLABSI Collaborative demonstrated this in practice. Standardized definitions, redesigned work systems, and the deliberate inclusion of patient and caregiver narratives in governance discussions led to more reliable processes, greater caregiver confidence, and sustained reductions in CLABSI rates.

The lesson is straightforward but often overlooked: durable improvement depends not only on technical tools, but on embedding meaning into daily practice. When education reflects real home environments rather than idealized clinical settings, and when escalation norms are reinforced through story as well as policy, safety interventions become easier for teams to explain, adapt, and sustain.

## CONCLUSION

Sustaining improvement in healthcare requires more than reliable processes and well-designed metrics. It depends on an organization's ability to preserve meaning over time. This chapter has shown that technical solutions alone rarely endure unless they remain connected to the lived experience of patients, caregivers, and staff.

Storytelling emerged as a critical mechanism for linking data to purpose, reinforcing why safeguards exist, and preventing the gradual drift that often follows early success.

Through examples such as the Home Infusion CLABSI Collaborative, the chapter illustrates how pairing human factors principles with implementation science allows teams to design systems that reflect real-world conditions and evolve as those conditions change. When narratives, system design, and leadership routines are intentionally aligned, improvement becomes part of daily work rather than something dependent on project timelines or individual champions. Sustained reliability grows in organizations that treat safety as both a technical and human endeavor; one in which meaning is continually renewed through stories, routines, and structures that keep the patient at the center of the work.

## REFERENCES


Berwick, D. M. (1989). Continuous improvement as an ideal in health care. *The New England Journal of Medicine*, *320*(1), 53–56. DOI: 10.1056/NEJM198901053200110 PMID: 2909878

Cowie, J., Nicoll, A., Dimova, E. D., Campbell, P., & Duncan, E. A. S. (2020). The barriers and facilitators influencing the sustainability of hospital-based interventions: A systematic review. *BMC Health Services Research*, *20*(1), 588. DOI: 10.1186/s12913-020-05434-9 PMID: 32594912

Deming, W. E. (1986). *Out of the crisis*. MIT Press.

Foster, M., Edwards, A., . . .. (2023). Impact of leadership walkarounds on operational, cultural, and clinical outcomes: A systematic review. *Journal of Patient Safety*. https://pmc.ncbi.nlm.nih.gov/articles/PMC10582976/

Glasgow, R. E., Vogt, T. M., & Boles, S. M. (1999). Evaluating the public health impact of health promotion interventions: The RE-AIM framework. *American Journal of Public Health*, *89*(9), 1322–1327. DOI: 10.2105/AJPH.89.9.1322 PMID: 10474547

Holden, R. J., Carayon, P., Gurses, A. P., Hoonakker, P., Hundt, A. S., Ozok, A. A., & Rivera-Rodriguez, A. J. (2013). SEIPS 2.0: A human factors framework for studying and improving the work of healthcare professionals and patients. *Ergonomics*, *56*(11), 1669–1686. DOI: 10.1080/00140139.2013.838643 PMID: 24088063

Institute for Healthcare Improvement. (n.d.). *4 steps to sustaining improvement in health care*. https://www.ihi.org/library/publications/four-steps-sustaining-improvement-health-care

Institute of Medicine. (2000). *To err is human: Building a safer health system*. National Academies Press.

Keller, S. C., Salinas, A., Williams, D., McGoldrick, M., Gorski, L. A., Alexander, M., Norris, A., Charron, J., Stienecker, R. S., Passaretti, C. L., Maragakis, L. L., & Cosgrove, S. E. (2020). Reaching consensus on a home infusion central line–associated bloodstream infection surveillance definition via a modified Delphi approach. *American Journal of Infection Control*, *48*(9), 993–1000. DOI: 10.1016/j.ajic.2019.12.015 PMID: 31982215

Lennox, L., Antonacci, G., Harris, M., & Reed, J. (2023). Unpacking the 'process of sustaining'—identifying threats to sustainability and the strategies used to address them: A longitudinal multiple case study. *Implementation Science Communications*, *4*(1), 68. DOI: 10.1186/s43058-023-00445-z PMID: 37337274

Murray, J. S., Clifford, J., Scott, D., Kelly, S., & Hanover, C. (2024). Leader rounding for high reliability and improved patient safety. *Federal Practitioner : for the Health Care Professionals of the VA, DoD, and PHS*, *41*(1), 16–21. DOI: 10.12788/fp.0444 PMID: 38835357

Tawfik, D. S., Adair, K. C., Palassof, S., Sexton, J. B., Levoy, E., Frankel, A., Leonard, M., Proulx, J., & Profit, J. (2023). Leadership behavior associations with domains of safety culture, engagement, and healthcare worker well-being. *Joint Commission Journal on Quality and Patient Safety*, *49*(3), 156–165. DOI: 10.1016/j.jcjq.2022.12.006 PMID: 36658090

Vehviläinen, E., Charles, A., Sainsbury, J., Stacey, G., Field-Richards, S. E., & Westwood, G. (2024). Influences of leadership, organizational culture, and hierarchy on raising concerns about patient deterioration: A qualitative study. *Journal of Patient Safety*, *20*(5), e73–e77. DOI: 10.1097/PTS.0000000000001234 PMID: 39028433

## KEY TERMS AND DEFINITIONS

**CLABSI (Central Line–Associated Bloodstream Infection):** A preventable infection associated with central venous access devices; in home infusion, CLABSIs require definitions and surveillance methods that reflect real-world environments and caregiver involvement.

**Hardwiring Safety:** The deliberate integration of safe practices, routines, and narrative reinforcement into everyday work so improvement becomes part of organizational identity rather than a temporary initiative.

**Human Factors Engineering:** An approach that designs systems around real human capabilities and constraints, increasing the likelihood that safety interventions can be reliably used in everyday practice.

**Leadership Presence:** The visible, consistent engagement of leaders through behaviors such as storytelling, inquiry, and recognition, which signals priorities and supports sustainment.

**Modified Delphi Method:** A structured, iterative consensus-building process used in the collaborative to establish an evidence-based, home-infusion CLABSI definition.

**Normalization of Risk:** A gradual erosion of vigilance in which teams become accustomed to unsafe conditions or deviations, making harm more likely unless purpose and meaning are continually reinforced.

**RE-AIM:** An implementation science framework used to evaluate the reach, effectiveness, adoption, implementation, and maintenance of interventions to ensure improvements are scalable and sustainable.

**Safety Storytelling:** The structured use of patient, caregiver, or staff narratives to contextualize data, reinforce purpose, and maintain attention on the human experience behind metrics.

**SEIPS 2.0:** A human factors framework that examines how people, tasks, tools, environments, and organizational conditions interact to shape safety outcomes, guiding the design of safer work systems.

**Sustainment:** The ongoing ability of an organization to maintain and adapt improvement gains over time by preserving meaning, purpose, and shared routines, not just processes or metrics

# APPENDIX

## Practice-Based Vignette 1. When the Story Prevented Drift

Six months after the launch of a new home infusion CLABSI prevention toolkit, performance dashboards continued to show strong bundle adherence and declining infection rates. Leadership attention had begun to shift toward new organizational priorities, and the toolkit was no longer a standing agenda item in governance meetings. On paper, the work appeared complete. During a routine nursing huddle, a clinician shared a brief story about a patient receiving home infusion therapy whose caregiver struggled to maintain sterile technique due to limited workspace and poor lighting in the home. The caregiver had followed the written instructions correctly, yet environmental constraints introduced risk that was not immediately visible in the checklist. The nurse described how she paused, adapted the setup, and used a QR-coded video to reinforce technique in the actual home environment.

The story prompted discussion among the team. Leaders recognized that while bundle compliance remained high, environmental variability posed a latent risk not fully captured by existing measures. Rather than revising the metric, the team adjusted the process: environmental safety checks were elevated in training refreshers, and home setup examples were added to ongoing education materials. The dashboard remained unchanged, but its meaning deepened. In subsequent months, leaders intentionally paired outcome data with brief caregiver or patient stories during governance reviews. These narratives reinforced why safeguards existed and helped teams recognize early signs of drift before performance declined. Over time, staff no longer referred to the CLABSI toolkit as a "new initiative," but as "how we do home infusion safely."

This vignette illustrates a central lesson of sustainment: improvement endures not because metrics are stable, but because meaning is continuously renewed. When stories are embedded into routine practice and linked to system design, organizations are better equipped to adapt without losing reliability. Figure 12.2 illustrates how strong performance signals (e.g., a low or declining CLABSI rate) can mask emerging risk over time, and how a frontline safety story re-anchors attention to real-world conditions. A nurse's narrative reveals latent environmental vulnerabilities in the home, prompting team reflection, targeted system adjustments, and reinforced training. By pairing data with lived experience, organizations prevent drift, renew meaning, and sustain safer care as part of everyday practice rather than a time-limited initiative.

*Figure 2. Drift to discovery: How safety stories prevent improvement fatigue*

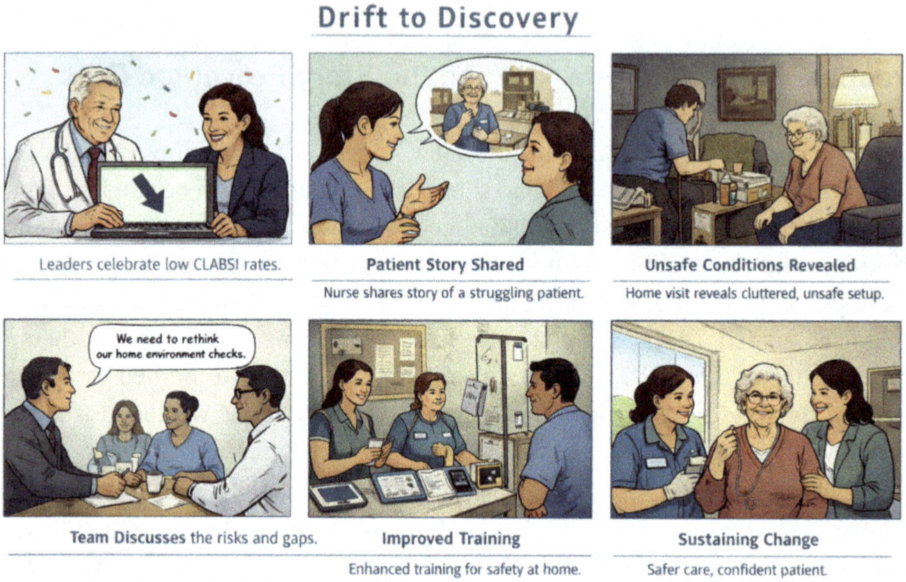
Drift to Discovery
Leaders celebrate low CLABSI rates.
Patient Story Shared
Nurse shares story of a struggling patient.
Unsafe Conditions Revealed
Home visit reveals cluttered, unsafe setup.
We need to rethink our home environment checks.
Team Discusses the risks and gaps.
Improved Training
Enhanced training for safety at home.
Sustaining Change
Safer care, confident patient.

## Practice-Based Vignette 2

A health system implemented a standardized medication reconciliation process for hospital-to-home transitions. Audits showed high checklist completion and fewer medication-related readmissions, suggesting success. Weeks later, a home care nurse found a patient taking both old and new blood pressure medications. Although reconciliation was documented correctly, the medications present in the home created confusion.

Using a SEIPS 2.0 lens, the team recognized a system issue: the process assumed understanding a list meant correct use at home. The workflow was redesigned to include a 48-hour post-discharge "medication reality check," verifying what medications were actually present and taken, supported by visual cues and teach-back. RE-AIM was applied to track reach, adoption, implementation of fidelity, and maintenance over time. Medication reconciliation shifted from a discharge task to a reinforced transition process. Readmission remained low not because the checklist endured, but because the system was designed for real use and evaluated for sustainability, demonstrating how SEIPS and RE-AIM together turn compliance into lasting safety practice. Implementation sustainment using a SEIPS 2.0 informed view is illustrated in Figure 3, which shows how tasks, tools, environment, people, and organizational processes interact to support durable medication reconciliation practices across the transition from hospital to home. Adapted from Holden et al. (2013).

*Figure 3. Medication reconciliation as an enduring system. A SEIPS 2.0–informed view of how tasks, tools, environment, people, and organizational processes interact to sustain medication reconciliation from hospital to home (Adapted from Holden et al. (2013)*

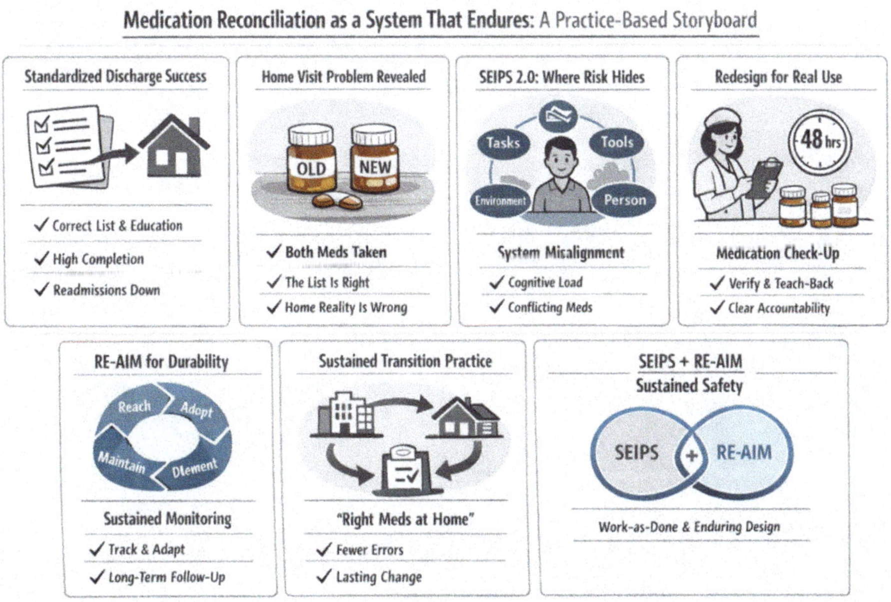

# Chapter 13
# When Policy Meets People:
## Translating Regulation Into Safer Care


## ABSTRACT

*Policies in healthcare are often treated as documents to update and store, yet their real value only becomes visible when care turns unpredictable. A policy is a promise an agreed upon path meant to guide decisions when clarity matters most. Its strength is not measured by formatting or regulatory alignment, but by whether people instinctively reach for it in moments of uncertainty. This chapter explores how policies move from written expectations to lived practice, drawing on situations where clear guidance prevented harm and others where aspirational wording quietly created risk. It argues that effective policy is written with intention that is clear enough to act on, honest enough to be followed, and grounded in how work actually unfolds.*


## INTRODUCTION

If you have spent time in quality and safety work, you have likely been asked to help with a policy. Sometimes it happens after an event, sometimes during a committee review, sometimes because someone realizes often urgently that "we don't have a policy for that yet." The request usually arrives with a familiar packet: a template outlining purpose, scope, definitions, procedures, responsibilities, and references. The mechanics are clear, and most of us know how to fill them in. And


DOI: 10.4018/979-8-3373-6496-4.ch013

yet, many people hesitate at the same point not at the template, but at the thinking. Where do you actually begin?

Policies are often treated as technical artifacts written, approved, filed. In practice, they are one of the most consequential tools in quality and safety work. A policy is where intent becomes expectation. It is where lessons from events, audits, and patient experiences are translated into guidance for everyday decisions. When a policy works, it quietly shapes behavior. When it doesn't, it exists on paper but not in practice. What is often missing from policy writing is time spent on the larger question: how will this guidance be experienced by the people expected to use it? Does it make sense in the flow of real work? Does it connect to existing systems, tools, and measures? Does it reflect the realities of patients, families, and frontline staff?

This chapter introduces the Four Lenses of Safety Translation: Language, Logic, Linkage, and Lived Experience as a way to approach policy writing differently. The framework is a conceptual model developed for this text, synthesizing principles from improvement science, human factors, safety communication, and experience based design. Rather than replacing existing templates, the lenses sit above them, shaping how each section is approached. They prompt policy writers to consider not only what must be included, but how policies are interpreted, applied, and sustained over time.

For those who have revised the same policy repeatedly without seeing change at the bedside or wondered why a well written policy failed to prevent recurrence, this framework offers a way to close that gap. Writing through these lenses helps policies do more than meet requirements; it helps them support safer care as it is actually delivered.

## Objectives of the Chapter

- Explain how policies move from written expectations to lived practice and influence real time safety decisions.
- Introduce the Four Lenses of Safety Translation: Language, Logic, Linkage, and Lived Experience as a framework for writing usable, reliable policies.
- Demonstrate how leadership presence, staff engagement, and continuous revision transform policies into tools that support readiness and trust.

## THE ANATOMY OF TRANSLATION: WRITING POLICY THROUGH THE LENS OF SAFETY

A well written policy does more than describe a process; it shapes how safety unfolds in real time. This becomes especially visible in the handling of critical laboratory results, where clarity can prevent harm and hesitation can cause it. Translating regulation into practice requires both structure and empathy. Policies must guide staff with precision while accounting for the unpredictability of clinical work rotating residents, after hours calls, and outside laboratories trying to reach the right provider when a potassium of 3.0 cannot wait until morning. Over time, I've relied on what I call the Four Lenses of Safety Translation, a framework that helps ensure a policy does more than meet a standard. It helps people act safely, confidently, and consistently.

The Four Lenses framework (Figure 13.1) synthesizes concepts from quality improvement, safety science, human factors, and narrative based approaches to explain how safety knowledge is translated into policy and sustained in practice. The Logic and Linkage lenses draw from systems thinking and improvement science, emphasizing cause and effect relationships, safeguard design, and alignment between measures and action (Berwick, 1989; Deming, 1986; Vincent et al., 2014). The Language lens reflects work in safety communication and organizational sensemaking, recognizing that technical requirements must be expressed in language that guides behavior under pressure (Reason, 2000; National Academies of Sciences, Engineering, and Medicine [NASEM], 2018).

The Lived Experience lens is informed by experience-based design and narrative medicine, which highlight the role of patient, family, and clinician perspectives in identifying risk and sustaining engagement (Bate & Robert, 2007; Charon, 2006). Applied to policy development, this integrated framework supports policies that are not only compliant, but understandable, actionable, and grounded in real-world conditions. By connecting formal requirements to system logic, operational workflows, and lived experience, the framework aligns safety policy with how care is actually delivered—improving consistency and long-term reliability.

*Figure 1. Four lenses of safety translation*

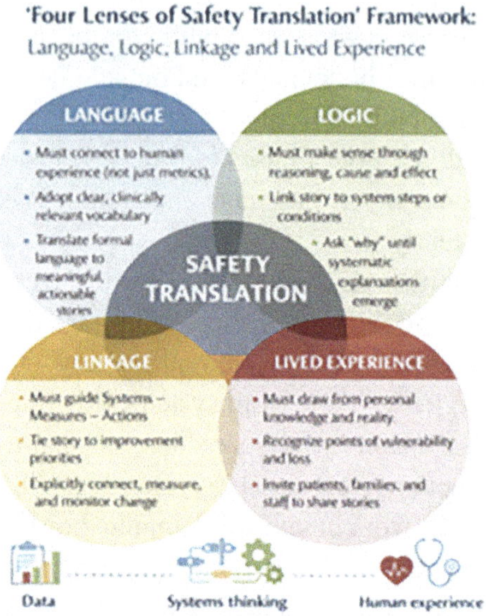

'Four Lenses of Safety Translation' Framework:
Language, Logic, Linkage and Lived Experience
LANGUAGE
• Must connect to human experience (not just metrics).
• Adopt clear, clinically relevant vocabulary
• Translate formal language to meaningful, actionable stories
LOGIC
• Must make sense through reasoning, cause and effect
• Link story to system steps or conditions
• Ask "why" until systematic explanations emerge
SAFETY TRANSLATION
LINKAGE
• Must guide Systems – Measures – Actions
• Tie story to improvement priorities
• Explicitly connect, measure, and monitor change
LIVED EXPERIENCE
• Must draw from personal knowledge and reality
• Recognize points of vulnerability and loss
• Invite patients, families, and staff to share stories
Data
Systems thinking
Human experience


To make the lenses concrete, the framework is applied to a familiar, high risk process: communicating critical laboratory results. Walking through this example shows how Language, Logic, Linkage, and Lived Experience reshape a policy from a compliance document into a practical safety tool.

1. Language: Write for Clarity, Not Assumption

Safety begins with words people can act on. Many critical labs result policies state: *"The licensed staff receiving a critical lab value will immediately notify the ordering provider."* It sounds clear until you are in a teaching hospital with rotating residents and unclear call schedules. In one tracer, we found laboratory staff unsure who the "ordering provider" actually was, leading to delays and misdirected calls.

We revised the policy to read: *"Laboratory staff must immediately contact the ordering provider listed on the lab requisition. If that provider cannot be reached, the responsible attending or covering on-call physician must be contacted without delay. The staff member who receives or communicates the result will document the time, name, and method of notification."* The change replaced assumption with precision. "Immediate" became actionable. Responsibility became explicit. Clear language turns policy from a statement into a safety tool.

2. Logic: Design Safety into the Communication Chain

A policy can be technically correct and still fail in practice. In ambulatory settings, critical results from outside laboratories often arrive after hours and are routed through answering services. During one review, we discovered results left overnight not because staff were inattentive, but because the system did not clearly direct who to call next. We redesigned the process to include redundancy. Answering service scripts now verify the ordering provider, confirm backup contacts, and require continued outreach until direct communication occurs. The logic became simple: a critical result is never left as a message; it must reach a licensed provider in real time. This design aligns with Joint Commission PC.02.01.03 which requires immediate reporting of critical test results to the responsible caregiver (Joint Commission. (2024).

3. Linkage: Connect Policy to Its Safety Purpose

Every line in a critical results policy should answer a single question: *How does this prevent harm?* When we revised our policy, we added a sentence to the purpose section: *"This policy ensures that all critical test results are communicated directly and immediately to a licensed provider who can act to prevent patient harm."*That one sentence changed how the policy was received. It reminded technicians, nurses, and physicians that the policy existed not for compliance, but for protection. A timely phone call can mean the difference between stabilization and decline.

4. Lived Experience: Let Practice Inform the Policy

Policies must reflect how care actually happens. In home infusion programs, outside laboratories sometimes list the referring physician rather than the managing provider on requisitions. Results go to the wrong office while patients wait. After several near misses, we added a simple line: *"The clinician obtaining the specimen must confirm that the lab requisition lists the correct treating provider and agency contact information. Incorrect or incomplete information must be corrected before submission."*

Those few words closed a long standing safety gap by placing accountability at the start of the process. This approach reflects the intent of Joint Commission LD.04.01.05, which calls for leadership to involve staff in designing processes that support safe, high quality care Joint Commission. (2024).

## Measuring What Matters

When policies are written through the lenses of Language, Logic, Linkage, and Lived Experience, effectiveness is measured not only by audit results, but by what does *not* happen: no missed calls, no unacknowledged results, no preventable harm. Most communication failures arise not from negligence, but from unclear direction. By applying human factors principles, writing for how people think and act under pressure, we build safety into every sentence. Metrics tell us whether policies work; stories reveal why they matter. A potassium of 3.0 cannot wait until morning.

### A Moment That Tested the Policy

I once stood beside a Joint Commission surveyor during a home care visit when fall prevention came up. A week earlier, an elderly patient had slipped while transferring from a recliner to her walker. It wasn't catastrophic, but it prompted close review. The surveyor asked, "Walk me through what happened and how your policy guided your response." I described how the clinician followed our Fall Prevention and Post Fall Assessment policy: reassessing the home, notifying the provider, and initiating a rapid debrief. What impressed the surveyor was not the paperwork, but the reflection. Within 24 hours, the case had been discussed in a safety huddle and a revised checklist; co-designed with frontline staff was already in use. "That's exactly what the standard is asking for," the surveyor said. The policy had not just protected the patient; it had protected the integrity of the care.

### When Policy Overpromised

Not every policy story resolves neatly. During a pressure injury tracer, our policy promised a 24-hour follow up after any noted skin change. The care had been delivered, but documentation occurred two days later. The surveyor observed, kindly, "This policy promises something you don't consistently do. You've written commitment, not capability." We rewrote the policy to reflect reality: *"For patients at high risk, a skin assessment will be completed and documented at least weekly, and sooner if clinical changes or new risks are observed."* The next audit commended its clarity. A perfect policy had once made us look uncertain. An honest one made us look ready.

## SHAPING SAFETY THROUGH POLICY

Policy is more than instruction; it is intention. The strongest policies do not just direct behavior, they shape belief. When staff see their experience reflected in words, policy stops feeling imposed and starts feeling owned. This participatory approach mirrors Joint Commission LD.04.01.05 (Joint Commission, 2024), and the principles of Gemba: safety is designed where work actually happens.

## Bridging Compliance and Compassion

Compliance and compassion are often framed as opposites, but in practice they depend on one another. The safest organizations are those where people feel safe enough to follow policy naturally. When language leaves room for judgment *"as soon as safely possible" accountability* is preserved without denying reality. As one nurse told me, "It gave me permission to act, and I knew leadership would understand. "That is where policy finds its purpose.

## From Readiness to Reliability

Regulatory readiness is not a checklist; it is the byproduct of alignment between safety and compliance in daily work. Policies written for auditors become rulebooks. Policies written for clinicians become guides. The difference shows up not in binders, but at the bedside. Reliability begins with words. Every sentence signals intent and accountability. Policy writing is not administrative work; it is one of the most powerful safety tools leaders have.

## FROM READINESS TO RELIABILITY: WRITING POLICY FOR SAFETY AND COMPLIANCE

Regulatory readiness is often described as being "survey ready every day." But readiness isn't a checklist. It's the visible sign that safety and compliance are already living in daily practice. When a policy is written clearly, used consistently, and reinforced through trust, readiness shows up naturally. Policies that focus only on compliance may pass a survey and still fail a patient. Policies that focus only on safety may inspire people and still fall apart under scrutiny. The goal is balance; language and structure that satisfy regulatory intent while keeping patient protection at the center.

Writing policy for both safety and compliance means designing systems that work when conditions aren't ideal. Every word should guide staff toward the safest next step while still meeting the intent of standards like Joint Commission LD.04.01.05, IC.02.02.01, and PC.02.01.03 (Joint Commission, 2024). Over time, writing policies across hospital, ambulatory, and home care settings taught me something that sounds obvious but is easy to forget: how we write determines how people act.

If a policy is written for auditors, it becomes a rulebook. If it's written for clinicians, it becomes a guide. The difference doesn't show up in the binder. It shows up at the bedside, in the hallway, in the patient's living room. Reliability begins with words. Every sentence signals accountability and intent, shaping what people do when it matters most. The next section looks at why policy writing isn't just administrative work; it is one of the most powerful safety tools leaders have.

## Lesson 1: Safety First, Compliance Always

When we write a policy, we may begin with regulations, but we should end with risk. During one internal review, our medication storage policy met every Joint Commission requirement, yet staff still reported temperature excursions that risked drug integrity. On paper, we were compliant. In practice, we were vulnerable. We rewrote the purpose to lead with safety: "This policy ensures safe storage of medications to prevent patient harm and maintain compliance with applicable standards." That shift from rule to reason changed how staff talked about the work. Safety became the story; compliance became the structure.

## Lesson 2: Write Policy for the People Who Live It

Policies have to sound like the people expected to use them. When the tone feels distant from practice, staff disengage. In rewriting the critical lab results policy, we replaced "notify the provider without delay" with "laboratory staff must immediately contact the ordering provider listed on the requisition." Simple. Direct. Human. People understood exactly what to do. During the next audit, team members could explain the process without flipping through the document. Readiness wasn't memorized; it was lived.

## Lesson 3: Integrate Reflection into the Policy Lifecycle

Readiness doesn't end at approval. Policies have to be observed, tested, and revised. During a documentation audit, a therapist pointed out that our home safety check required entry at every visit—even when a patient refused a walk-through. She wasn't being noncompliant; she was identifying a design flaw. We updated the policy to include: "If a home-safety check cannot be completed, staff will document the reason and patient refusal, and notify the supervisor if risk persists." One sentence turned a compliance problem into an accountability safeguard.

## Lesson 4: Make Readiness a Shared Habit, not a Leadership Event

When readiness becomes part of the daily rhythm, it starts to feel less like preparation and more like pride. We began each huddle with a question: "Which policy helped you keep someone safe this week?" At first, people hesitated. Then the stories came: infusion pump cleaning, oxygen tank transport, patient identification, secure order communication. Policy stopped being "inspection material" and started feeling like a shared safety net. That's when it clicked for me: readiness is sustained by ownership, not oversight. When people can see themselves in the policies guiding their work, compliance becomes culture, and safety becomes second nature.

## THE WRITING BEHIND READINESS

Policy writing can look administrative from the outside, but it's one of the most powerful safety tools we have. Each word signals accountability and intent. Over time, I've come to see policy as both a mirror and a map mirror of organizational values, and a map toward safer, more reliable care. The lesson is simple: write for safety, and compliance will follow. Write only for compliance, and both will fail. Readiness, in its truest form, is what you can see when policies are written with clarity, lived with compassion, and refined through learning. Even the best written policies can't remain static. Healthcare is dynamic, and the documents guiding it have to move with it. The next section explores how policies evolve through observation, feedback, and revision transforming from fixed rules into living systems that learn.

## WHEN POLICIES LEARN

A good policy teaches; a great policy learns. The most reliable organizations aren't the ones that write flawless policies, they're the ones that rewrite them when reality exposes a gap. Every audit, near miss, or staff concern is a chance for a policy to evolve. When leaders treat revision not as correction but as conversation, policy becomes something closer to a living system. We saw this with fall prevention. Despite full compliance with written steps, incidents persisted. Field clinicians surfaced what the document missed. "The checklist doesn't reflect how I actually teach patients about fall safety," one nurse said. "It feels like reading a script." Another added, "The home hazards section doesn't mention clutter or pets. "Together, we revised the policy to include flexible teaching prompts and documentation for environmental risks. Within three months, post-fall reviews showed fewer contributing hazards and more consistent notes. The policy didn't just survive revision. It evolved through it.

## LISTENING BEFORE REWRITING

During a Joint Commission mock tracer, a surveyor noted our medication reconciliation policy lacked clarity about follow-up when discrepancies were discovered after discharge. We didn't rush to edit. We gathered a cross disciplinary group and talked through what actually happened. Within minutes, the missing piece was obvious: sequence. Everyone assumed the steps; no one had written who initiated or confirmed communication. We added: "When a medication discrepancy is identified, the discovering clinician will document the variance, notify the prescribing provider, and confirm reconciliation before the next patient encounter." That single sentence unified practice and reduced confusion in later audits.

## REVISING WITH RESPECT

Each revision is an act of respect. It acknowledges imperfection and honors those who live the process daily. Inviting frontline staff into policy review strengthens psychological safety and signals that leadership listens. When home infusion nurses explained why documenting every port flush slowed emergency response, we redesigned the process. When delivery technicians suggested clearer oxygen-tank documentation, we listened. Each revision made the policy more credible and the system more reliable.

## WHEN POLICIES TEACH US BACK

Patterns of variance are messages from the system. Repeated deviations or workarounds are not just failures; they are data. The question isn't "Why didn't they follow it?" but "What did we miss in how we wrote it?" That mindset turns compliance into continuous improvement. When policies start to "teach us back," readiness becomes ongoing, and compliance shifts from a fixed expectation into a living behavior.

## THE COURAGE TO REVISE

The hardest part of policy leadership is accepting that every document we write will someday need to change. Courage isn't defending our words. It's refining them with humility. When we treat policy as a living teacher, we create an organization that is both compliant and compassionate where rules serve people, not the other way around. That's when regulation becomes reliability, and policy becomes one of the most practical learning tools in healthcare.

As policies adapt, they become more credible and more connected to practice. Yet words alone can't sustain trust. Leadership presence brings those words to life. The following section shows how showing up, listening, asking, and engaging turns policy from a document into a shared promise.

## WHERE POLICY MEETS PRESENCE

At its best, policy isn't bureaucracy; it's a promise. A quiet commitment to every patient, family, and employee: you are safer here because we've anticipated what could go wrong and agreed on how we will respond. That promise becomes real when leaders show up. Presence, being there, asking, listening, closes the gap between policy and practice. During one rounding visit, a nurse said, "It helps just seeing you out here. It reminds me these aren't just rules; they're about people." She wasn't thanking me for an audit. She was thanking me for presence. Presence doesn't change the words on the page, but it changes how those words feel. When leaders show up without judgment, accountability shifts from surveillance to shared responsibility. A policy that once felt like enforcement can become a symbol of trust.

The real test of policy isn't whether staff can quote it. It's whether they live it when no one is watching. When words reflect values and presence reinforces them, safety becomes more instinctive. Policy is presence in written form; presence is policy in human form. One gives structure. The other gives soul. Together, they create reliability where safety isn't performed for auditors but practiced for people. That is where policy truly meets presence: in ordinary, unannounced moments when someone makes the safe choice and not because it's written, but because it's right.

### Key Takeaways

- **Write for safety first.** Start with the harm you're trying to prevent, not the citation you're trying to satisfy.
- **Use the Four Lenses.** *Language, Logic, Linkage,* and *Lived Experience* keep policy clear, usable, and grounded in real conditions.
- **Make staff co-authors.** Involvement improves accuracy and builds ownership, the policy starts to sound like work, not paperwork.
- **Hold accountability with empathy.** The right wording supports judgment under pressure without lowering the bar.
- **Keep policies alive.** Review them, learn from drift and workarounds, revise them in the open.

- **Lead with presence.** Visibility and curiosity turn "the policy" into "how we do it here."
- **Let safety pull compliance along.** When people understand the "why," readiness becomes routine.

## PRACTICE IMPACT

Policies built through clarity and lived experience change what happens in the moment, especially when the situation is moving fast. Precise, actionable language reduces ambiguity and helps staff respond under pressure, shifting compliance away from box-checking and toward instinctive safe practice (Reason, 2016; Dekker, 2020). Leadership presence amplifies that effect. When leaders involve staff in policy development and show up without a punitive edge, accountability starts to feel shared rather than surveilled. That shift supports psychological safety and makes it easier for people to speak up about gaps, workarounds, and near misses before they harden into "the way we do things" (Carroll & Edmondson, 2021; Wears, Hollnagel, & Braithwaite, 2015). This participatory approach aligns with Joint Commission expectations for leadership engagement and supports sustainable readiness by embedding policy behaviors into daily routines rather than episodic audits (Joint Commission, 2024).

Over time, integrating human factors principles into policy writing and revision helps move readiness from a reactive sprint to a steady habit. Organizations that treat policies as living systems observed, tested, and refined tend to build reliability where compliance follows naturally because safety is already designed into the work (Vincent et al., 2023; Dekker, 2020). The practical payoff is fewer preventable harms, stronger staff confidence, and better alignment between regulatory expectations and compassionate, patient-centered care.

## CONCLUSION

Policies are more than compliance tools; they are instruments of safety, trust, and culture. This chapter shows how organizations can translate regulations into usable standards that protect patients and support staff especially in the moments when care gets messy and time is thin. Across the real-world examples, the same point keeps resurfacing: a policy's strength isn't just in how it reads, but in how instinctively people reach for it when something goes sideways.

The Four Lenses of Safety Translation: Language, Logic, Linkage, and Lived Experience offer a practical way to write policies that are clear, workable, and honest about the conditions of care. When policies reflect frontline reality, they stop feeling like rules imposed from above and start functioning as shared safety commitments. Leadership presence and participatory development are what keep those commitments from fading. Continuous measurement and iterative revision ensure policies remain living systems able to adapt as work changes and risks evolve. Ultimately, readiness is not an event but a habit. When policies are written for safety first, refined through collaboration, and reinforced through visible leadership engagement, compliance follows naturally. In that way, policy becomes more than a document; it becomes a promise lived every day.

## REFERENCES


Bate, P., & Robert, G. (2007). *Bringing user experience to healthcare improvement: The concepts, methods and practices of experience-based design*. Radcliffe Publishing.

Berwick, D. M. (1989). Continuous improvement as an ideal in health care. *The New England Journal of Medicine, 320*(1), 53–56. DOI: 10.1056/NEJM198901053200110 PMID: 2909878

Carroll, J. S., & Edmondson, A. C. (2021). *Learning from failure in healthcare: Systems that learn, people who care*. Harvard Business Review Press.

Charon, R. (2006). *Narrative medicine: Honoring the stories of illness*. Oxford University Press. DOI: 10.1093/oso/9780195166750.001.0001

Dekker, S. (2020). *Foundations of safety science: A century of understanding accidents and disasters*. CRC Press.

Deming, W. E. (1986). *Out of the crisis*. MIT Press.

Joint Commission. (2024). *Comprehensive Accreditation Manual for Hospitals (CAMH): The official handbook*. Joint Commission Resources.

Joint Commission. (2024). *Comprehensive Accreditation Manual for Home Care (CAMHC): The official handbook*. Joint Commission Resources.

National Academies of Sciences, Engineering, and Medicine. (2018). *Crossing the global quality chasm: Improving health care worldwide*. National Academies Press.

Reason, J. (2000). Human error: Models and management. *BMJ (Clinical Research Ed.), 320*(7237), 768–770. DOI: 10.1136/bmj.320.7237.768 PMID: 10720363

Reason, J. (2016). *Managing the risks of organizational accidents* (2nd ed.). Routledge. DOI: 10.4324/9781315543543

Vincent, C., Burnett, S., & Carthey, J. (2014). *The measurement and monitoring of safety*. Health Foundation.

Vincent, C., Burnett, S., & Carthey, J. (2023). *The measurement and monitoring of safety: A new framework for improvement*. Health Foundation.

Wears, R. L., Hollnagel, E., & Braithwaite, J. (2015). *Resilient healthcare (Vol. 2): The resilience of everyday clinical work*. CRC Press.

## KEY TERMS AND DEFINITIONS

**Four Lenses of Safety Translation:** Language, Logic, Linkage, and Lived Experience as criteria for writing effective policy.

**Gemba:** "The real place" where work happens; observing it helps connect policy to reality.

**Human Factors Engineering (HFE):** Designing systems that support real human performance under stress.

**Just Culture:** A framework balancing accountability with system learning.

**Leadership Presence:** The visible, empathetic engagement of leaders that connects written policy to lived behavior.

**Lived Experience:** Frontline input ensuring policies match real workflow and conditions.

**Policy Lifecycle:** The continuous development, implementation, and revision of policies.

**Policy Translation:** Turning regulations into practical, context-specific procedures staff can reliably follow.

**Regulatory Readiness:** Continuous preparedness where daily practice aligns naturally with standards.

**Safety-Centered Policy:** A policy written primarily to prevent harm, with compliance as an outcome.

# APPENDIX I

## Translating a Patient Identification Policy Through Four Safety Lenses

After a near-miss involving two patients with similar names scheduled for outpatient infusion, the organization initiated a review of its Patient Identification policy. While the existing policy met regulatory requirements, leaders recognized that compliance alone was not ensuring consistent practice across settings. Using the *Language* lens, the policy was rewritten in plain, clinically relevant terms. Instead of regulatory phrasing, the policy clearly stated the expectation: staff must verify two patient identifiers at specific points in care, using language patients could understand. Visual examples were added to illustrate correct and incorrect practices, and frontline staff were involved in refining terminology so it aligned with everyday workflow.

The *Logic* lens guided the rationale for the policy. Leaders mapped where identification failures were most likely to occur; handoffs, specimen collection, and medication administration and explicitly linked each policy requirement to the type of harm it was intended to prevent. This helped staff understand not just what to do, but why it mattered. Through the *Linkage* lens, the policy was connected to operational systems. Patient identification steps were embedded into the electronic health record, barcode scanning workflows, and audit tools. Ownership was assigned to specific roles, and performance metrics were tied to unit-level dashboards with clear escalation pathways for noncompliance. Finally, the *Lived Experience* lens ensured the policy reflected real-world conditions. Patient and family advisors reviewed the policy and training materials, highlighting situations where identifiers were confusing or difficult to confirm. Their feedback led to changes in wristband design and patient-facing education, reinforcing the patient's role in identification.

By applying all four lenses, the Patient Identification policy moved beyond a written requirement. It became a shared practice that staff understood, patients participated in, and leaders could monitor and sustain over time (Figure 2).

*Figure 2. Application of the four lenses of safety translation to a patient identification policy, illustrating how language, logic, linkage, and lived experience work together to translate policy requirements into clear, reliable, and patient-engaged practice that can be implemented and sustained across care settings*

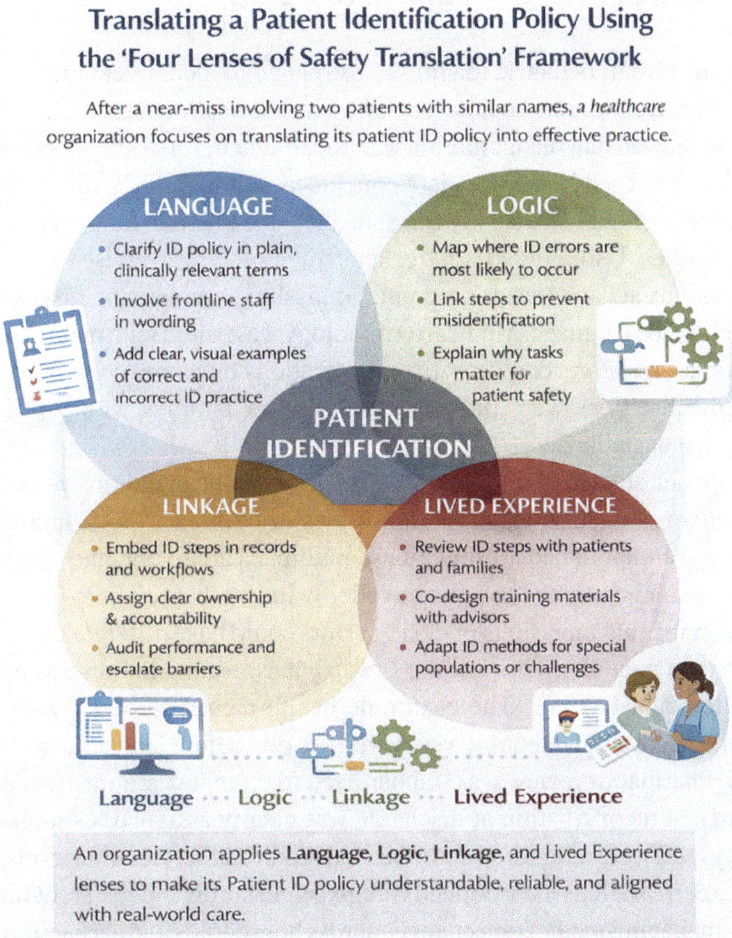

## APPENDIX II

### Translating a Pediatric Medication Reconciliation Policy Through the Four Lenses of Safety

Following several pediatric readmissions related to incomplete medication lists after discharge, a children's hospital reviewed its Medication Reconciliation policy. Chart audits showed that reconciliation was documented, yet discrepancies persisted once children returned home. Leaders concluded that the policy met technical requirements but did not consistently translate into safe practice for pediatric patients and their families. Using the *Language* lens, the policy was revised to clearly define expectations at each transition point: admission, transfer, and discharge using caregiver-centered language. Medical terminology was paired with plain descriptions so parents and caregivers could confirm medications by name, dose, and schedule. Visual medication lists were introduced to support families with limited health literacy or language barriers.

The *Logic* lens clarified why pediatric medication reconciliation required additional safeguards. Leaders mapped common pediatric risk factors, including weight-based dosing, compounded formulations, multiple caregivers, and school-based medication administration. The policy explicitly linked these risks to reconciliation steps, reinforcing that omissions or dosing errors could have different consequences in children than in adults. Through the *Linkage* lens, reconciliation was embedded into workflow and systems. The electronic health record was configured to flag high-risk medications and require weight verification before reconciliation could be completed. Pharmacist review was standardized for complex regimens, and responsibility for final reconciliation at discharge was clearly assigned. Compliance and discrepancy rates were monitored and reviewed at unit and service-line levels. Finally, the *Lived Experience* lens incorporated caregiver and family input. Parents described challenges managing medication changes across households and care settings. Their feedback led to improvements in discharge education, including teach-back and follow-up calls within 48 hours. Families were explicitly encouraged to speak up if something did not match what they gave at home. By applying the Four Lenses of Safety Translation, the pediatric Medication Reconciliation policy evolved from a documentation requirement into a practical, family-centered safety practice that supported accurate medication management beyond the hospital setting (Figure 3).

*Figure 3. Application of the four lenses of safety translation to a medication reconciliation policy, illustrating how language, logic, linkage, and lived experience work together to translate policy requirements into clear, reliable, and patient-engaged practice that can be implemented and sustained across care settings*

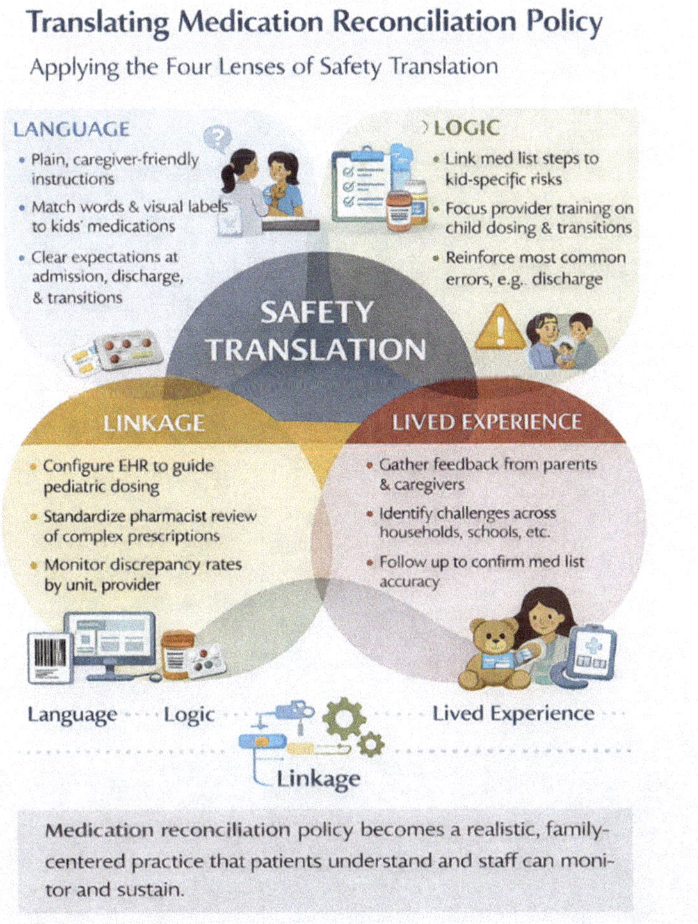

# Chapter 14
# Equity in Every Step: Building Safer Systems Through Inclusion


## ABSTRACT

*Equity is increasingly recognized as a core dimension of patient safety, yet many healthcare organizations struggle to move equity from policy statements into everyday quality and safety work. This chapter frames equity as a practical way of identifying risk through the lenses of quality, safety, and service rather than as a separate domain. It introduces the Equity Review Cycle—Observe, Listen, Act, Reflect—as an operational approach grounded in health equity scholarship, quality improvement, and safety science. The cycle supports the use of stratified data, patient and caregiver experience, system redesign, and leadership accountability within routine workflows. Through real-world examples, the chapter shows how equity concerns often emerge as early safety signals, particularly during transitions of care and in home based settings. By reframing disparities as indicators of preventable harm, equity is positioned as integral to reliable, patient centered care.*


## INTRODUCTION: SEEING WHAT WE MISS

In many safety conversations, there is a moment when the room goes quiet. It often happens after someone asks a simple question: "Safe for whom?" The question does not accuse, but it unsettles. It shifts attention away from performance metrics and toward presence. Over time, I have come to understand that equity is not something added to safety work. It is what determines whether safety is real or selective. When harm or improvement consistently bypasses certain groups, the system may


DOI: 10.4018/979-8-3373-6496-4.ch014

look reliable on paper, but it is not reliable in practice (Equity is essential to patient safety, 2023).

I do not come to this work as a health equity expert. My training and my day to day practice live in quality, safety, and service operations. Equity entered my work not through theory, but through patterns I could not ignore. Early in my leadership roles, equity often appeared at the margins. It showed up as a final slide, a required field in a report, or a checkbox in a compliance review. We tracked rates and outcomes carefully, yet something felt incomplete.

That discomfort grew as I listened more closely to staff and patients. Near misses, complaints, and readmissions carried stories that did not align neatly with our dashboards. The inequities were rarely dramatic. More often, they were embedded in routine assumptions. Discharge instructions written above a patient's reading level. Interpreter needs addressed inconsistently. Care plans that assumed someone would be home to help, or had transportation, or could navigate follow up on their own. These were not edge cases. They were everyday conditions that shaped whether care was safe once the visit ended.

I began to see that safety depends on visibility. Risks that remain unseen are not neutral. They accumulate. Invisibility is one of the most dangerous conditions a system can tolerate.

This shift in perspective is no longer optional. Equity is now embedded in national standards and accreditation frameworks. Organizations are expected to stratify outcomes, identify disparities, and demonstrate leadership accountability for addressing them (Centers for Medicare & Medicaid Services, 2023; The Joint Commission, 2023; National Committee for Quality Assurance, 2024). These expectations move equity from aspiration to operational requirement, influencing reimbursement, certification, and public trust.

Policies that incorporate equity checkpoints, such as language access, health literacy assessment, and social determinant screening, extend safety work beyond clinical protocols and into the realities of patients' lives (World Health Organization, 2023; Institute for Healthcare Improvement, 2022). When aligned thoughtfully, these frameworks offer more than compliance. They provide an opportunity to redesign systems that anticipate risk rather than react to harm, particularly for populations who have historically been least visible within safety metrics (Equity is essential to patient safety, 2023).

## Chapter Objectives

1. Describe how equity functions as a core component of patient safety by examining how disparities in language, access, and environment contribute to preventable harm across care settings.

2. Apply the Equity Review Cycle (Observe–Listen–Act–Reflect) to translate stratified data and lived experience into equity informed system redesign and sustained quality improvement.
3. Demonstrate practical strategies for embedding equity into routine quality and safety work through real world case examples in pediatric discharge and home based care.

## FROM EVIDENCE TO ACTION: SYNTHESIZING EQUITY CONCEPTS FOR REAL WORLD SAFETY PRACTICE

My work in quality and safety has placed me at the intersection of data, policy, frontline experience, and patient outcomes. That position carries both a vantage point and a responsibility. Concepts that live comfortably in separate bodies of literature rarely arrive in practice as tidy frameworks. Instead, equity, safety, and quality challenges surface through partial signals. A disparity becomes visible only after data are stratified. A patient story emerges during a committee discussion. A workflow works well for some populations and quietly fails others (Institute for Healthcare Improvement, 2017; National Academies of Sciences, Engineering, and Medicine, 2018).

The Equity Review Cycle did not emerge as a new theory or a claim of conceptual ownership. It took shape over time, informed by repeated engagement with established guidance and by the practical need to make that guidance usable in daily work. Many organizations know what the literature recommends. Measure inequities. Engage affected stakeholders. Redesign systems. Monitor outcomes. What is often missing is a coherent, repeatable way to hold these actions together without turning equity into a parallel project (Bate & Robert, 2007; Vincent et al., 2014).

The four steps, Observe, Listen, Act, and Reflect, draw directly from well established sources across disciplines. Observing inequities through stratified data aligns with national and regulatory expectations for transparency and equity focused measurement (Institute for Healthcare Improvement, 2017; National Academies of Sciences, Engineering, and Medicine, 2018; The Joint Commission, 2023). Listening to patients, caregivers, and frontline staff reflects experience based design and community engaged improvement approaches that center lived experience as a source of system insight rather than anecdote (Bate & Robert, 2007). Acting through system redesign mirrors foundational quality improvement methods, while making explicit the risk that well intentioned interventions can reinforce inequity if structural conditions are ignored (Berwick, 1989; Deming, 1986). Reflecting through governance review, leadership oversight, and feedback loops aligns with learning health system models that sustain change beyond initial implementation (Vincent et al., 2014).

Figure 1 illustrates how these elements are sequenced in practice through the Equity Review Cycle. The figure shows how organizations can move from identifying inequities through observation, to understanding lived barriers through listening, to implementing equity informed system changes, and finally to sustaining progress through structured review and accountability. Together, the narrative and the figure demonstrate how fragmented equity recommendations can be translated into a practical cycle that supports learning, harm prevention, and sustained improvement.

*Figure 1. The equity review cycle: Turning insight into action*

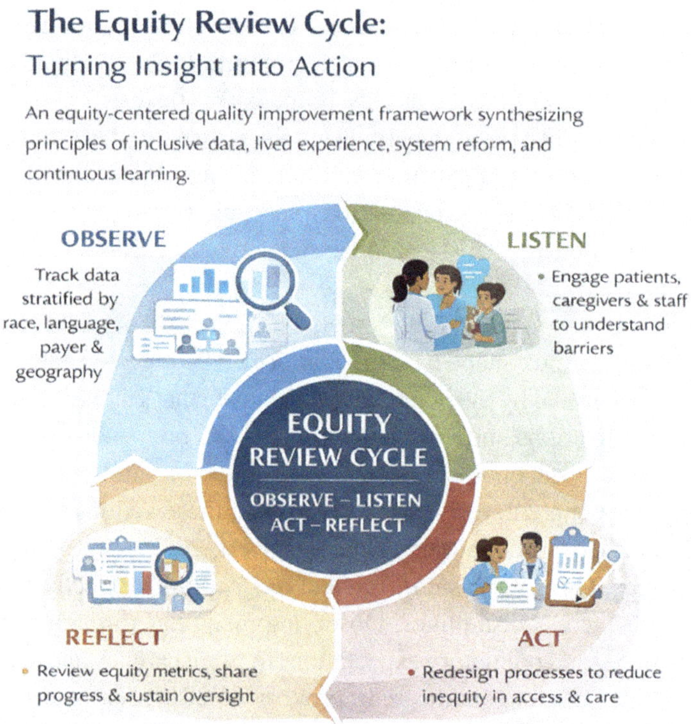


Because this book focuses on real world strategies for implementing quality and safety, the Equity Review Cycle is offered as a translation tool rather than a prescriptive model. It reflects how equity concepts have been applied in practice through quality, safety, and service work, not a claim of disciplinary expertise in health equity. The cycle intentionally synthesizes ideas that already exist across multiple bodies of literature and reframes them into a structure that teams can use to move from insight to action. Its purpose is practical. It helps organizations close equity gaps and prevent harm using approaches that are familiar, feasible, and grounded in the realities of care delivery rather than theoretical ideal states.

## How to Use the Equity Review Cycle in Practice

The Equity Review Cycle is designed as a guide for teams, not as a fixed sequence that must be followed exactly. It can be applied at multiple levels, including unit based improvement work, organizational quality initiatives, and policy review processes. Teams may enter the cycle at any point depending on what brings attention to a concern. Triggers often include a safety event, a disparity in outcomes, a regulatory finding, or a concern raised by patients or staff.

In practice, Observe begins with making inequities visible. This typically involves disaggregating data and presenting it transparently so patterns that are hidden in aggregate reporting can be seen. **Listen** follows by engaging those most affected, including patients, caregivers, interpreters, and frontline staff, to understand barriers that data alone cannot explain. Act focuses on redesigning systems, workflows, or communication practices in ways that reduce inequity rather than shifting responsibility to individuals. Reflect ensures that changes are reviewed over time, with leadership oversight, clear accountability, and ongoing monitoring of equity related outcomes.

When used consistently, the cycle supports learning rather than one time fixes. It helps teams avoid fragmented efforts by providing a shared structure for decision making, prioritization, and sustainment. Most importantly, it reinforces equity as a core component of patient safety, embedded in everyday improvement work rather than treated as a parallel initiative. Equity does not sit alongside safety. It shapes whether safety practices reach everyone. When inequities are made visible, prevention becomes possible. The Observe–Listen–Act–Reflect cycle offers a structured way to move from identifying disparities to embedding equity into routine quality and safety practice.

## OBSERVE: MAKING INEQUITY VISIBLE

Initial signals of inequity rarely appear as isolated events. More often, they emerge as patterns across dashboards, complaints, and follow up data. In one pediatric discharge review, overall compliance with discharge processes appeared strong. At first glance, the system looked reliable. Once the data were stratified, a different picture emerged. Thirty day readmission rates were higher among children from families with limited English proficiency. Further disaggregation showed that missed follow up appointments clustered among families who required interpreter services.

Similar patterns surfaced in other settings. Communication related complaints increased after evening hours. Missed appointments rose among patients receiving English only reminders. Home safety events were linked to factors not routinely addressed in clinical protocols, including electricity access and broadband reliability. Each data slice raised the same underlying question: safe for whom? Over time, invisibility itself became a measurable risk. Language, literacy, and environment were not peripheral variables. They were predictors of harm that remained hidden by aggregate reporting (Equity Is Essential to Patient Safety, 2023; Disparity Dashboards, 2023).

## LISTEN: UNDERSTANDING LIVED BARRIERS

Data clarified where inequities existed, but it did not explain why they persisted. That understanding emerged through structured listening with patients, caregivers, interpreters, and frontline staff. In the pediatric discharge example, families described confusion about follow up instructions and difficulty navigating scheduling systems after discharge. Interpreter access was inconsistent, and written materials were not always accessible.

In other settings, listening efforts surfaced assumptions embedded in routine care processes. Teams assumed instructions would be translated by family members. Printed materials were assumed to be readable. Technology based communication was assumed to work equally well for all patients.

When patients and staff were asked to demonstrate how care plans actually functioned at home rather than simply describing them, barriers became tangible. Interpretation was delayed. Print was unreadable. Technology was inaccessible. Workflows had been designed for efficiency rather than comprehension. Listening translated abstract disparities into specific design flaws that could be addressed through system change (Disparity Dashboards, 2023).

## ACT: REDESIGNING SYSTEMS, NOT REMINDING PEOPLE

Action focused on redesigning systems rather than reinforcing compliance expectations. In the pediatric discharge workflow, standardized teach back with interpreters was implemented. Written instructions were simplified. Proactive scheduling support was provided before discharge, and clear ownership was assigned for confirming follow up appointments.

Across care settings, language flags were embedded into electronic records so interpretation became part of routine workflows rather than an exception. Teach back evolved into show back, allowing teams to verify understanding through demonstration. Educational materials were redesigned using plain language, larger fonts, and visual cues. Interpreter access was extended into evening hours, reducing communication related complaints. Ambulatory clinics piloted multilingual reminders that were tested directly with patients, leading to improved appointment adherence.

For conditions such as heart failure, equity checkpoints were embedded across the care continuum. Language and literacy were flagged on admission. Comprehension was verified at discharge. Follow up reach was stratified by ZIP code and language. Home based risks were addressed through partnerships with community agencies. When patients with limited English proficiency were found to be significantly less likely to answer post discharge calls, scripts were rewritten, language routing was added, and new templates were tested with frontline staff. Within months, follow up completion improved across groups.

## REFLECT: SUSTAINING EQUITY AS A SAFETY PRACTICE

Sustained improvement depended on how results were reviewed and discussed. Disparities were treated as feedback rather than fault. Leadership reviews paired stratified metrics with patient stories. Equity focused huddles became routine. During rounds and handoffs, teams began asking two questions more consistently: Who might not understand this process? Whose voice has not been heard? Over time, interpreter utilization increased and language related readmissions declined. More importantly, the culture shifted. Safety moved away from a compliance exercise and toward a practice grounded in presence and protection. Reflection did not close the loop. It sharpened the next Observe step by improving how risks were identified, interpreted, and addressed (Equity Is Essential to Patient Safety, 2023).

## EQUITY IN MOTION ACROSS THE CARE CONTINUUM

Equity challenges often arise not from lack of effort, but from systems designed for uniformity rather than diversity. In ambulatory care, efficiency driven workflows amplified exclusion when communication tools assumed a single language or level of digital access. Introducing multilingual reminders and testing them with patients reduced missed appointments without adding complexity. In home based care, safety depends on conditions beyond clinical walls. Patients reliant on power dependent equipment faced increased risk during utility disruptions. Partnering with utility providers and social service agencies reframed safety as a shared ecosystem rather than a checklist, allowing environmental risks to be addressed alongside clinical ones.

## MAKING FAIRNESS MEASURABLE, THE EQUITY DASHBOARD

Sustaining equity work required moving it out of narrative alone and into something teams could see together. We developed a Heart Failure Equity Dashboard to make disparities visible in real time. The dashboard displayed a small set of signals that mattered operationally:

- Readmission rates by language, race, and payer type
- Telehealth visit completion by ZIP code
- Home visit timeliness by geography

Once these patterns were visible, conversations began to change. Fairness was no longer discussed as an abstract value. It became something measurable and actionable. Teams started using the dashboard to anticipate risk rather than respond after harm occurred. Some departments introduced brief "equity huddles," short check ins where staff discussed what the data revealed that week and what might need attention before the next patient encounter.

The dashboard did more than report metrics. It shaped how people thought. Visibility shifted equity from a special initiative to part of routine safety culture (Disparity dashboards, 2023). Over time, the data told a quieter story. Language related readmissions declined, and interpreter utilization increased. The more meaningful change, however, showed up in everyday dialogue. During safety rounds, questions like "Who might not understand this process?" or "Whose voice have we not heard yet?" became increasingly common. When those questions are normalized, safety begins to resemble justice.

## ALIGNING WITH THE NATIONAL MOVEMENT

Regulatory expectations around equity now extend beyond moral aspiration. They are embedded in accreditation and oversight. CMS requires inclusive quality review cycles. The Joint Commission integrates leadership accountability and community engagement into its equity certification. NCQA frames cultural responsiveness as a measurable dimension of quality (Centers for Medicare & Medicaid Services, 2023; The Joint Commission, 2023; National Committee for Quality Assurance, 2024).

Compliance alone, however, does not create meaningful change. Progress occurs when leaders begin to use equity as a method rather than a mandate. Stratification becomes a way to understand risk more precisely, not simply a reporting requirement. A physician leader once said to me, "When we stratify our data, we are not just finding disparities. We are finding opportunities to care better." That observation stayed with me. When practiced intentionally, equity restores a human dimension to improvement work. Safety without equity is incomplete. Equity without safety is unsustainable. Each depends on the other to endure.

Figure 14. 2 presents a practical, single page view of how the Equity Review Cycle can be used to translate equity standards into everyday quality and safety work. Rather than treating equity requirements as separate or additive, the figure aligns each step of the cycle, Observe, Listen, Act, and Reflect, with relevant standards and concrete actions that teams can apply in routine operations.

By moving horizontally across the figure, leaders and frontline teams can see how expectations related to data stratification, patient and staff engagement, system redesign, and leadership oversight connect directly to specific behaviors and workflows. The figure is intended to support shared understanding across disciplines and roles, offering a common reference point for policy development, improvement planning, and regulatory readiness. In doing so, it reinforces equity not as an adjunct to safety, but as an integral part of how safety is practiced.

*Figure 2. Equity review cycle mapped to standards and practical actions, illustrating how equity-focused expectations can be translated into routine quality and safety practice*

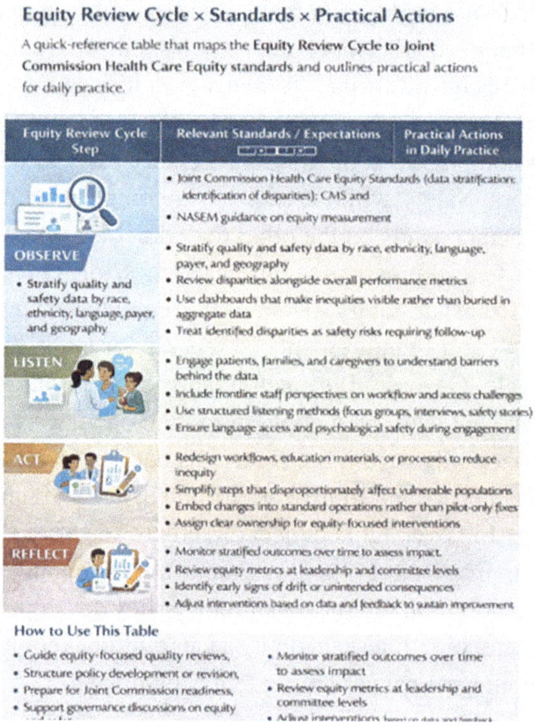
Equity Review Cycle × Standards × Practical Actions

A quick-reference table that maps the **Equity Review Cycle to Joint Commission Health Care Equity standards** and outlines practical actions for daily practice.

| Equity Review Cycle Step | Relevant Standards / Expectations | Practical Actions in Daily Practice |
|---|---|---|
| | • Joint Commission Health Care Equity Standards (data stratification; identification of disparities); CMS and<br>• NASEM guidance on equity measurement | |
| OBSERVE<br>• Stratify quality and safety data by race, ethnicity, language, payer, and geography | • Stratify quality and safety data by race, ethnicity, language, payer, and geography<br>• Review disparities alongside overall performance metrics<br>• Use dashboards that make inequities visible rather than buried in aggregate data<br>• Treat identified disparities as safety risks requiring follow-up | |
| LISTEN | • Engage patients, families, and caregivers to understand barriers behind the data<br>• Include frontline staff perspectives on workflow and access challenges<br>• Use structured listening methods (focus groups, interviews, safety stories)<br>• Ensure language access and psychological safety during engagement | |
| ACT | • Redesign workflows, education materials, or processes to reduce inequity<br>• Simplify steps that disproportionately affect vulnerable populations<br>• Embed changes into standard operations rather than pilot-only fixes<br>• Assign clear ownership for equity-focused interventions | |
| REFLECT | • Monitor stratified outcomes over time to assess impact.<br>• Review equity metrics at leadership and committee levels<br>• Identify early signs of drift or unintended consequences<br>• Adjust interventions based on data and feedback to sustain improvement | |

How to Use This Table

- Guide equity-focused quality reviews,
- Structure policy development or revision,
- Prepare for Joint Commission readiness,
- Support governance discussions on equity
- Monitor stratified outcomes over time to assess impact
- Review equity metrics at leadership and committee levels

## WHERE SAFETY MEETS THE SOCIAL DETERMINANTS OF HEALTH

Patient safety and the social determinants of health are inseparable in practice. Safety does not live only in protocols or checklists. It lives in housing stability, food access, reliable transportation, digital connectivity, and the predictability of daily life. A patient who loses power and cannot operate an oxygen concentrator faces a risk no less serious than a patient who receives the wrong medication. In both cases, the harm is preventable. What differs is not the severity of risk, but where the system failed. One failure occurs inside clinical care. The other occurs at the intersection of care and daily living.

Evidence from the World Health Organization and the Institute for Healthcare Improvement consistently shows that many preventable adverse outcomes are shaped more by social context than by medical error alone (World Health Organization, 2023; Institute for Healthcare Improvement, 2022). When social instability overlaps with clinical complexity, risk compounds. For this reason, contemporary safety programs cannot stop at the bedside. They must extend into neighborhoods, into discharge planning, and into the conditions patients return to once formal care ends.

Shifting the question from what went wrong to what made this possible requires safety leaders to treat social determinants as part of routine surveillance and system design. This means incorporating questions about housing, income, food access, transportation, and digital connectivity into incident reviews and improvement planning. When teams ask, "What in this person's life increased the likelihood of this event?" the focus moves away from individual fault and toward prevention. Equity, in this sense, becomes a safety strategy rather than a social abstraction. When organizations routinely ask, "For whom is this safe?" and respond to what they find, safety moves closer to its purpose. Fairness becomes observable. Improvement becomes personal. Safety becomes more widely shared.

## PRACTICE IMPACT

Embedding equity into patient safety work changes how care is designed, not just how it is delivered. Integrating tools such as equity dashboards, language flag alerts, and visibility mapping allows teams to detect risks that traditional metrics overlook. Stratifying readmission data by language and payer type, for example, often reveals patterns hidden by aggregate reporting. Once visible, those patterns can be addressed through targeted interventions that improve comprehension and reduce avoidable readmissions.

Inclusive education practices further strengthen safety. Techniques such as show back, translated materials, and simplified communication allow teams to confirm understanding rather than assume it. These approaches build trust while reducing error risk, particularly during transitions of care (Disparity dashboards, 2023). Over time, such practices move safety beyond compliance. Fairness becomes embedded in routine workflows, and improvement work begins to reflect compassion as well as accountability (Equity is essential to patient safety, 2023).

Leadership plays a critical role in sustaining this shift. When leaders integrate equity metrics into dashboards, conduct equity focused walk rounds, and normalize conversations about disparities, they communicate that fairness is foundational to safety, not optional. This posture moves organizations away from reactive compliance and toward proactive design. Inequities are treated as signals for improvement rather than as individual failures (Equity is essential to patient safety, 2023).

Leadership accountability also matters in how safe teams feel raising concerns. Visibility mapping, recognition programs, and inclusion of equity metrics in Quality and Safety Council reviews help create psychological safety. Teams are more willing to surface hidden risks when they trust that the response will be curiosity rather than blame (Disparity dashboards, 2023). Through modeling attentiveness and responsiveness, leaders transform equity from an external mandate into a shared organizational value, ensuring that improvement efforts reflect the lived realities of diverse patient populations.

## CONCLUSION

The work across this chapter returns to a simple but defining truth. Equity is not an addition to safety. It is the condition that allows safety to exist. The Equity Review Cycle offers a practical way to bring that understanding into everyday quality and safety work.

By observing stratified data, teams move beyond averages and make visible the disparities that standard reporting conceals. By listening to patients, families, and frontline staff, organizations uncover the lived experiences that give context to those disparities. Through action, systems redesign workflows, communication tools, and care processes so that responsibility shifts from individuals to structures. Through reflection, leaders create the governance and accountability needed to sustain progress.

What emerges is not another initiative layered onto existing work, but a shift in how safety is approached. Equity becomes part of the rhythm of improvement. The alignment between the Equity Review Cycle and The Joint Commission's Health Care Equity standards reinforces this point. Equity is not a separate compliance task. It is a lens through which core operations, decisions, and care processes are viewed.

When teams adopt this mindset, data becomes more than measurement. It becomes insight. Listening becomes more than courtesy. It becomes method. Action becomes more than correction. It becomes redesign. Reflection becomes more than reporting. It becomes culture.

## REFERENCES


Bate, P., & Robert, G. (2007). *Bringing user experience to healthcare improvement: The concepts, methods and practices of experience-based design*. Radcliffe Publishing.

Berwick, D. M. (1989). Continuous improvement as an ideal in health care. *The New England Journal of Medicine, 320*(1), 53–56. DOI: 10.1056/NEJM198901053200110 PMID: 2909878

Centers for Medicare & Medicaid Services. (2023). *Quality Assurance and Performance Improvement (QAPI) and Health Equity Framework: Guidance for Home Health and Post-Acute Settings*. U.S. Department of Health and Human Services.

Dashboards, D. (2023)... *Healthcare Executive, 38*(6), 24–27.

Deming, W. E. (1986). *Out of the crisis*. MIT Press.

Equity is essential to patient safety. (2023). *The Joint Commission Sentinel Event Alert,* (67), 1–6.

Institute for Healthcare Improvement. (2017). *Achieving health equity: A guide for health care organizations*. Institute for Healthcare Improvement.

Institute for Healthcare Improvement. (2022). *Improving health equity through patient safety: The intersection of social determinants and harm prevention*. Institute for Healthcare Improvement.

National Academies of Sciences, Engineering, and Medicine. (2018). *Crossing the global quality chasm: Improving health care worldwide*. National Academies Press.

National Committee for Quality Assurance. (2024). *Health Equity Accreditation 2024 Standards*. NCQA.

The Joint Commission. (2023). *Health care equity standards*. The Joint Commission.

Vincent, C., Burnett, S., & Carthey, J. (2014). *The measurement and monitoring of safety*. The Health Foundation.

World Health Organization. (2023). *Social determinants of health: Key concepts*. World Health Organization.

## KEY TERMS AND DEFINITIONS

**Disparity Dashboard:** A visualization tool that displays stratified metrics so teams can spot inequities in real time and guide improvement efforts.

**Environmental Safety Risks:** Non-clinical conditions—such as electricity, broadband, housing, or transportation—that shape health outcomes and require attention to ensure equitable safety.

**Equity Checkpoint:** A deliberate pause in a workflow to confirm that processes are meeting diverse patient needs and preventing inequitable outcomes.

**Equity Informed System Redesign:** Workflow and communication changes that remove structural barriers and embed equity into routine operations.

**Equity Review Cycle:** A four-step iterative model—Observe, Listen, Act, Reflect—that identifies inequities, uncovers root causes, redesigns systems, and strengthens equitable safety practices.

**Language Flag Alert:** An EHR prompt that captures a patient's preferred language to improve access to interpreters and translated materials.

**Leadership Accountability:** Oversight structures that ensure equity efforts are implemented, measured, and sustained rather than treated as one-time projects.

**Lived Experience:** The on-the-ground insights of patients, families, and frontline staff that clarify why inequities persist beyond what data alone reveals.

**Show Back Method:** A communication approach in which patients demonstrate their understanding of care instructions to confirm comprehension across literacy and language levels.

**Stratified Data:** Quality and safety measures broken down by factors like language, race, payer, or geography to surface disparities hidden in aggregate results.

## APPENDIX I

### Case Example: Reducing Missed Follow Up After Pediatric Discharge

An organization identified higher 30-day readmission rates among pediatric patients from families with limited English proficiency. Aggregate discharge compliance appeared strong; however, stratified data revealed lower follow-up appointment completion in this population. Using the Equity Review Cycle, the team began with Observe, disaggregating readmission and follow-up data by language, race, and payer. This analysis showed that missed follow-up appointments clustered among families requiring interpreter services. During Listen, caregivers, interpreters, and frontline staff described barriers that were not visible in the data alone, including unclear discharge instructions, difficulty navigating scheduling systems, and inconsistent access to translated materials. In the Act phase, discharge workflows were redesigned to include standardized teach-back with interpreters, simplified written instructions, and proactive scheduling support before discharge. Clear responsibility for confirming follow-up appointments was assigned.

Through Reflect, leadership reviewed stratified outcomes and patient feedback monthly. Adjustments were made as new barriers emerged. Over time, disparities narrowed, and the redesigned process became part of routine discharge planning rather than a targeted intervention. *This case illustrates how applying Observe–Listen–Act–Reflect translates equity insights into sustained safety improvement.*

# APPENDIX B. CASE EXAMPLE: IMPROVING SAFETY IN HOME-BASED CARE THROUGH EQUITY-INFORMED REDESIGN

A home-based care program identified recurring safety concerns among patients using power-dependent medical equipment, including oxygen concentrators and infusion pumps. While equipment checks and maintenance met established standards, incident reviews revealed higher rates of service disruption and emergency visits among patients living in areas with unreliable power and limited broadband access.

Using the Equity Review Cycle, the team began with Observe, stratifying safety events and emergency visits by ZIP code and housing status. This analysis showed clustering of events in communities with higher rates of utility instability. During Listen, patients, caregivers, and home care staff described challenges not captured in standard assessments, including delayed notifications of power outages, difficulty accessing support services, and uncertainty about whom to contact when equipment failed.

In the Act phase, the organization redesigned intake and monitoring workflows to identify patients reliant on power-dependent equipment and proactively coordinate with utility providers and community agencies. Staff were trained to assess infrastructure risks alongside clinical needs, and escalation pathways were clarified. Through Reflect, leadership reviewed stratified safety events and follow-up outcomes at regular intervals. The process was refined based on patient feedback and operational experience. Over time, emergency visits related to equipment failure declined, and infrastructure risk screening became a routine component of home-based care planning.

This case demonstrates how equity informed system redesign can extend patient safety beyond clinical settings and into the environments where care is delivered. Figure 3 illustrates the application of the Equity Review Cycle (Observe–Listen–Act–Reflect) across care settings. The pediatric discharge and home-based care vignettes demonstrate how stratified data, lived experience, system redesign, and leadership review work together to translate equity insights into sustained safety improvements.

*Figure 3. Application of the equity review cycle (observe–listen–act–reflect) across care settings*

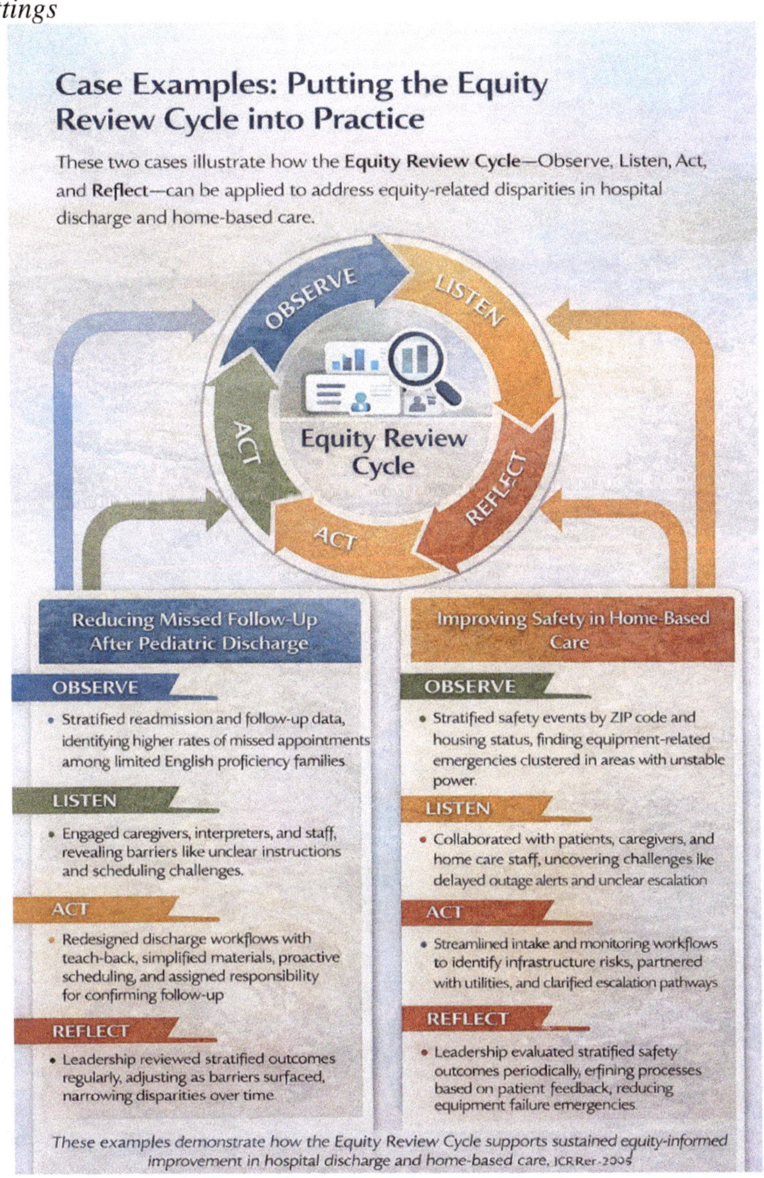

# Chapter 15
# The Likelihood to Recommend as a Signal of Safety


## ABSTRACT

*Safety and patient experience are often discussed as separate concerns, one focused on systems and safeguards, the other on how care is perceived. In practice, they are closely intertwined, meeting at the bedside, during discharge teaching, in follow-up calls, and in moments of care delivered at home. This chapter reframes patient experience not as satisfaction, but as an early signal of safety. Drawing on evidence and real-world examples, it examines how listening to patients sharpens organizational awareness, exposes communication gaps, and reveals risk before harm occurs. National surveys such as HCAHPS, HHCAHPS, and CG-CAHPS are explored not as service metrics, but as lenses for understanding safety and guiding action. When patient voices inform improvement cycles, organizations move from reacting to events toward recognizing early signals and protecting both safety and dignity.*


## INTRODUCTION

Safety and patient experience are often treated as parallel domains. One is grounded in systems, protocols, and outcomes, the other in perception and sentiment. In practice, however, they are tightly intertwined. Patients do not experience safety through dashboards, policies, or committee reports. They experience it through explanations


DOI: 10.4018/979-8-3373-6496-4.ch015

that make sense, follow up that happens when promised, and the confidence they carry after clinicians leave the room or the home.

Likelihood to Recommend (LTR) sits squarely at this intersection. When patients are asked whether they would recommend a service to someone they care about, they are not rating hospitality. They are making a judgment about trust. Would I send my spouse here? My parent? My child? In that sense, LTR functions less as a satisfaction score and more as a reflection of perceived reliability and safety.

Likelihood to Recommend is a patient reported measure that captures whether an individual would recommend a healthcare organization or service to family or friends (Centers for Medicare & Medicaid Services, 2023). While often categorized as a patient experience metric, LTR reflects a broader assessment of trust, consistency, and perceived safety rather than satisfaction alone (Doyle et al., 2013). It compresses multiple aspects of care; communication, confidence in clinicians, preparedness to manage care, and follow-through into a single global judgment about whether the system feels dependable (Anhang Price et al., 2014).

For decades, Press Ganey has shaped how patient experience data are collected and interpreted, emphasizing LTR as a meaningful indicator of the human experience of care and its relationship to quality and safety (Press Ganey, 2023). In quality and safety work, LTR is increasingly understood as a leading indicator and not of comfort, but of vulnerability. Declines often precede documented safety events, surfacing communication gaps, coordination failures, and unmet expectations before harm is formally recognized (Reader et al., 2014).

What gives LTR its power is not the score itself, but the conditions beneath it. Patients judge safety through clarity of instructions, consistency of information, and predictability of follow up features clinicians may label as "experience," but patients interpret as markers of risk. When communication falters or expectations are unclear, unease appears early. Long before an incident report is filed, patients feel something isn't steady. In this way, LTR operates as an early signal of system strain, reflecting whether care feels coordinated and reliable enough to recommend to someone they love.

Listening at this level is not optional or abstract; it is embedded in the national frameworks that shape how patients experience care. Among these, the Hospital Consumer Assessment of Healthcare Providers and Systems (HCAHPS), the Home Health Care Consumer Assessment of Healthcare Providers and Systems (HHCAHPS), and the Clinician and Group Consumer Assessment of Healthcare Providers and Systems (CG-CAHPS) provide some of the most consistent and structured views. When examined closely, these surveys translate lived experience into early indicators of safety risk.

## Hospital Consumer Assessment of Healthcare Providers and Systems (HCAHPS)

HCAHPS captures how patients experience hospitalization whether communication was clear, whether staff were responsive, and whether patients felt prepared to leave. Viewed through a safety lens, each question points toward a potential failure mode.

- *Did nurses and doctors explain things in a way you could understand?* → health literacy and medication safety.
- *Did you get help when you needed it?* → response time and fall prevention.
- *Was the hospital room quiet at night?* → rest, fatigue, and recovery.

One HCAHPS comment came from a patient recovering after heart surgery: "They explained everything when I was awake, but after anesthesia I didn't remember a thing. I wish someone had written it down." That single sentence led the unit to introduce a standardized teach-back sheet; brief, written, and aligned with verbal instruction. Within three months, readmissions related to medication confusion declined.

Another patient, an older woman admitted for pneumonia, circled "no" next to *Did you get help when you needed it?* and added, "I was afraid to get up by myself, but I didn't want to bother anyone." That response prompted a review of overnight call light response times. The delays were longer than leadership realized. Adjusting rounding patterns reduced falls and improved HCAHPS responsiveness scores at the same time.

High performing hospitals treat these responses as signals of reliability, not courtesy. When patients understand instructions and trust that help will come, they ask questions sooner, follow plans more accurately, and make fewer errors after discharge (Agency for Healthcare Research and Quality, 2023).

## Home Health Care Consumer Assessment of Healthcare Providers and Systems (HHCAHPS)

In home based care, the survey often becomes more revealing because the home is both the care environment and the patient's life. HHCAHPS asks whether clinicians listened carefully, explained medications clearly, and communicated with physicians about care. These questions map directly onto the conditions that prevent home-based harm.

One HHCAHPS comment read, "The nurse seemed rushed and left before my husband finished his questions." When reviewed alongside scheduling data, the pattern became clear: evening visits were routinely compressed, leaving little time for teaching. After redistributing visits and reinforcing teach-back at the close of each encounter, medication adherence improved alongside HHCAHPS scores. Another patient wrote, "My nurse always listens, but she calls my doctor before I even have to ask." That small observation revealed the value of proactive communication. Patients who answered "always" to *nurses communicated with my doctor about my care* had lower rates of unplanned emergency visits.

Each home visit carries quiet hazards; oxygen near heat sources, medications stored improperly, fall risks from clutter, or isolation that masks depression. HHCAHPS brings these realities forward. A note about "dim lighting in the hallway" may seem minor until it aligns with a pattern of falls. In home care, experience and safety are rarely separate; they reflect the same priorities through different lenses.

## Clinician and Group Consumer Assessment of Healthcare Providers and Systems (CG-CAHPS)

In ambulatory care, experience often shapes the earliest and most durable impression of the system. CG-CAHPS asks whether patients felt heard, whether time was sufficient, and whether they understood what to do next.

One parent wrote after an asthma visit, "The doctor explained the inhaler but didn't show me how to use it." Reviewing similar comments revealed a gap between documentation and demonstration. A visual education protocol was introduced, and staff now show and verify technique at every visit.

Another patient managing hypertension wrote, "I felt rushed. I didn't want to bring up my dizziness because the nurse had already opened the door for the next person." That hesitation pointed to a diagnostic near miss. A simple pause "Is there anything else you're worried about before we finish?" was added to the close of visits. Within months, clinicians identified multiple early cardiac symptoms that might otherwise have gone unnoticed.

## Listening as a Safety System

Together, HCAHPS, HHCAHPS, and CG-CAHPS form a national listening post for safety. They translate patient emotion into operational insight, revealing where reliability frays and where empathy repairs it. When reviewed with humility rather than defensiveness, CAHPS data become less about comparison and more about care.

Patients do not separate safety from experience. They understand safety through the steadiness of interactions surrounding their care. When asked whether they would recommend an organization, they are answering whether those interactions felt coherent, predictable, and safe. In this way, Likelihood to Recommend functions as a meaningful proxy for safety itself; capturing trust long before traditional safety indicators begin to move. Figure 1 depicts Likelihood to Recommend (LTR) as a patient reported indicator shaped by trust, consistency, and perceived safety. Rather than reflecting satisfaction alone, LTR captures whether care feels dependable, clearly communicated, and emotionally secure. When viewed through this lens, willingness to recommend becomes an early signal of system reliability and patient confidence, offering insight into conditions that support safe, coordinated care.

*Figure 1. Likelihood to recommend as a signal of safety and reliability*

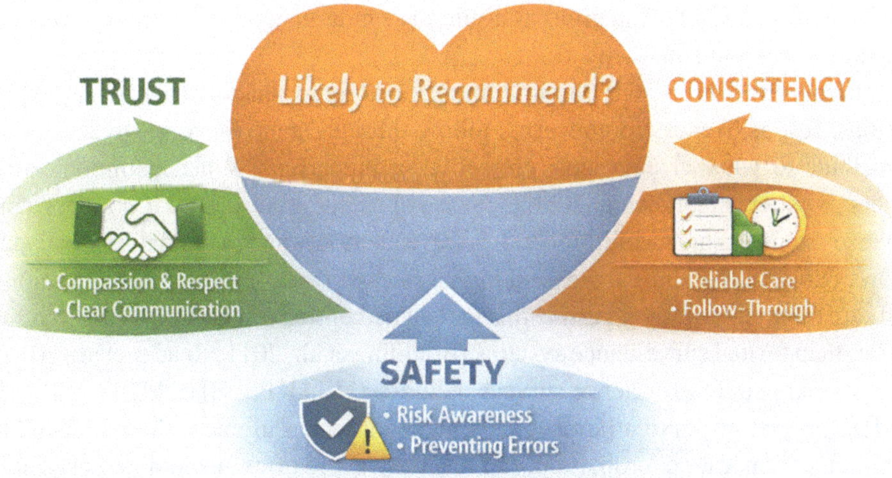


## Objectives

This chapter advances three related aims:

- Show how patient experience, particularly Likelihood to Recommend (LTR) can function as an early signal of safety risk rather than a retrospective satisfaction score.
- Explore how trust and emotional safety shape whether harm is prevented, surfaced, or silently carried forward.
- Offer practical strategies for integrating experience, safety, and quality into a single learning system rather than treating them as parallel domains.

## HOW LIKELIHOOD TO RECOMMEND REVEALS SAFETY

Likelihood to Recommend (LTR) is often categorized as a patient experience or satisfaction measure, yet in practice it reflects something more fundamental: a patient's perception of safety and trust. When patients are asked whether they would recommend a healthcare organization to a family member or friend, they are implicitly weighing whether the care feels reliable enough to place someone they love in its hands. Research consistently shows that trust, communication, and perceived reliability shape willingness to recommend care more strongly than technical measures patients cannot directly observe (Anhang Price et al., 2014; Doyle et al., 2013). In this way, LTR functions as a summary judgment of safety as experienced; not safety as documented.

Patients encounter safety through interactions rather than metrics. Clear explanations, responsiveness to concerns, follow through, and respectful treatment all contribute to whether care feels protective or precarious. When communication falters or patients feel dismissed, their sense of safety erodes, even if no reportable adverse event occurs. Multiple studies have demonstrated associations between poorer patient experience scores and higher rates of safety incidents, readmissions, and care fragmentation, suggesting that patient perception often detects vulnerability earlier than formal surveillance systems (Boulding et al., 2011; Reader et al., 2014).

National patient experience surveys including HCAHPS, HHCAHPS, and CG-CAHPS, therefore serve a purpose beyond service measurement. Items related to communication, care coordination, and responsiveness offer insight into how safely care is perceived across settings. Both the Centers for Medicare & Medicaid Services and the Agency for Healthcare Research and Quality have increasingly emphasized patient experience data as a source of risk identification and improvement guidance, recognizing that patients are uniquely positioned to observe gaps in continuity and reliability (Centers for Medicare & Medicaid Services, 2023).

When organizations treat Likelihood to Recommend as a safety signal rather than a branding metric, patient feedback becomes a proactive source of learning. Listening closely to why patients would or would not recommend care surfaces risks that may not yet appear in incident reports or outcome dashboards. In this way, patient experience data supports a shift from reactive safety management toward anticipatory learning systems. Safety is no longer defined solely by the absence of harm, but by the presence of trust, dignity, and confidence; conditions patients must feel in order to recommend care to those they love.

## LTR: The Hidden Compass of Safety and Quality

At first glance, Likelihood to Recommend appears to be a marketing question. In practice, it functions as a proxy for safety and trust, a brief prompt that captures complex judgments about quality, reliability, and psychological safety (Figure 2).

Patients do not recommend care that feels uncertain. They recommend care that feels safe. Behind every affirmative response is usually a story of reassurance; someone who felt listened to, respected, and protected. Behind every negative response is often a moment where trust frayed: communication broke down, expectations were unclear, or empathy was missing. LTR does not simply measure loyalty; it reflects whether patients believe the system will keep them, or those they care about most, safe.

*Figure 2. Likelihood to recommend sits at the intersection of safety and quality*

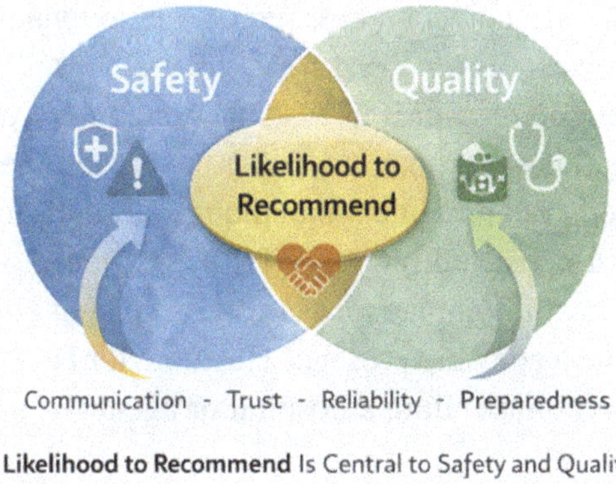


1. WHY "LIKELIHOOD TO RECOMMEND" REFLECTS SAFETY

Research consistently shows that patients who report higher likelihood to recommend also describe fewer adverse events and medication errors, stronger teamwork and communication, and greater adherence to care plans and follow-up recommendations (AHRQ, 2023). These associations exist because patients tend to equate safety with predictability and coordination. When communication feels steady and staff appear aligned, care is interpreted as safe. When it feels fragmented, rushed, or disjointed, patients sense risk; even when no harm has occurred.

2. LINKING LTR TO QUALITY AND RELIABILITY

Quality improvement efforts traditionally focus on indicators such as infection rates, readmissions, or medication reconciliation compliance. Likelihood to Recommend offers something different: a real time reliability signal that often precedes those outcomes. Sudden declines in LTR frequently coincide with operational strain, staffing instability, documentation inconsistency, or emerging communication gaps. When LTR trends are examined alongside safety data, organizations often find that experience scores begin to drop one to two months before adverse event rates rise.

In one hospital, for example, a downward trend in LTR comments referencing "delays" and "waiting for results" prompted further review. Leadership soon identified an unreported diagnostic turnaround delay linked to staffing gaps. Addressing workflow and communication early helped avert potential downstream harm.

3. Emotional Safety and the Trust Equation

Recommending care to someone else requires emotional confidence. Patients implicitly ask themselves: *Would I trust this team with the person I love most?* That moment of reflection measures not satisfaction, but psychological assurance. It captures whether patients felt heard, whether the environment felt orderly rather than chaotic, and whether communication among staff appeared cohesive.

Organizations with consistently high LTR scores tend to demonstrate strong safety culture and teamwork climate measures, transparent communication during uncertainty, and visible leadership presence (Institute for Healthcare Improvement, 2022). In this sense, recommending a hospital or agency is not a transaction; it is a testimonial of trust.

4. Using Likelihood to Recommend as a Learning Metric

Treating LTR as a learning indicator rather than a public score creates space for deeper inquiry. Practical strategies include linking LTR themes to root cause analyses when patients reference communication or confidence, integrating LTR trends into QAPI dashboards alongside safety indicators, discussing LTR patterns during leadership rounding debriefs, and recognizing staff when patients explicitly describe safety related behaviors such as careful medication checks or calming explanations.

Viewed this way, Likelihood to Recommend becomes a safety temperature check; a measure of how coordinated, trustworthy, and protective care feels to those living within it. Recognizing LTR as a learning metric is only part of the work; understanding whose voices are captured and whose are missing is equally critical.

## WHO SPEAKS, AND WHO DOESN'T

Every survey tells at least two stories. One appears neatly in numbers and trend lines. The other lives between the lines in fragments of language, pauses, and sometimes in silence. Behind every score is a human voice, sometimes confident, sometimes hesitant, trying to describe what safety feels like from the other side of care.

In one round of HHCAHPS feedback, a patient wrote, *"Everyone was kind, but I never knew who to call when I had questions."* Another noted, *"The nurse was wonderful, but the medicine instructions looked different every time."* Neither comment used the word *safety*. Yet both described the conditions that quietly increase the likelihood of harm: unclear handoffs, inconsistent information, and uncertainty about what to do next. This is the understated power of patient experience surveys. They do more than measure satisfaction. They reveal where communication and safety intersect. The Agency for Healthcare Research and Quality (2023) has shown that when patient experience data are examined alongside safety outcomes, they consistently surface issues of system reliability; particularly around communication, coordination, and readiness for transitions. Patients may not label these as safety failures, but they feel them.

Surveys such as HCAHPS, HHCAHPS, and CG-CAHPS rely on people being both willing and able to share their experiences. Not everyone is. Those who feel heard are more likely to respond. Those who felt invisible often remain silent. When participation drops, it is rarely about indifference. More often, it signals barriers, access, comfort, trust. Sometimes the quietest patients are the ones carrying the greatest risk.

Low response rates, then, are not merely a data quality problem. They are a safety signal. They prompt uncomfortable but necessary questions: Who did not respond, and why? Was the survey too long, the language too formal, the timing too distant from the care experience? Did patients believe their feedback would matter, or did they assume nothing would change?

The Institute for Healthcare Improvement (2022) describes this practice as *listening for risk*. Silence, they argue, often conceals system level vulnerabilities where patients felt uncertain, dismissed, or excluded. Every unanswered survey represents a missed safety report waiting to be interpreted.

One organization began pairing patient experience feedback with safety data to see what the numbers alone could not explain. Words like *confusing*, *waited*, and *rushed* appeared repeatedly in patient comments, echoing patterns already present in incident reports and near misses. Units struggling with communication also showed higher rates of medication clarification calls and follow up requests for instruction errors. Once these connections became visible, leaders redesigned patient education materials for clarity, strengthened teach-back practices, and added 24-hour follow-up calls. Within months, medication safety improved, and the tone of patient comments shifted from uncertainty toward reassurance.

A truly safe organization does not stop at celebrating favorable scores. It looks harder, asking who has not spoken and what their silence might be telling us. In patient experience data, silence rarely signals satisfaction. More often, it marks unseen risk.

## Changing Habits, Shifting Voices

The way people share feedback is changing as rapidly as healthcare itself. A generation ago, surveys arrived by mail, long, formal, and easy to set aside. Today, most people live in a world of brief messages and immediate responses. They text family members, confirm appointments online, and expect to offer feedback in the same way: quickly, while the experience is still fresh. In many organizations, participation in paper based surveys has declined sharply. Not because patients no longer care, but because the process feels outdated and inconvenient. Paper surveys often arrive weeks after care has ended. By then, details blur and emotional urgency fades.

When we piloted a short digital survey in Pediatrics, response rates nearly tripled. One parent wrote, *"I like this because I can answer while it's fresh in my mind."* That immediacy mattered. It captured emotion and specificity that a month old paper form never could. According to AHRQ (2023), timeliness of feedback is one of the strongest predictors of actionable improvement because it allows organizations to connect perception with process in near real time. Yet digitization introduces new equity challenges. Older adults, rural patients, and those with limited data access may struggle with online formats. Translation software can flatten tone or misinterpret meaning, stripping emotion from a patient's words.

A hybrid approach, combining text, email, phone, and when necessary, paper offers broader access. The format matters less than the message it sends; that feedback is welcomed and will be used. Each organization will find its own balance, but the aim remains the same; to listen early, listen inclusively, and act quickly. Every additional voice strengthens the safety net. Every unheard story leaves risk unseen. In the end, the completeness of our listening shapes the completeness of our care (Institute for Healthcare Improvement, 2022).

## From Recommendation to Relationship

"Likelihood to Recommend" is often treated as a marketing metric. In practice, it reveals the emotional architecture of safety. It captures what dashboards struggle to show: the interplay of trust, empathy, and reliability. Every affirmative response reflects a moment when care felt coordinated, transparent, and humane. Every negative response points to a fracture; an instant where confidence wavered, even if no technical error occurred. When this question is approached as a story rather than a score, it becomes a compass, pointing toward the deeper forces that shape safety: human factors, emotional security, and presence.

Patients rarely separate emotional experience from physical outcome. They may not speak in the language of reliability engineering or process improvement, but they sense alignment when it exists and fragmentation when it does not. Willingness to recommend care is not a brand endorsement. It is a verdict on consistency and compassion. It is also predictive. Units with higher LTR scores often report fewer near misses, stronger teamwork climate scores, and more timely error disclosure. The pattern is straightforward: where trust is present, silence recedes. When patients believe their voice matters, they speak up about missed doses, side effects, or new symptoms before those concerns evolve into harm. In this way, Likelihood to Recommend becomes the first ripple in a larger story about emotional safety and human factors. It marks the beginning of partnership.

## From Experience to Partnership

If Likelihood to Recommend signals trust, partnership is how trust is sustained. Partnership emerges when patients and families are not merely recipients of care, but contributors to safety design. I recall inviting a patient to join an infusion safety workgroup. As we reviewed medication labeling, she paused and said quietly, *"I can't tell which one is my antibiotic and which one is the flush."* That single observation led to a redesign of labeling across the program; something no policy review had surfaced.

Partnership shifts power into presence. When patients are included as collaborators, safety becomes something created *with* them rather than *for* them. Organizations that integrate Patient and Family Advisory Councils into safety work report higher engagement and fewer preventable events. Partnership also redistributes accountability. It requires asking, *"How do you define safety?"* and remaining open to answers that challenge professional assumptions. Listening without interruption is among the most advanced safety practices available.

## Seeing the Whole Picture

In my current role, I oversee quality, safety, regulatory readiness, and patient experience. These domains are often managed separately, each with its own dashboards and meetings. Holding them together has altered how I understand the work. It no longer feels like parallel efforts; it feels like a single ecosystem.

I have sat in meetings where patient experience leaders present Likelihood to Recommend scores, some rising, some dipping below target. In other rooms, safety teams report declining event rates. Elsewhere, quality leaders review incentive performance. Each group speaks its own language, confident in its slice of the truth. Rarely do those stories converge. Yet they describe the same lived experience. A low LTR score often mirrors what safety data already knows that something felt uncertain, communication faltered, or trust weakened. A regulatory citation may reflect not a compliance failure, but the same communication gaps that confuse staff and frustrate patients. The dashboards may live in different folders, but the experience belongs to the same people.

Integration, then, is not simply structural. When safety, quality, and experience are viewed as one conversation, patterns emerge. A dip in "staff listened carefully" may precede a rise in medication clarification calls by weeks, offering a window for early intervention (Institute for Healthcare Improvement, 2022).

An integrated dashboard is less a new tool than a shared language. It replaces fragmented reporting with collective meaning. When patient experience anchors the conversation, safety gains context and quality gains purpose. The goal is not to demonstrate performance, but to understand how care feels to those who trust us with their lives and to make that feeling of safety visible, measurable, and real.

## PRACTICE IMPACT

This chapter moves Likelihood to Recommend out of the realm of sentiment and into daily safety practice. Rather than treating LTR as a reputational score, it shows how patient feedback, especially comments about communication, medication understanding, and follow up, can be used as an early learning signal within quality and safety work. When patient experience data are traced back to care processes and leadership decisions, they reveal risk sooner than traditional outcome measures.

In home care, this signal is particularly important. Once the visit ends, patients and caregivers carry much of the responsibility for safety. Whether patients feel confident managing medications, recognizing warning signs, and knowing how to get help often determines whether they would recommend care. When that confidence is missing, LTR scores tend to fall even when no adverse event has been reported. Seen through a safety lens, these declines function as early warnings rather than performance failures.

One home care organization encountered this when HHCAHPS Likelihood to Recommend scores stagnated despite stable clinical indicators. Deeper review revealed a persistent gap in one measure, whether clinicians visually reviewed medications with patients. Scores averaged well below target. Patient comments clarified the issue. Many felt unsure about medication changes after hospitalization. Medications were discussed, but not always reviewed in a way that felt concrete or reassuring.

Instead of chasing survey improvement, leaders reframed the issue as a medication safety opportunity. They strengthened visual medication reconciliation, clarified expectations before visits, reinforced teach-back, and physically reviewed each medication with patients. A simple visual cue, a green medication sheet, signaled shared review and reinforced understanding after the visit ended.

The impact was practical and measurable. Clinicians reported fewer discrepancies and clarification calls. Patients described greater confidence managing medications. HHCAHPS scores on visual medication review rose from the high sixties to the high eighties, followed by corresponding gains in Likelihood to Recommend. These improvements were not driven by scripting or service recovery tactics. They reflected the downstream effects of strengthening a safety critical process.

The lesson is straightforward. Likelihood to Recommend reflects whether care feels safe, clear, and dependable. When patient experience data are treated as safety signals and patient stories are folded into improvement cycles, organizations move from reacting to harm toward anticipating risk, reinforcing reliability, and sustaining trust where care actually happens.

## CONCLUSION

This chapter reframes patient experience as more than satisfaction. It positions experience as an early warning system for safety risk. Declines in experience scores often surface communication breakdowns that precede serious safety events. Emotional safety for both patients and staff emerges as a foundational condition for harm prevention, shaping whether concerns are raised or remain unspoken.

Likelihood to Recommend is treated not as a marketing measure, but as a predictive signal of trust and reliability. Its relationship to operational consistency shows how perception often precedes performance. The chapter makes the case for integrated dashboards that bring together patient experience, safety, and quality data to support earlier risk detection and real-time learning. Leadership presence and rounding are highlighted as practical ways to strengthen psychological safety and reinforce confidence across care settings. Equally important is partnership with patients and families, whose insights often reveal risks that structured data miss. The chapter also acknowledges the value of digital feedback tools for timeliness, while cautioning against equity gaps. Together, these insights underscore a simple conclusion. Safety, quality, and experience are not separate goals. They function as one system. When aligned, organizations see risk sooner, respond with greater clarity, and sustain trust where it matters most.

## REFERENCES

Agency for Healthcare Research and Quality. (2023). *Patient safety culture surveys: User guide and resources.* U.S. Department of Health and Human Services. https://www.ahrq.gov/sops/index.html

Anhang Price, R., Elliott, M. N., Zaslavsky, A. M., Hays, R. D., Lehrman, W. G., Rybowski, L., Edgman-Levitan, S., & Cleary, P. D. (2014). Examining the role of patient experience surveys in measuring health care quality. *Medical Care Research and Review : MCRR, 71*(5), 522–554. DOI: 10.1177/1077558714541480 PMID: 25027409

Boulding, W., Glickman, S. W., Manary, M. P., Schulman, K. A., & Staelin, R. (2011). Relationship between patient satisfaction with inpatient care and hospital readmission within 30 days. *The American Journal of Managed Care, 17*(1), 41–48. PMID: 21348567

Centers for Medicare & Medicaid Services. (2023). *Framework for health equity 2022–2032: A 10-year vision to advance equity in the pursuit of improved health outcomes for all people.* U.S. Department of Health and Human Services. https://www.cms.gov/about-cms/agency-information/omh/equity-initiatives/framework-for-health-equity

Doyle, C., Lennox, L., & Bell, D. (2013). A systematic review of evidence on the links between patient experience and clinical safety and effectiveness. *BMJ Open, 3*(1), e001570. DOI: 10.1136/bmjopen-2012-001570 PMID: 23293244

Institute for Healthcare Improvement. (2022). *Establishing measures: The Model for Improvement.* https://www.ihi.org/library/model-for-improvement/establishing-measures

Press Ganey. (2023). *Human experience in healthcare: 2023 performance insights report.* Press Ganey Associates. https://www.pressganey.com

Reader, T. W., Gillespie, A., & Roberts, J. (2014). Patient complaints in healthcare systems: A systematic review and coding taxonomy. *BMJ Quality & Safety, 23*(8), 678–689. DOI: 10.1136/bmjqs-2013-002437 PMID: 24876289

## KEY TERMS AND DEFINITIONS

**Care Coordination:** The clarity and consistency of information shared across settings, essential for preventing gaps that lead to error.

**Communication Breakdown:** A failure in information exchange—between staff, or between staff and patients that often precedes adverse events.

**Emotional Safety:** The sense of being heard, respected, and supported—conditions that influence whether patients and staff speak up about concerns.

**Integrated Dashboard:** A unified view of patient experience, safety, and quality metrics that reveals patterns and enables proactive learning.

**Likelihood to Recommend (LTR):** A patient's expression of trust and perceived safety, often functioning as an early reliability signal rather than a satisfaction metric.

**Near Miss:** An event that could have caused harm but did not, offering an important opportunity for learning and prevention.

**Patient and Family Advisory Council (PFAC):** A structured partnership where patients and caregivers contribute to system-level improvements and safety design.

**Patient Experience:** How patients perceive their care, including communication, respect, and trust, offering early insight into safety risks.

**Safety Culture:** The shared behaviors, attitudes, and expectations that determine how reliably an organization prevents harm.

**Teach-Back Method:** A communication approach where patients repeat information in their own words to confirm understanding and reduce safety risks.

# APPENDIX I

## Building an Integrated Dashboard for Patient Experience, Safety, and Quality

This appendix offers a practical roadmap for organizations seeking to integrate **patient experience, safety, and quality** data into one unified learning system. The goal is to transform fragmented metrics into shared meaning turning feedback into forward motion.

This tool helps leaders build one cohesive dashboard that reflects how patients experience safety and quality in real time (Figure 3). Instead of treating patient experience, safety, and quality as three separate reports, this approach merges them into one conversation; one that starts with how care feels and ends with how reliably it is delivered.

1. Why Integration Matters

In most organizations, each domain has its own metrics:

- **Patient Experience:** CAHPS scores and comments
- **Safety:** Incident rates, near misses, harm events
- **Quality:** Clinical outcomes, compliance, performance incentives

*Figure 3. Example of an integrated patient experience, safety, and quality dashboard that displays CAHPS feedback alongside safety events and clinical performance measures to support shared learning and proactive risk identification*

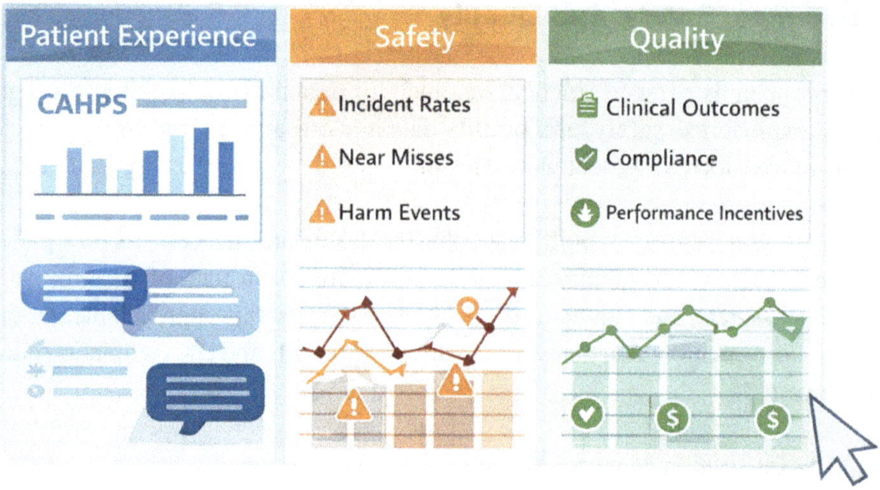


Example of an integrated Patient experience; safety and quality dasboard

# APPENDIX II

## Using Likelihood to Recommend as a Learning Signal

During an ambulatory quality review, a multispecialty clinic noticed a modest drop in its Likelihood to Recommend scores. Operational and safety indicators such as medication discrepancies, follow up failures, and urgent return visits remained steady, but the shift in patient sentiment caught the team's attention. Instead of treating it as a satisfaction issue, they decided to use LTR as an early learning signal.

They began reviewing recent comments from patients who had expressed lower confidence. Several described uncertainty after visits, especially when medication plans changed or when they weren't sure how to schedule follow-up tests. The concerns mirrored themes that had surfaced in near miss reviews, where incomplete communication rather than technical errors had created preventable confusion. The team added LTR trends to the ambulatory dashboard, placing them alongside metrics for after visit summary completeness, timely test result communication, and call back volumes. A pattern emerged: clinics with lower LTR also had more clarification calls from patients after appointments. During leadership walk rounds, leaders asked staff a simple question: "What helps patients leave a visit feeling confident enough to recommend our care?"

Clinicians and medical assistants offered grounded examples; reviewing medication changes in plain language, using teach-back, taking an extra minute to confirm follow-up steps, and pausing to ask, "What questions do you have before you go?" These observations were woven into team huddles and recognition efforts, using patient comments that highlighted clear, safety supporting behaviors. Over the next few months, LTR gradually improved, but the more notable shift was earlier detection of communication gaps and stronger patient trust at the clinic level. What began as a slight drop in a single metric became a lens for understanding how patients experience safety in real time.

Figure 4 illustrates how using Likelihood to Recommend as a learning metric shifts the focus from scoring to improvement by linking patient feedback to root cause analysis, QAPI dashboards, leadership dialogue, and staff recognition to strengthen trust, safety, and quality.

*Figure 4. Using likelihood to recommend as a learning metric*

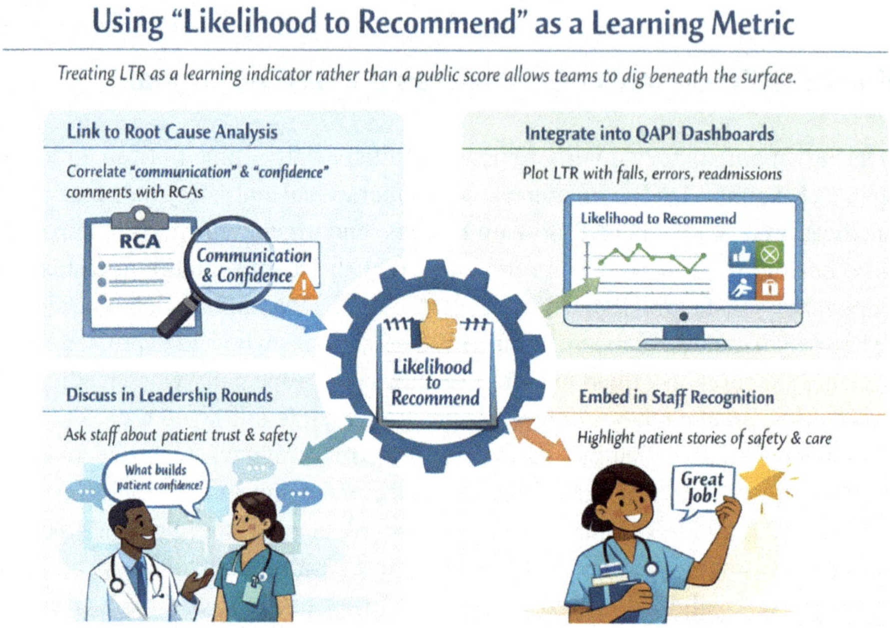

# Chapter 16
# When Things Go Wrong: Failure Modes and Effects Analysis, Root Cause Analysis, and Apparent Cause Analysis


## ABSTRACT

*Every healthcare system carries at least two stories. One emerges after something goes wrong. The other remains embedded in routines, handoffs, and workarounds, waiting to surface. This chapter explores how leaders and teams turn error into understanding through three analytic approaches commonly used in healthcare. Failure Modes and Effects Analysis (FMEA) offers a forward-looking method for anticipating where processes may fail. Root Cause Analysis (RCA) looks backward to understand how conditions align to produce harm. Apparent Cause Analysis (ACA) provides a rapid, focused review of near misses and operational disruptions. Rather than treating these methods as technical exercises, the chapter examines them as acts of organizational sensemaking. Their value lies not in assigning fault, but in uncovering the conditions that allow risk to emerge or remain hidden. Through concrete examples, the chapter illustrates how disciplined analysis can restore trust, support learning, and strengthen system resilience before harm recurs.*


## INTRODUCTION

Every safety event reveals something about how care is actually delivered. That insight extends beyond the bedside into the layers of policy, technology, staffing, and leadership decisions that shape everyday work. In healthcare organizations, analytic tools such as Failure Modes and Effects Analysis (FMEA), Root Cause Analysis (RCA), and Apparent Cause Analysis (ACA) do not arise spontaneously. They are activated, shaped, and constrained by regulatory expectations, accreditation

DOI: 10.4018/979-8-3373-6496-4.ch016

standards, internal governance structures, and prevailing norms about accountability and learning. This chapter examines not only what these tools are, but how they come to be recognized, selected, and used in real organizational settings.

For many organizations, exposure to these methods begins through external requirements. Accrediting bodies such as Joint Commission and regulatory agencies including the Centers for Medicare & Medicaid Services (CMS) mandate structured investigation of serious safety events, most often through RCA, while also encouraging proactive approaches such as FMEA to reduce risk before harm occurs (The Joint Commission, 2023; Agency for Healthcare Research and Quality, 2022). Over time, these expectations become codified in policy. Thresholds are established for reportable events. Escalation pathways to senior leadership are defined. Timelines for analysis are standardized. In this environment, safety analysis can easily become associated with compliance rather than learning. This chapter reframes these tools as practices of organizational understanding, ways of making sense of how risk is produced rather than simply how it is recorded.

In day-to-day operations, decisions about which analytic method to use often begin with harm classification. Events involving serious injury or death typically trigger formal RCA processes, executive oversight, and board level reporting. Near misses, equipment failures, and workflow disruptions may lead to ACA or other focused reviews. FMEA is most often applied during new program launches, technology implementations, or major workflow redesigns. These pathways are not neutral. They reflect how organizations define urgency, allocate authority, and balance foresight against hindsight. While severity appropriately drives immediacy and support needs, it should not be the sole determinant of analytic approach. Learning is strongest when the method is matched to the question being asked, not only to the outcome that occurred.

Across healthcare settings, the visibility of these tools has evolved unevenly. FMEA has gained prominence through patient safety organizations, quality improvement initiatives, and high reliability frameworks, particularly in technology enabled and transitional care environments where anticipation of risk is essential (Agency for Healthcare Research and Quality, 2022). RCA remains the dominant retrospective method for serious events, though its effectiveness varies widely. Leadership engagement, psychological safety, and follow-through often matter more than the tool itself (National Patient Safety Foundation, 2015). ACA, while less standardized across institutions, has gained traction as organizations seek faster learning cycles that prevent small failures from compounding into major harm. Taken together, these approaches form a continuum of learning that spans anticipation, response, and rapid adaptation.

Before turning to analytic methods, it is essential to center the experience of patients and families. When harm occurs, the organization's first responsibility is to address the patient's immediate clinical needs. This must be followed by timely, transparent, and compassionate communication. Communication and Resolution Programs (CRPs), including the Communication and Optimal Resolution (CANDOR) framework, provide structured approaches for disclosure, apology when appropriate, and ongoing engagement with patients and families after adverse events (Mello et al., 2014). These programs emphasize listening, acknowledgment of harm, and support for healing while maintaining accountability. Analytic investigation should never precede or replace these responsibilities. Inquiry comes after safety, disclosure, and support have been established.

At the same time, organizations must attend to the impact of adverse events on the clinicians and staff involved. Such events often give rise to the "second victim" phenomenon, characterized by emotional distress, professional self doubt, and fear of blame (Scott et al., 2009). In response, many healthcare systems have implemented structured support programs, including Caring for the Caregiver initiatives and peer response models such as the Resilience in Stressful Events (RISE) program at Johns Hopkins, to provide timely emotional and professional support following safety events (Scott et al., 2009; Wu et al., 2017). Addressing patient harm and workforce well being in parallel reinforces a central insight of safety science. Investigation without care can retraumatize patients and staff, erode trust, and undermine the psychological safety required for meaningful learning (National Patient Safety Foundation, 2015). When analytic tools such as FMEA, RCA, and ACA are intentionally paired with workforce support programs like RISE, organizations create the conditions for honest reflection and system focused improvement (Dekker, 2016; Wu & Connors, 2018).With these supports in place, organizations are better positioned to move from response to learning. Analytic methods can then be applied to understand how harm emerged and how future risk might be reduced in durable ways.

This chapter introduces a decision logic grounded in how healthcare systems actually function, linking harm recognition with regulatory triggers, leadership escalation, workforce support, and clearly articulated learning goals. It illustrates how RCA is applied in high acuity settings where multiple system defenses have failed, how FMEA supports proactive design across programs and transitions of care, and how ACA enables rapid insight in fast moving operational environments. Throughout, the emphasis remains on purposeful use of analytic tools, not their completion as an end in itself.

Culture remains inseparable from technique. Psychological safety allows staff to describe work as it is actually done. Just Culture frameworks clarify accountability without defaulting to blame (Dekker, 2016). Human factors thinking shifts attention from individual vigilance to system conditions. Measurement and feedback loops translate insight into sustained reliability. The aim is not simply to satisfy investigative requirements, but to strengthen the system's capacity to detect, absorb, and adapt to risk. By the end of this chapter, readers will be able to recognize how analytic tools are activated within healthcare organizations, select methods based on learning need rather than outcome severity, and integrate investigation with caregiver support and system redesign. These principles are carried forward as analytic findings are translated into proactive risk mitigation and sustainment strategies across complex care environments (Figure 1).

*Figure 1. This figure compares FMEA, RCA, and ACA, highlighting how each method varies in timing, purpose, and depth from proactive risk prevention to detailed investigation of harm events and rapid learning from near misses*

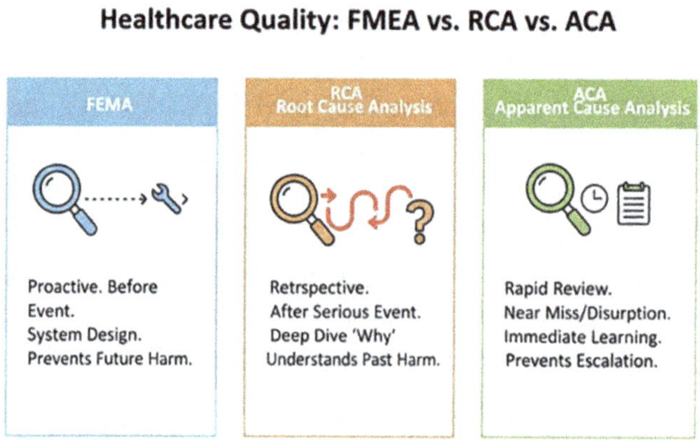


## INTEGRATED DECISION LOGIC: HARM INFORMS RESPONSE, NOT METHOD

In mature safety programs, investigative decisions tend to follow a recognizable logic. Harm classification establishes urgency and clarifies accountability. The analytic method, however, is selected based on what the organization needs to learn. In this framing, harm functions as context rather than constraint. Harm describes the outcome. Investigation examines how the system performed. When severity alone dictates the scope or method of analysis, inquiry often narrows prematurely, and vulnerabilities that extend beyond a single event may remain unexamined.

Near misses frequently surface the same system weaknesses as events involving serious injury. Conversely, high harm outcomes may result from an uncommon alignment of conditions rather than a broadly embedded design flaw. Effective safety programs make a deliberate distinction between what happened and how best to learn from it. This separation allows organizations to pursue insight without being anchored solely to outcome severity, a distinction illustrated in Figure 2 (Tool Selection by Harm Level).

Many organizations rely on Press Ganey's HPI framework to standardize how safety events are labeled, reviewed, and trended. The Safety Event Classification (SEC®) focuses on whether care deviated from expected performance, whether that deviation reached the patient, and the degree of harm involved. Paired with this classification, the Serious Safety Event Rate (SSER®) tracks preventable serious harm over a rolling period. Together, these measures help leaders understand urgency, assign accountability, and monitor reliability while preserving flexibility in how learning is pursued.

The Serious Safety Event Rate (SSER®) extends this approach by following serious, preventable harm over time using a rolling, volume adjusted measure. Its value lies less in external comparison than in internal reflection. Patterns emerge. Progress toward zero harm becomes visible. The impact of system-level interventions can be assessed with greater fidelity. In this way, SSER® shifts attention away from isolated outcomes and toward organizational reliability. Taken together, SEC® and SSER® provide the governance and measurement foundation for the decision logic depicted in Figure 16.2. They anchor leadership accountability while leaving space for analytic judgment, ensuring that investigative depth is guided by learning need rather than dictated solely by harm severity.

*Figure 2. Tool selection by harm level*

Tool Selection by Harm Level

| Harm Identification (SEC® Context) | Primary Learning Need | Recommended Analytic Tool | Purpose in Practice |
| --- | --- | --- | --- |
| **Serious Safety Event** (serious, preventable harm) | Understand how multiple system defenses failed | **Root Cause Analysis (RCA)** | Conduct a comprehensive, retrospective analysis with leadership oversight to |
| **Near Miss or Low-Harm Event** | Learn quickly before risk escalates | **Apparent Cause Analysis (ACA)** | Enable rapid, focused learning from operational disruptions or close calls without delaying |
| **Anticipated Risk, New Process, or Recurrent Pattern** | Prevent failure before harm occurs | **Failure Modes and Effects Analysis (FMEA)** | Proactively identify vulnerabilities and redesign processes to reduce the ine and impact of failure |

**Note.** Serious Event Classification (SEC®) establishes urgency and accountability, while the Serious Safety Event Rate (SSER®) tracks serious, preventable harm over time to assess organizational reliability. Analytic tools are selected based on learning need rather than outcome severity alone.

Within this context, analytic tool selection remains deliberate and adaptive. As summarized in Figure 2, events classified as serious safety events appropriately trigger Root Cause Analysis (RCA) to examine how multiple system defenses failed and to guide leadership level corrective action. Near misses and low harm events are well suited for Apparent Cause Analysis (ACA), enabling rapid insight and early correction before risk escalates. Failure Modes and Effects Analysis (FMEA) extends learning forward by proactively identifying vulnerabilities in new processes, transitions, or recurring patterns and redesigning systems to prevent future harm.

Together, the decision logic and tool pathways shown in Figure 2 demonstrate how harm classification informs response while analytic method remains intentionally aligned with learning need rather than outcome severity alone. Figure 2 illustrates how analytic tools are *envisioned* to be selected based on harm identification within the Serious Event Classification (SEC®) context. Harm classification establishes urgency and accountability while preserving flexibility in analytic approach: serious safety events prompt comprehensive Root Cause Analysis (RCA), near misses and low harm events are suited to rapid Apparent Cause Analysis (ACA), and anticipated risks or recurring patterns are addressed proactively through Failure Modes and Effects Analysis (FMEA). The framework reflects intended use to support system learning and organizational reliability rather than prescriptive or regulatory mandate.

## TURNING ANALYSIS INTO UNDERSTANDING

In healthcare, we often talk about "learning from mistakes." But real learning requires more than documentation; it requires translation. FMEA, RCA, and ACA aren't checklists. They are languages of understanding; ways of asking, *what is this event trying to teach us?* Over the years, it has been observed that the most powerful investigations begin not with data, but with empathy. Sitting beside a nurse, listening to what made an action seem reasonable at the time, often reveals more truth than any spreadsheet. Patterns emerge not from punishment, but from patience. The next sections explore how these tools, FMEA, RCA, and ACA work in different settings: the hospital that learns through deconstruction, the clinic that learns through conversation, and the home care team that learns through trust. Each one shows that when leaders approach "what went wrong" with humility, they find something far greater: what can still go right.

## THE THREE LENSES OF LEARNING: HOW SYSTEMS REVEAL THEMSELVES

### 1. The Hospital: Seeing Patterns Beneath Pressure

Hospitals are extraordinary places of healing and pressure. Every beep, checklist, and handoff carry the weight of urgency. It's where most of us in quality and safety first learn what "investigation" really means. One of my earliest root cause reviews took place after a delayed antibiotic administration in the emergency department. The patient recovered, but the event exposed a deeper truth: what seemed like a single error was really a pattern of workflow overload. As I sat with the team, the charge nurse, pharmacist, and ED tech, I asked them to walk me through what happened minute by minute. The timeline looked messy, overlapping, and human. A lab result had been printed, placed under another chart, and the clock kept ticking. In the old days, this would have ended with a policy reminder. But that day, we mapped the process instead.

We used RCA not to assign fault, but to *see the system through the eyes of the people living it.* Three key insights surfaced:

- **Information congestion:** The printer was shared between four bays, causing constant interruptions.
- **Priority conflicts:** Nurses were juggling triage and medication prep simultaneously.
- **Communication gaps:** The electronic alert appeared on one screen but not another.

The fix was simple, a dedicated printer for stat results and a visual cue on the triage board. But what mattered most was what came after. The team asked to repeat the mapping exercise for all high-risk meds. That moment told me something powerful: when people are treated as learners instead of suspects, they start leading their own solutions. Hospitals will always be complex. RCA doesn't remove that complexity, but it gives it shape. It turns chaos into conversation and conversation into change.

### 2. The Clinic: Discovering the Everyday FMEA

Ambulatory care looks calmer on the surface, but risk hides in its routines. In the clinic setting, I often found that the most useful tool wasn't RCA, but FMEA, a way to predict failure before it happens. A few years ago, we were preparing to launch a new vaccine storage process. Instead of waiting for a temperature excursion to teach us a lesson, we gathered the team, medical assistants, nurses, and the clinic manager around a whiteboard. "Let's imagine this goes wrong," I said. "Where could failure sneak in?" At first, the room was quiet. Talking about hypothetical problems felt uncomfortable. But once we listed the steps, the insights poured out:

- *What if the sensor battery dies?*
- *What if the back-up fridge is on a different circuit?*
- *What if the alarm goes off after hours and no one's on call?*

By the end of the hour, the team had created a risk priority table: each possible failure mode, its likelihood, and its potential impact. They ranked the top three and wrote simple mitigations of fresh batteries logged monthly, a weekend alert rotation, and dual circuits for refrigeration. The exercise took less than 90 minutes, but it built something larger: shared ownership. The following month, when a brief power outage occurred, the back-up system activated flawlessly. A medical assistant later said, "It worked because we imagined it first." That's what FMEA really does. It replaces surprise with foresight and turns anxiety into preparedness. And in that process, people begin to trust not only their systems, but their own ability to prevent harm before it starts.

## 3. Home Care: The Power of Rapid Learning

In home care, the environment itself becomes part of the equation. You can't control every variable weather, pets, lighting, family stress but you can build quick learning systems that keep up with reality. That's where Apparent Cause Analysis (ACA) comes in. ACA is like a speedboat beside the larger RCA ship, nimble, focused, and responsive. We used it often in home health to respond to near misses or non-injury events that still carried lessons.

One case stands out. A delivery driver picked up several oxygen cylinders from the warehouse for routine home deliveries. When he lifted one cylinder labeled as full, it felt noticeably light; far too light for a full tank. His experience told him something wasn't right. Instead of continuing his route, he stopped, returned to the warehouse, and raised the concern with his supervisor. That single observation triggered a rapid ACA. Within hours, the supervisor gathered a small group: the driver, the respiratory therapist overseeing home oxygen services, and the warehouse lead. Because the organization had recently transitioned to a new oxygen vendor, the team also brought the vendor's quality representative into the review. The group centered the ACA on two simple questions:

1. What happened, and how close were we to harm?
2. What made this seem reasonable at the time?

Within 30 minutes, a pattern emerged. The vendor had changed its cylinder filling and labeling workflow during the contract transition. On the vendor's side, the quality assurance step meant to catch misfilled cylinders was inconsistently applied that week due to onboarding of new staff. No one was blamed. The miss belonged to the system, not the individuals doing their best within it. The group moved quickly to reinforce safeguards:

- **Vendor corrections:** Reinstituted mandatory fill checks and standardized label placement across all cylinders.
- **Staff education:** Brief refresher for drivers and warehouse technicians on weight cues, escalation signals, and how to document discrepancies.
- **Shared learning:** The vendor and DME team agreed on a weekly quality check huddle for the first 90 days of the new contract.

A potentially dangerous misfilled cylinder never made it into a patient's home. What could have been an unnoticed close call instead became a system level improvement; because a driver trusted his instincts, paused the process, and spoke up.

## PUTTING THE TOOLS TO WORK: BRINGING STRUCTURE TO REFLECTION

Years of leading patient safety investigations have reinforced a central lesson: structure does not replace empathy, it sustains it. When emotions run high and the demand for answers is immediate, structured methods such as RCA, FMEA, and ACA help teams remain inquisitive rather than reactive. Although each method prompts different questions, all serve the same purpose: organizational learning that reduces the likelihood of recurrence, a principle emphasized by both Joint Commission and the Agency for Healthcare Research and Quality (AHRQ). What matters most is not the sophistication of the template, but the quality of the dialogue it enables. One facilitation principle consistently anchors this work: *start with listening, not labeling*. When psychological safety is present, staff describe work as it is actually performed, not as it is imagined in policy. From that shared understanding, meaningful analysis can begin.

## SELECTING INVESTIGATIVE TOOLS: LEARNING OVER LABELS

Once harm is recognized and classified including identification of a Serious Safety Event (SSE) organizations must determine how best to learn from the event. At this stage, harm level informs urgency, escalation, and leadership oversight, but it should not independently dictate the investigative method. The purpose of analysis is not to match tool to severity, but to select the approach most likely to reveal system risk, support learning, and prevent recurrence.

## CORE STEPS OF FAILURE MODES AND EFFECTS ANALYSIS (FMEA) IN PRACTICE.

Failure Modes and Effects Analysis unfolds as a deliberate sequence that helps teams see where a process is most vulnerable. It begins with choosing and mapping the workflow, so everyone shares an accurate understanding of how the work is actually performed. From there, the team identifies potential failure modes, places where the process could break down and explores their possible causes and effects. Each failure mode is then evaluated for severity, likelihood, and detectability to distinguish routine nuisances from the risks most likely to cause harm. Those insights guide the design of targeted preventive actions aimed at reducing risk at its source rather than relying on vigilance alone. The final step, often the most overlooked, is monitoring teams track whether the changes are working, recalibrate as needed, and reinforce improvements until they become part of everyday practice. This progression turns FMEA from a one time exercise into an ongoing method for strengthening reliability.

Figure 3 illustrates the sequential application of FMEA as a proactive risk assessment method, moving from selection and mapping of a high-risk process to identification and prioritization of potential failure modes, design of preventive system controls, and ongoing monitoring. When applied consistently, FMEA enables teams to anticipate vulnerabilities, strengthen defenses, and reduce the likelihood of harm before failures reach patients or caregivers.

*Figure 3. Steps of Failure Modes and Effects Analysis (FMEA)*

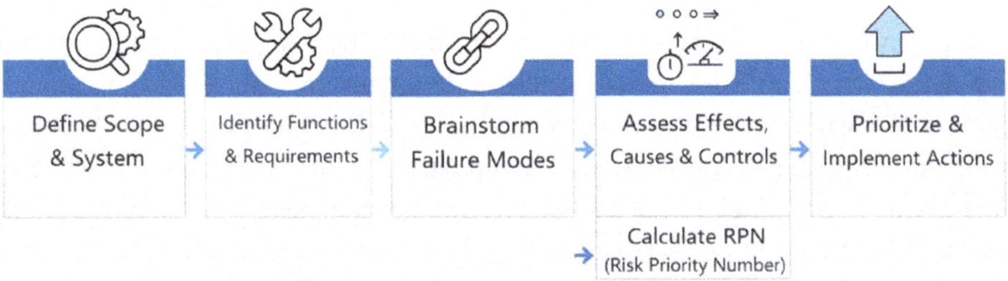


## CORE STEPS OF ROOT CAUSE ANALYSIS (RCA) IN PRACTICE

Root Cause Analysis unfolds through a structured series of steps designed to understand how system factors contributed to an adverse event and to translate that insight into sustainable redesign. The process begins by assembling a review team that includes those closest to the work, ensuring a grounded view of how the event unfolded. Establishing psychological safety early allows participants to speak honestly about conditions and constraints without fear of blame. With that foundation in place, the team reconstructs a clear, factual timeline from preconditions through outcome to surface gaps, delays, and points of ambiguity. Contributing factors across communication, design, technology, environment, workload, and human factors are then examined to reveal where the system was most vulnerable. Using structured questioning to probe deeper, the team identifies the underlying root causes, those conditions that allowed defenses to fail. From there, corrective actions are developed that focus on system-level change rather than individual remediation. The final step is monitoring, tracking outcomes and process measures to confirm that the interventions reduce risk over time. Together, these steps transform RCA from a retrospective exercise into a disciplined path toward reliability (Figure 4).

*Figure 4. Core steps of Root Cause Analysis (RCA) in practice*

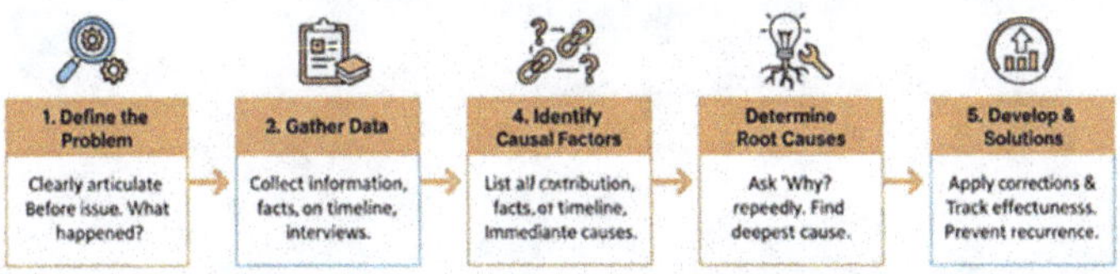

## Apparent Cause Analysis in Practice

Apparent Cause Analysis is a rapid, practical method that helps teams learn quickly from near misses and lower-harm events while details are still vivid. The process begins with a timely review usually within 24 to 72 hours to preserve context and ensure the narrative reflects what actually happened. Frontline staff directly involved in the event are brought into the conversation so the analysis stays grounded in real work rather than assumptions. Together, the group briefly reconstructs what occurred and gauges how close the situation came to causing harm. They then explore why the actions taken made sense at the time, considering workload, competing priorities, design limitations, or implicit assumptions that shaped decisions. From that shared understanding, the team identifies one or two immediate, practical fixes that can be implemented without delay to reduce near term risk. The final step is broader sharing communicating key insights to peer teams so learning extends beyond a single incident. In this way, ACA functions as a fast, focused learning loop that strengthens reliability between larger investigations (Figure 5).

*Figure 5. Steps in Apparent Root Analysis (ACA) in practice*

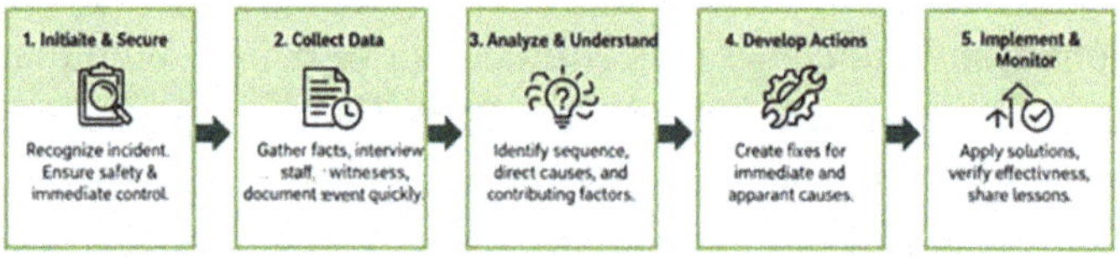


Taken collectively, FMEA, RCA, and ACA show distinct strengths. The following crosswalk outlines how these methods align with required standards and where leaders can extend learning beyond compliance. Figure 6 illustrates how common investigative approaches align with regulatory expectations while emphasizing that compliance requirements represent a baseline for action rather than a limit on organizational learning. The crosswalk highlights opportunities for leaders to extend analysis beyond minimum requirements to strengthen system reliability (Figure 6).

*Figure 6. Investigative tools across the safety learning continuum*

| Investigative Tool | Primary Purpose | Typical Use Case | Regulatory Alignment | Leadership Opportunity Beyond Compliance |
|---|---|---|---|---|
| Root Cause Analysis (RCA) | Retrospective system learning after harm | Serious Safety Events; Sentinel Events | Expected after Sentinel Events | Extend RCA to proactive redesign |
| Apparent Cause Analysis (ACA) | Rapid, focused learning | Near misses; Lower-harm events | Acceptable for Non-Sentinel Events | Use ACA trends for system analysis |
| Failure Modes & Effects Analysis (FMEA) | Prospective risk identification | New Processes; High-risk Workflows | Encouraged for Risk Assessment | Apply FMEA to prevent future SSEs |
| Combined / Iterative Use | Comprehensive learning cycle | Recurrent Events; System-wide Risk | Not Required by Regulation | Commitment to High Reliability |

## PRACTICE IMPACT

Implementing FMEA, RCA/HFMEA, and ACA in routine healthcare operations yields measurable safety gains: a longitudinal clinical laboratory study reported an 80% reduction in high risk pre-analytical errors over nine years after repeated FMEA cycles, underscoring the preventive power of proactive risk assessment (De Haro, Papay Ramirez, & Garcia Chileme, 2024). In hospital medication systems, HFMEA-guided interventions produced relative risk reductions in prescription errors (−22%), validation errors (−19%), and dispensing errors (−38%), demonstrating how structured analysis translates into fewer downstream failures (Vélez-Díaz-Pallarés, Delgado-Silveira, Carretero-Accame, & Bermejo-Vicedo, 2013). Rapid learning from near misses via enhanced ACA processes has also improved reliability and shortened turnaround time in one pediatric center, average ACA action-plan reliability increased while cycle time decreased, reinforcing the role of timely, multidisciplinary reflection in sustaining safety culture (Crandall, Sten, Almuhanna, Fahey, & Shah, 2017).

## CONCLUSION

This chapter explored how healthcare organizations can transform adverse events and near misses into opportunities for learning and improvement through three key tools: Failure Modes and Effects Analysis (FMEA), Root Cause Analysis (RCA), and Apparent Cause Analysis (ACA). FMEA provides a proactive lens to anticipate failure before harm occurs, RCA offers a structured retrospective approach to uncover systemic contributors to adverse events, and ACA enables rapid, context-rich learning from near misses. Across hospital, clinic, and home care settings, the chapter emphasized that these tools are most effective when grounded in empathy, psychological safety, and collaboration. Rather than assigning blame, the goal is to understand how design, communication, and human factors interact to create risk and then redesign systems to prevent recurrence. By integrating FMEA, RCA, and ACA into a continuous learning cycle, leaders can foster a culture of curiosity, resilience, and shared accountability, ensuring that safety becomes a reflexive habit rather than a reactive response.

## REFERENCES


Agency for Healthcare Research and Quality. (2022). *Strategies and approaches for investigating patient safety events (RCA, FMEA, etc.)*. Patient Safety Network (PSNet). https://psnet.ahrq.gov/primer/strategies-and-approaches-investigating-patient-safety-events

Crandall, K. M., Sten, M.-B., Almuhanna, A., Fahey, L., & Shah, R. K. (2017). Improving apparent cause analysis reliability: A quality improvement initiative. *Pediatric Quality & Safety*, *2*(3), e025. DOI: 10.1097/pq9.0000000000000025 PMID: 30229162

De Haro, T., Papay Ramirez, L., & Garcia Chileme, S. (2024). Failure Mode and Effects Analysis (FMEA) methodology as a strategy to increase patient safety. *Clinical Chemistry*, *70*(Supplement 1), hvae106.186. Advance online publication. DOI: 10.1093/clinchem/hvae106.186

Dekker, S. (2016). *Just culture: Restoring trust and accountability in your organization* (3rd ed.). CRC Press. DOI: 10.4324/9781315251271

Mello, M. M., Boothman, R. C., McDonald, T., Driver, J., Lembitz, A., Bouwmeester, D., Dunlap, B., & Gallagher, T. H. (2014). Communication-and-Resolution Programs: The challenges and lessons learned from six early adopters. *Health Affairs*, *33*(1), 20–29. DOI: 10.1377/hlthaff.2013.0828 PMID: 24395931

National Patient Safety Foundation. (2015). *RCA$^2$: Improving root cause analyses and actions to prevent harm*. Author.

Press Ganey. (n.d.). *The HPI SEC® and SSER® patient safety measurement system for healthcare*. https://www.pressganey.com

Scott, S. D., Hirschinger, L. E., Cox, K. R., McCoig, M., Hahn-Cover, K., Epperly, K. M., Phillips, E. C., & Hall, L. W. (2009). The natural history of recovery for the healthcare provider "second victim" after adverse patient events. *Quality & Safety in Health Care*, *18*(5), 325–330. DOI: 10.1136/qshc.2009.032870 PMID: 19812092

The Joint Commission. (2023). *Root cause analysis in health care: A Joint Commission guide to analysis and corrective action of sentinel and adverse events* (7th ed.). Joint Commission Resources.

Vélez Díaz Pallarés, M., Delgado Silveira, E., Carretero Accame, M. E., & Bermejo Vicedo, T. (2013). Using Healthcare Failure Mode and Effect Analysis to reduce medication errors in the process of drug prescription, validation and dispensing in hospitalized patients. *BMJ Quality & Safety*, *22*(1), 42–52. https://qualitysafety.bmj.com/content/22/1/42. DOI: 10.1136/bmjqs-2012-000983 PMID: 22976504

Wu, A. W., & Connors, C. (2018). Supporting clinicians after adverse events: The second victim phenomenon. *BMJ (Clinical Research Ed.)*, *363*, k4149. DOI: 10.1136/bmj.k4149

Wu, A. W., Shapiro, J., Harrison, R., Scott, S. D., Connors, C., Kenney, L., & Etchegaray, J. (2017). The impact of adverse events on clinicians: What's needed to support second victims. *BMJ Quality & Safety*, *26*(11), 878–882. DOI: 10.1136/bmjqs-2016-005987

## KEY TERMS AND DEFINITIONS

**Apparent Cause Analysis (ACA):** A rapid review for near misses or recurring issues to enable quick learning.

**Drift:** The gradual, unnoticed shift from safe practice toward unsafe norms.

**Failure Modes and Effects Analysis (FMEA):** A proactive method to identify and mitigate potential process failures before harm occurs.

**Human Factors:** The study of how people interact with systems to design processes that anticipate error.

**Just Culture:** An approach that balances accountability with learning by distinguishing human error from reckless behavior.

**Learning Loop:** A continuous cycle of noticing, analyzing, and adapting processes based on feedback.

**Moral Residue:** The emotional weight left when professionals cannot reconcile expectations with real-world limitations.

**Psychological Safety:** A shared belief that people can speak up without fear of blame or retribution.

**Root Cause Analysis (RCA):** A structured review to uncover underlying system factors after an event.

**Serious Safety Event (SSE):** A preventable patient safety event that results in significant harm, requiring immediate escalation and system-level learning.

**Signal-to-Noise Problem:** Difficulty distinguishing meaningful alerts from background distractions.

## APPENDIX I

## Practical Toolkits for FMEA, RCA, and ACA

You've just explored how structured learning transforms errors into insight. Now it's time to make it real. The following tools are designed to help leaders translate FMEA, RCA, and ACA into daily practice, simple enough for a huddle, but rigorous enough to build a system of reliability.

## Applying FMEA to Patient Identification: Practical Example

A near miss involving home infusion labels, correctly applied but inconsistently verified during a weekend shift prompted the organization to conduct a focused FMEA. The concern wasn't the single event itself but the possibility of a broader pattern the team hadn't yet seen. The FMEA examined the entire labeling and verification process, from printing the label to confirming it with the patient in the home. The goal was simple: understand where the process could fail, how likely those failures were, and how easily they would be detected. The team brought together a home infusion pharmacist, a field nurse, a DME technician, a scheduler, and a quality facilitator. Their perspectives grounded the review in the realities of home care, where workflows often look different in practice than they do on paper.

By walking step-by-step through the process and scoring each potential failure mode, the team identified points where reliability relied too heavily on human vigilance. The FMEA made those vulnerabilities visible and became the foundation for targeted, practical improvements that strengthened the system overall.

## How to Score an FMEA Sheet

Scoring an FMEA involves rating each potential failure mode across three dimensions:

1. **Severity (S)** – How serious the impact would be if the failure reached the patient.

   Score 1–10: 1 = negligible; 10 = catastrophic.

2. **Occurrence (O)** – How likely the failure is to happen.

   Score 1–10: 1 = rare; 10 = frequent.

3. **Detection (D)** – How likely the failure would be detected before causing harm.

Score 1–10: 1 = very detectable; 10 = not detectable.
Once each category is scored, the Risk Priority Number (RPN) is calculated:
RPN = Severity × Occurrence × Detection
The higher the RPN, the greater the need for immediate mitigation.
Typical prioritization:

- **High risk (RPN ≥ 50):** Address immediately.
- **Moderate risk (30–49):** Improve as resources allow.
- **Low risk (< 30):** Monitor and maintain.

Teams score collaboratively to reduce bias, then revisit and rescore after implementing improvements to verify that risk has been reduced. Figure 6 illustrates a step-by-step FMEA identifying potential failure modes across the labeling and packaging workflow, their causes and effects, associated risk priority numbers (RPNs), and targeted mitigation strategies to reduce misidentification and delivery errors before harm occurs (Figure 7).

*Figure 7. Example Failure Modes and Effects Analysis (FMEA) for medication labeling and packaging*

| Step | Possible Failure Mode | Cause | Effect | Severity (1–5) | Likelihood (1–5) | RPN | Mitigation / Control |
|---|---|---|---|---|---|---|---|
| Label printing | Duplicate or incorrect labels | Hardware glitch; no auto-refresh | Wrong label attached | 5 | 3 | 45 | Auto-refresh; printer maintenance; alerts |
| Label transport | Label smudges or detaches | Condensation | Patient misidentific-cation | 4 | 3 | 36 | Waterproof labels; sealed transport |
| Barcode scan | System fails to refresh | Software lag | Missed alert | 4 | 4 | 64 | Auto-refresh; visual confirmation |
| Verification | Second identifier skipped | Workload pressure | Wrong bag delivered | 5 | 3 | 60 | Reinforce two identifiers; coaching |
| Final packaging | Label obscured | Non-standard process | Delivery confusion | 3 | 2 | 24 | Label zone; standardized packaging |

## Interpreting and Prioritizing RPN Scores

- **High RPN (50–75):** Immediate focus

*Example:* Barcode lag (RPN 64), skipped verification (RPN 60)

- **Moderate RPN (30–49):** Monitor and improve as feasible

*Example:* Printer issues (RPN 45)

- **Low RPN (<30):** Acceptable risk; monitor without overcorrection

*Example:* Label tape overlap (RPN 24)

## Why Scoring Matters

Scoring transforms emotion into evidence. It helps teams:

- Balance severity and likelihood
- Justify sequencing of fixes
- Communicate risk clearly to leadership

*Example:* Label smudging (RPN 24) is less urgent than skipped verification (RPN 60), even if both feel concerning in discussion.

## Practical Tips for Leaders

- Score risks as a team to reduce bias
- Recalculate RPNs after mitigation
- Visualize progress over time
- Pair FMEA with live observation (Gemba)
- Share reductions in RPN as success stories

## Root Cause Analysis (RCA)

Case Vignette: Hospital-Acquired Pressure Injury

A patient admitted for cardiac monitoring developed a Stage 3 pressure injury on the sacrum after five days in the ICU. The injury was identified during routine rounding, requiring wound care consultation and extended hospitalization. While the patient recovered, the event raised concerns about prevention practices in high acuity settings.

## How RCA Was Conducted

- **Assemble the Team:** ICU nurse, wound care specialist, charge nurse, and quality leader participated to ensure multiple perspectives.
- **Establish Psychological Safety:** The facilitator acknowledged the emotional impact and emphasized learning over blame.
- **Reconstruct the Timeline:**
    - Patient admitted with limited mobility and high Braden risk score.
    - Initial skin assessment documented; repositioning plan noted.
    - Staffing shortages led to missed turns during peak hours.
    - Pressure-relieving mattress ordered but delayed due to supply constraints.
- **Identify Contributing Factors:**
    - **Workload pressure:** High nurse-to-patient ratio during surge.
    - **Equipment availability:** Delay in specialized mattress delivery.
    - **Communication gaps:** Repositioning reminders not integrated into EHR alerts.
- **Root Cause (5 Whys):**
    - Why did the injury occur? → Repositioning was inconsistent.
    - Why inconsistent? → Competing priorities and staffing shortages.
    - Why shortages? → Surge planning lacked contingency for high-risk patients.
    - Why no contingency? → No predictive model for resource allocation.
    - Why no model? → Absence of structured escalation for pressure injury risk.
- **Corrective Actions:**
    - Implement EHR-based repositioning alerts.
    - Create surge staffing protocol prioritizing high-risk patients.
    - Maintain a buffer stock of pressure-relieving mattresses.

Figure 8 illustrates a three-phase process in which investigation reconstructs events and reveals operational barriers, analysis applies the 5 Whys to identify the true root cause, and resolution focuses on system redesign to hard-wire safety through structured escalation, EHR alerts, and buffer stocks.

*Figure 8. From investigation to resolution: Translating analysis into system design*

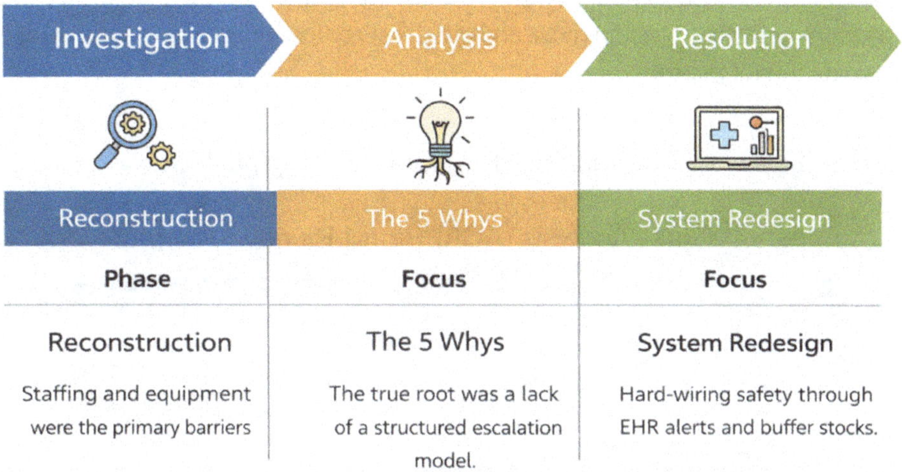


## Apparent Cause Analysis (ACA) Rapid Review Template

Case Vignette: Vaccine Storage Alarm Near Miss

During a routine morning check in an ambulatory clinic, a medical assistant noticed that the vaccine refrigerator temperature had briefly exceeded the safe range overnight. The alarm had triggered but was silenced automatically after 30 seconds, and no one on the weekend rotation received an alert. No vaccines were compromised, but the event exposed a gap in the monitoring process.

How ACA Was Used:

- **Small Group Review:** Within 48 hours, the clinic manager, two medical assistants, and the nurse lead met for a 30-minute discussion.
- **Guiding Questions:**
    - o *What happened?* The alarm activated during off-hours but did not sustain or notify staff.
    - o *What made it seem reasonable?* Staff assumed the system would escalate alerts automatically; no one realized the silence feature was active.
- **Immediate Fix:** Added persistent alarm settings, implemented a weekend alert rotation, and posted a quick-reference guide near the unit.
- **Learning Shared:** Changes and lessons were communicated across all ambulatory sites within the same week.

Figure 9 illustrates how a brief, team-based ACA was used to examine a vaccine storage alarm near miss, identify why the failure seemed reasonable at the time, implement immediate system fixes, and rapidly share learning to prevent recurrence across ambulatory sites.

*Figure 9. Apparent Cause Analysis (ACA) rapid review in practice*

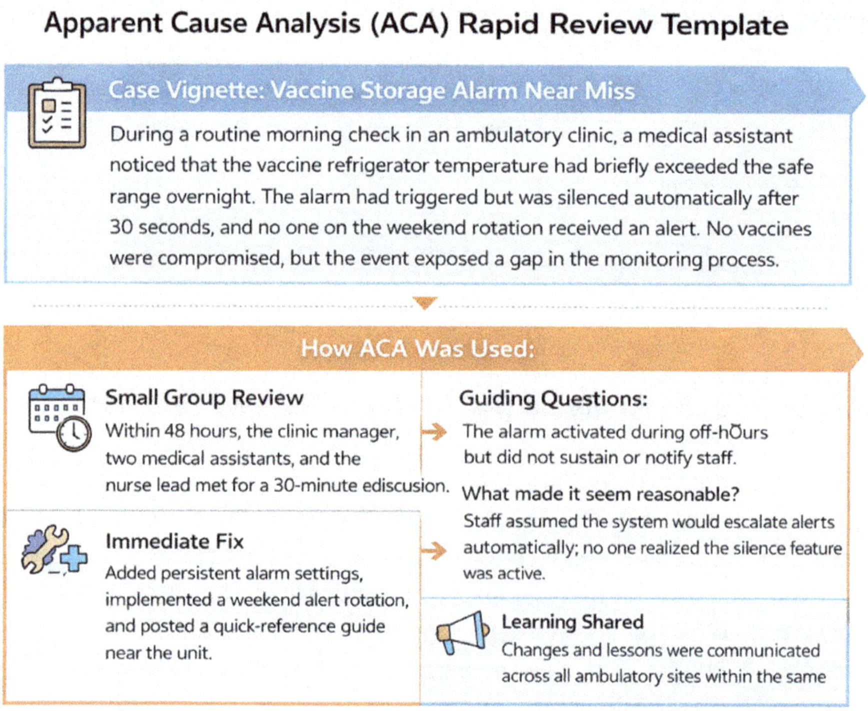

# Chapter 17
# Invisible Failures:
## Algorithmic Bias as a New Category of Safety Risk


## ABSTRACT

*Artificial intelligence is increasingly embedded in clinical decision making, introducing safety risks that are often subtle, distributed, and difficult to detect in real time. Algorithmic bias functions as a latent safety condition, distorting risk assessment, masking early signs of clinical deterioration, and quietly reproducing inequities without triggering traditional indicators of harm. This chapter frames algorithmic bias as a patient safety concern requiring the same rigor applied to other high-risk clinical systems. It demonstrates how established safety science methods, including Root Cause Analysis, Failure Mode and Effects Analysis, and Just Culture, can be adapted to AI-supported workflows. Drawing on national principles for responsible AI use in healthcare, the chapter emphasizes governance, transparency, continuous monitoring, and human accountability, and offers practical tools to support equitable, operational, and survey ready AI oversight in everyday safety practice.*


## INTRODUCTION

Artificial intelligence is no longer peripheral to healthcare work. It now shapes routine clinical decisions by prioritizing risk, flagging potential deterioration, and influencing how care is delivered across settings. Much of this occurs quietly, through algorithms that process large volumes of data faster than any human can. Over time, organizations begin to trust these outputs as signals of where to look, who to worry about, and what requires action. That trust introduces a new kind of safety challenge.

Traditional patient safety efforts have focused on events that are visible and traceable. Medication errors, falls, infections, equipment failures, and communi-


DOI: 10.4018/979-8-3373-6496-4.ch017

cation breakdowns tend to leave evidence. They show up in incident reports, chart reviews, patient complaints, or direct observation. Algorithmic bias often does not. When an algorithm produces a confident but flawed output, it can appear technically sound while still masking risk. If clinicians and leaders accept that output without questioning how it was generated or whom it reflects, harm may occur without triggering familiar safety alarms. This chapter argues that algorithmic bias should be understood as a distinct category of safety event. It arises when data driven tools inherit inequities embedded in historical data, design assumptions, or incomplete representations of patient populations. The resulting harm is rarely dramatic. More often it appears as delay rather than error, underestimation rather than miscalculation, or missed escalation rather than overt failure. These patterns are systemic and distributed, which makes them difficult to detect using conventional surveillance methods alone.

The risk increases when organizations rely too heavily on AI to analyze trends, identify hazards, and explain events without maintaining meaningful human oversight. Algorithms do not pause to question their assumptions. They do not recognize who is missing from the data or whose experiences are poorly represented. When AI becomes the primary lens through which risk is interpreted, organizations may gradually lose sight of harm that falls outside the model's frame.

## Objectives

- Define algorithmic bias as a patient safety risk by positioning it as a preventable, often invisible form of harm within AI enabled care.
- Apply established safety science approaches to AI by demonstrating how RCA, FMEA, ACA, and Just Culture can be used to detect, interpret, and mitigate bias in clinical algorithms.
- Review the seven core elements of responsible AI use identified by The Joint Commission and CHAI, showing how each aligns directly with the safety concepts explored in this chapter.

## A NEW KIND OF HARM

It began with a home visit. A nurse arrived to check on Mrs. Green, a 63-year-old woman recovering from COVID related respiratory complications. Her pulse oximeter, gleaming on the nightstand, displayed a reassuring 98 percent. Yet Mrs. Green sat forward, struggling to complete a sentence. The nurse hesitated, should she trust the device or her instincts? Minutes later, paramedics confirmed what the nurse's intuition already knew: the patient's true oxygen saturation was 86 percent on arterial blood gas.

That day, the event was documented as equipment malfunction. But the failure was not mechanical; it was algorithmic. The oximeter's calibration algorithm had never been properly validated across darker skin tones (Martin et al., 2024). For those of us who lead in quality, safety, and patient experience, such moments demand a redefinition of harm. We used to think of safety as tangible, falls, medication errors, infections. Now, harm can emerge from information itself. When AI systems misclassify patients or perpetuate gaps in representation, the outcome is not a glitch, it is preventable, systemic harm (Obermeyer et al., 2019).

AI's brilliance lies in pattern recognition and predictive precision, but its danger hides in what it cannot see. The same mathematics that improve care can also conceal inequity. Just as we investigate a retained surgical sponge, we must learn to investigate *retained bias in code* (Amann et al., 2020).

When I first read the FDA's pulse oximetry advisory, I realized the problem was not only technological, but it was also cultural. We have built vast infrastructures to prevent physical harm, yet digital harm often escapes our notice because it doesn't fit our incident taxonomy. Patients, however, experience care as one continuous story. To them, the algorithm's accuracy is inseparable from the clinician's compassion. When a model's output contradicts human observation and the human defers to the machine, trust fractures. Mrs. Green's story reminds us that bias can hide inside the tools we trust most.

## Mapping Algorithmic Bias to Joint Commission and CMS Safety Expectations

Although neither Joint Commission nor CMS currently uses the term *algorithmic bias* explicitly in their standards, the risks associated with biased or opaque algorithms fall squarely within existing patient safety, quality, and equity expectations. When viewed through a safety lens, algorithmic bias represents a latent system failure; one that meets established definitions of preventable harm, variation in care, and inequitable outcomes.

Why it matters to event review teams: when risk scoring tools underperform for a subgroup, that is a latent condition that belongs in the same queue as medication safety signals. Joint Commission already expects leaders to identify such system risks under LD/QPS/PI. A practical test is simple: ask whether the alert performs similarly after stratification by race/language/sex; if not, queue an RCA/FMEA cycle.

## JOINT COMMISSION: PATIENT SAFETY AND LEADERSHIP STANDARDS

1. Systems Based Risk Identification (LD, PI, and QPS Standards)

Joint Commission requires organizations to identify and mitigate risks arising from systems, processes, and technology. Algorithms that influence clinical decisions such as risk scoring, deterioration alerts, or diagnostic support are part of the care delivery system. If these tools perform differently across patient populations or obscure true clinical risk, they represent a system vulnerability that warrants formal review under quality and patient safety standards.

Algorithmic bias aligns with the Joint Commission's expectation that organizations proactively identify *latent conditions* that could contribute to harm, even in the absence of a sentinel event. Failure to examine how algorithms perform across race, language, sex, or socioeconomic groups constitutes a gap in system risk assessment.

2. Data Integrity and Use in Performance Improvement (QPS/PI)

Joint Commission expects organizations to use data responsibly to drive improvement. When AI tools rely on historical data that reflect inequitable care patterns, the resulting outputs may perpetuate those inequities. Treating algorithmic outputs as unquestioned "truth" conflicts with standards requiring leaders to understand the limitations of their data and ensure it supports safe, effective care. In this context, algorithmic bias is a performance improvement issue: the data source itself may be introducing harm.

3. Health Care Equity Standards (2023)

Joint Commission's Health Care Equity standards explicitly require organizations to identify disparities and take action to reduce them. Algorithms that under detect deterioration, under prioritize risk, or misclassify patients from certain populations directly undermine this requirement. Equity focused stratification must therefore extend beyond outcomes to include how digital tools perform across populations. Failing to assess algorithmic impact on equity is functionally equivalent to failing to stratify outcomes data. (Joint Commission (Health Care Equity), 2023).

## CMS: CONDITIONS OF PARTICIPATION AND QUALITY PROGRAMS

1. Conditions of Participation (CoPs): Quality Assessment and Performance Improvement (QAPI)

CMS requires organizations to maintain an effective QAPI program that identifies adverse events and high risk processes. Algorithms used in clinical decision making are high risk processes by definition when they influence triage, diagnosis, monitoring, or treatment decisions. Algorithmic bias fits within CMS's expectation that organizations analyze *process failures*, not just outcomes. When AI-driven tools systematically miss risk in certain populations, this constitutes a QAPI issue even if no single event triggers an immediate investigation.

2. Patient Safety and Non-Discrimination Expectations

CMS programs emphasize equitable access, non-discrimination, and consistent quality across populations. Algorithms trained on incomplete or biased datasets may unintentionally violate these principles by producing differential care recommendations. In this way, algorithmic bias creates exposure not only to safety risk but also to compliance and civil rights concerns.

3. Value Based Purchasing and Outcome Measurement

CMS increasingly ties reimbursement to outcomes and patient experience. If algorithms contribute to delayed recognition of harm or diminished patient confidence particularly among marginalized populations those effects may surface in publicly reported measures such as readmissions, complications, or Likelihood to Recommend. Algorithmic bias thus becomes both a safety risk and a financial risk under CMS programs.

## REFRAMING ALGORITHMIC BIAS AS A REPORTABLE SAFETY RISK

Mapped to existing expectations, algorithmic bias should be treated similarly to other system failures:

- As a **latent safety risk** subject to proactive assessment
- As a **process failure** appropriate for RCA or FMEA

- As an **equity gap** requiring stratified analysis
- As a **leadership accountability issue** within governance structures

This framing allows organizations to apply familiar safety science tools: Root Cause Analyşis, Failure Mode and Effects Analysis, Just Culture without waiting for new regulations or technology specific standards. By integrating algorithm oversight into existing Joint Commission and CMS aligned safety infrastructure, organizations can detect harm they cannot easily see and ensure that digital tools support, rather than silently distort, safe and equitable care.

## HOW BIAS GETS BUILT IN

Bias rarely begins with intent; it begins with inheritance. Every algorithm reflects the data that trained it, the collective memory of past choices and omissions. When datasets mirror inequitable access or incomplete documentation, the algorithm learns those patterns as truth. In safety language, that is a *latent condition*: an error waiting silently within design (Wachter, 2023).

Several common types of bias emerge along this path:

**Sampling bias** occurs when datasets over-represent some groups and under-represent others. For example, a sepsis prediction model trained primarily on patients from large tertiary academic hospitals may misjudge severity or delay alerts when applied in rural critical access hospitals, where baseline acuity, transfer thresholds, and resource availability differ substantially.

**Measurement bias** arises when devices or data capture methods perform differently across populations. A well-documented example is pulse oximetry, where light-based sensors have been shown to overestimate oxygen saturation in individuals with darker skin tones, leading to missed hypoxemia and delayed escalation of care (Sjoding et al., 2020).

**Label bias** develops when outcome definitions rely on subjective, contextual, or socially mediated judgments. For instance, classifying hospital readmissions as indicators of poor quality without accounting for housing instability, caregiver availability, or access to outpatient services can systematically mislabel socially vulnerable patients and the teams caring for them.

**Deployment bias** occurs when models built for one setting are applied in another without recalibration. A common example is deploying a hospital-trained deterioration or medication-risk algorithm into home-based care or remote monitoring environments, where data frequency, patient behavior, and response pathways differ, increasing false alarms or masking true risk.

Each of these biases behaves like an unreported near miss: silent, cumulative, and invisible until damage is done (Buolamwini & Gebru, 2018).

In future reviews of AI-assisted risk alerts, safety analysts may find that predictive models perform best for those already best served. A pressure injury algorithm, for example, could trigger earlier for patients with complete documentation but later for those with sparse records, often individuals from marginalized communities. The algorithm, in such cases, would not be malfunctioning; it would be performing exactly as designed. Recognizing bias is not an act of accusation but one of vigilance.

## From Transparency to Trust: The Black Box Problem

Trust is the quiet currency of safe care. Yet many AI systems still operate as black boxes, their logic hidden from those who rely on them. A clinician may receive an alert reading *"High risk for deterioration"* without understanding why. When these tools fail, reactions often swing between distrust, abandoning AI entirely, or blind reliance to avoid blame. Both extremes are unsafe (Wachter, 2023).

True transparency extends beyond open code; it requires transparency of reasoning. A responsible model should be able to articulate which data points shaped its output, its confidence level, and plausible alternative explanations. The next generation of clinical systems may feature interactive "rationale windows" that display these elements in real time, transforming algorithms from opaque oracles into conversation partners (Amann et al., 2020). In our sentinel reviews, the 'Was AI involved?' entry is now a standard header; if yes, we attach model version + data slice alongside the MAR and device logs.

## Embedding Explainability into Just Culture

As AI becomes a co-participant in care, accountability must evolve. When an algorithm contributes to harm, the reflex should not be to punish clinicians for "following bad guidance" but to examine *why* the failure occurred. A Just Culture lens helps distinguish human error from design error: Was the harm due to model bias, lack of training, or unclear system limits? (Marx, 2001).

Future event reviews may routinely ask, *"Was AI involved?"* This simple question can surface systemic contributors hidden in data or code. For instance, studies have shown that outdated variables, such as over weighting white blood cell count over lactate, can skew sepsis predictions and delay escalation (Obermeyer et al., 2019).

Embedding explainability within Just Culture ensures shared accountability. When bias or error arises from an algorithm's blind spot, corrective action should target the system, not the individual. This fusion of ethical learning and technological transparency may define the next frontier of safety culture, where humans and machines learn accountability together.

As algorithmic bias emerges as a new category of patient safety risk, national accrediting bodies have begun to formalize expectations for how healthcare organizations govern, monitor, and learn from artificial intelligence. In 2025, Joint Commission, in partnership with the Coalition for Health AI (CHAI), released *Guidance on the Responsible Use of AI in Healthcare (RUAIH)*, a high level framework intended to help organizations safely deploy and oversee AI across clinical, operational, and administrative settings (Joint Commission, 2025).

The RUAIH guidance explicitly acknowledges that while AI holds transformative potential enhancing diagnostic precision, operational efficiency, and care coordination, it also introduces new forms of risk that traditional safety systems were not designed to detect. These include algorithmic bias, opaque decision logic, data drift, inappropriate reliance on automation, and privacy vulnerabilities. Importantly, the guidance frames these risks not as technical failures alone, but as patient safety, equity, and governance concerns that require structured oversight and human accountability

Joint Commission and CHAI identify seven core elements of responsible AI use. Each of which maps directly to the safety concepts explored throughout this chapter:

1. **AI Policies and Governance Structures**

Organizations are expected to establish formal governance mechanisms for AI oversight, including clear leadership accountability, multidisciplinary review, and routine reporting to governing bodies. As part of this structure, algorithm tiering should be integrated into the Medication Safety dashboard cadence, ensuring that higher-risk or patient-facing algorithms receive more frequent review, monitoring, and escalation. This approach aligns directly with the chapter's proposal for Algorithm Safety Review Committees, positioning algorithm oversight as a core function of safety leadership and medication safety governance rather than an isolated IT responsibility.

2. **Patient Privacy and Transparency**

RUAIH emphasizes that patient trust depends on transparency about when and how AI influences care. Patients should be informed when AI meaningfully affects clinical decisions, and consent should be obtained where appropriate. This reinforces the chapter's argument that invisible algorithmic influence undermines trust in ways patients experience as unsafe, even when no traditional error is recorded

3. **Data Security and Data Use Protections**

The guidance underscores strong data governance, including encryption, access controls, and strict limits on secondary data use. From a safety perspective, this reframes data misuse and re-identification risk as forms of organizational harm with ethical and legal consequences, expanding the scope of what safety leaders must oversee in AI-enabled environments

4. **Ongoing Quality Monitoring**

A central theme of RUAIH is that AI tools cannot be treated as static products. Algorithms evolve, data drift occurs, and performance can degrade unevenly across populations. Continuous, risk-based monitoring is therefore essential. This mirrors the chapter's emphasis on learning loops, bias audits, and the integration of algorithm performance into existing quality and safety dashboards. In practice, this includes building a fairness panel into the monthly harm huddle, enabling teams to routinely review algorithm performance across patient subgroups, identify emerging disparities, and trigger timely corrective action before harm occurs.

5. **Voluntary, Blinded Reporting of AI Safety Related Events**

The guidance encourages confidential reporting of AI-related near misses and harms through existing patient safety structures, such as Patient Safety Organizations (PSOs). In practice, this includes routing AI-related near misses through voluntary reporting systems to the PSO with an AI-specific tag, enabling aggregation, trend analysis, and learning across organizations. This approach reinforces the chapter's call to treat algorithmic bias as a reportable safety risk, even when harm is subtle, delayed, or distributed across populations rather than concentrated in a single event.

6. **Risk and Bias Assessment**

RUAIH explicitly recognizes that bias can arise at any stage of the AI lifecycle, from training data to deployment context and may not be apparent until outcomes are examined across subgroups. Organizations are encouraged to assess representativeness, validate tools on local populations, and monitor for differential performance over time. This directly supports the chapter's framing of bias as a latent condition that requires proactive detection rather than retrospective blame.

7. **Education and Training**

Finally, the guidance emphasizes AI literacy and role-specific training so clinicians and staff understand both the capabilities and limitations of AI tools. This aligns with the chapter's caution that new quality and safety leaders may mistake AI-generated completeness for correctness, underscoring the need to train leaders to validate, question, and contextualize algorithmic output rather than defer to it.

Collectively, Joint Commission and CHAI guidance affirms the central argument of this chapter: algorithmic bias is not a future concern or a technical edge case; it is a present day safety risk that fits squarely within existing quality, equity, and governance expectations. By embedding AI oversight into familiar safety infrastructure governance committees, event reporting systems, quality monitoring, and Just Culture organizations can address digital harm without waiting for entirely new regulatory frameworks.

In this way, RUAIH does not introduce a new safety paradigm so much as it extends safety science into the digital domain, reinforcing that human judgment, transparency, and accountability remain essential as AI becomes a routine participant in clinical decision making. Figure 1. translates the seven elements of Responsible Use of AI in Healthcare (RUAIH) articulated by Joint Commission and CHAI into concrete expectations for quality and safety event review. The crosswalk illustrates how governance, transparency, data stewardship, continuous monitoring, reporting, bias assessment, and education are operationalized during AI-assisted analyses, reinforcing that human judgment, accountability, and learning remain central to safe and equitable use of AI in healthcare.

*Figure 1. Operationalizing responsible use of AI in event review*

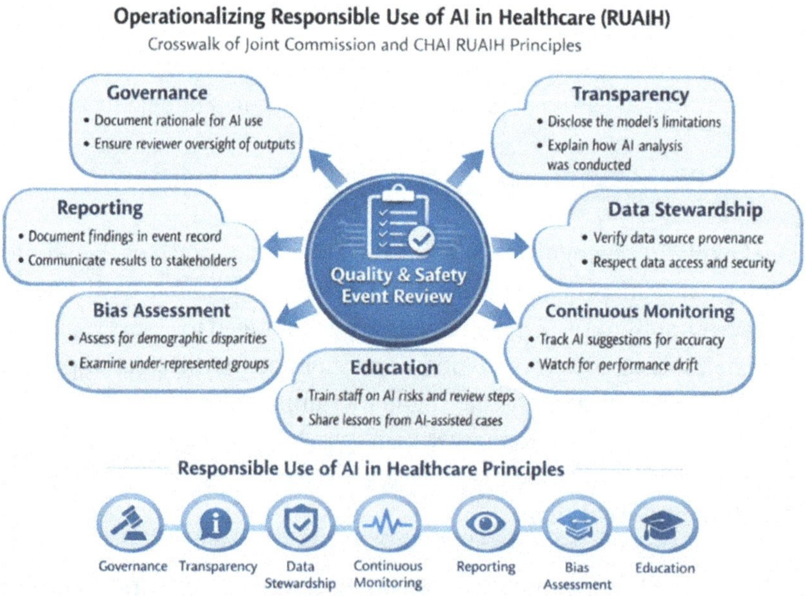

## ADAPTING SAFETY TOOLS FOR ARTIFICIAL INTELLIGENCE OVERSIGHT

Traditional safety frameworks can be reimagined to identify, prevent, and learn from algorithmic harm in healthcare.

- **Root Cause Analysis (RCA):** Traditionally used to analyze sentinel events; now adapted to trace the origin of bias within data or model design. *Example:* Detecting calibration bias in pulse oximetry readings.
- **Failure Mode and Effects Analysis (FMEA):** Originally applied to prevent process failures; now used to predict how bias might propagate through an algorithm. *Example:* Identifying missing subgroups in training data.
- **Apparent Cause Analysis (ACA):** Designed for rapid review of near misses; adapted as a short term bias audit to catch early warning signs. *Example:* Investigating false negatives in a fall risk prediction model

When clinicians and data scientists join the same RCA huddle, the focus shifts from *accuracy* to *accountability*. I recall a review of an image based wound-severity model. A nurse remarked, "It said low risk, but I could smell infection." The data scientist replied, "The model never saw infections that looked like this." That single conversation reframed how we defined algorithmic context. Safety science doesn't need reinvention; it needs translation. The discipline that once turned near misses into lessons can now turn model errors into insight (Marx, 2001).

### Strengthening Oversight Through an Algorithm Safety Committee

As artificial intelligence becomes inseparable from clinical decision making, healthcare will require a new form of oversight; one that treats algorithmic safety as an integral component of patient safety. Traditional committees focus on medication errors, infections, or occupational hazards; few are structured to examine the safety of algorithms that shape diagnosis, triage, or treatment. To support consistent identification and learning, organizations should adopt a house style definition of an "algorithmic event," explicitly defining when algorithm outputs influence clinical decisions, contribute to near misses, or introduce bias. These events should be logged within the Safety Intelligence Platform under a dedicated algorithmic safety category, ensuring visibility, trend analysis, and escalation alongside other safety signals.

In the near future, organizations may establish Algorithm Safety Review Committees (ASRCs) to review these events and ensure that algorithms remain transparent, fair, and clinically sound throughout their life cycle, embedding algorithm oversight within established quality and safety governance rather than treating it as an isolated technical function. Just as a medication safety committee evaluates a drug's indications, contraindications, and side effects, an ASRC would oversee algorithms with the same rigor, recognizing that software, too, can cause harm (Wachter, 2023).

A future-ready ASRC could:

1. Vet algorithms before deployment.
2. Monitor ongoing performance and retraining cycles.
3. Integrate algorithm related events into the patient-safety reporting system.
4. Educate clinicians on model limitations, escalation protocols, and safe override practices.

Membership would be deliberately diverse; clinicians, data scientists, human factors specialists, ethicists, and patient representatives, bridging the gap between data logic and bedside reality. In mature systems, each algorithm might receive a bias risk tier, prompting targeted safety analyses when a high impact tool is identified.

Research on pulse oximetry calibration revealed how underrepresentation of darker skin tones produced systematic error in oxygen readings (Sjoding et al., 2020). A committee attuned to algorithmic safety could translate such findings into procurement standards, vendor criteria, and staff training. Bias prevention, in this sense, becomes to data what infection prevention is to the body: an ongoing discipline of vigilance, learning, and adaptation. Algorithmic governance will not replace human judgment; it will refine and protect it.

## Integrating AI into Event Analysis Frameworks

As AI merges into daily workflows, traditional Root Cause Analysis (RCA) and Sentinel Event Review processes must expand. These methods were designed for human driven systems, miscommunication, handoff failures, or procedural errors, not for probabilistic reasoning or model drift. In the near future, AI-augmented event analysis will become a core safety discipline. Investigations may include:

- **Model version tracking**, linking an event to the specific algorithm iteration and training dataset.
- **Bias audits**, assessing whether underrepresentation contributed to error.
- **Explainability mapping**, translating each computational step into human-readable logic.
- **Feedback loops**, tying post event findings to model refinement and staff education.

These practices represent a cultural shift from viewing technology as a static tool to seeing it as a living system requiring surveillance, maintenance, and moral accountability. AI event analysis committees could sit beside existing safety bodies, ensuring algorithm related harms are examined with equal rigor. Over time, each investigation becomes part of the organization's collective intelligence, transforming algorithmic missteps into new safety knowledge (Friedman et al., 2017).

Figure 2 shows how traditional event analysis methods are expanded to account for AI-specific risks, illustrating the integration of model version tracking, bias audits, explainability checks, and structured feedback loops into established safety investigation frameworks. By visualizing these additional layers, the figure highlights how safety teams can systematically examine the digital contributors to harm and ensure that algorithm related failures are evaluated with the same rigor as human and process based events. This expanded framework underscores the need for continuous monitoring and transparent oversight as AI becomes embedded in routine clinical decision making.

*Figure 2. Expanding traditional event analysis to include AI-specific risks*

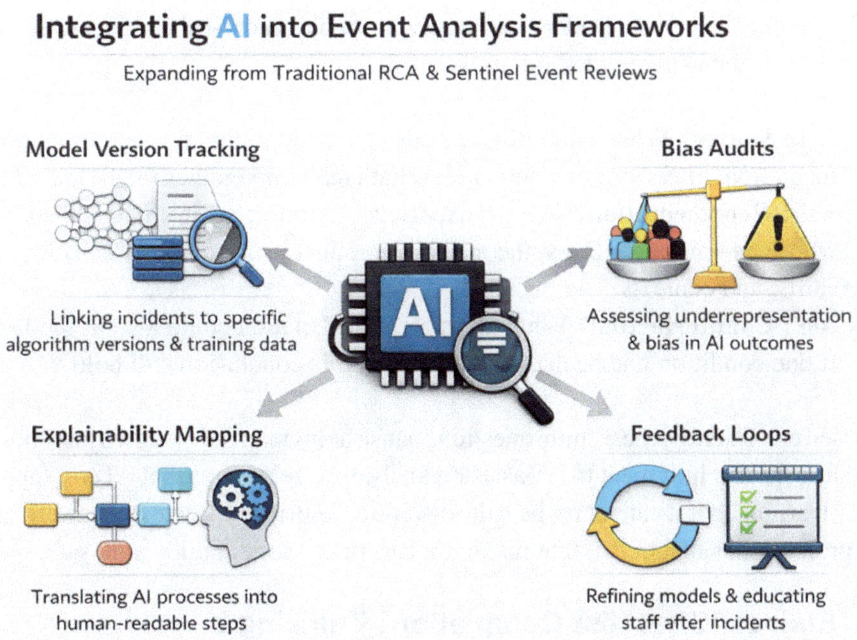

## Training New Quality and Safety Leaders to Detect Bias in AI-Assisted Event Reviews

As AI becomes more common in Root Cause Analyses (RCA), Failure Mode and Effects Analyses (FMEA), and Apparent Cause Analyses (ACA), many new quality and safety leaders encounter a subtle risk early in their development: mistaking completeness for correctness. AI-generated case reviews often appear thorough. They organize timelines, surface contributing factors, map causes to categories and produce language that aligns neatly with established frameworks. To a new leader, the output can feel authoritative, especially when it checks every required box. The danger is not that AI produces poor analysis. The danger is that it produces convincing analysis without discernment.

Experienced reviewers know that safety analysis is not just about structure; it is about judgment. It requires understanding how events unfold in real work, recognizing what is missing, and questioning assumptions embedded in the narrative. New leaders who rely solely on AI output without grounding in traditional review methods may unintentionally overlook bias, misclassify causes, or accept conclusions that feel logical but are incomplete or misleading.

To counter this risk, leaders can apply a simple micro-rubric during review, regardless of the analytic method used:

- **Ask: Source?** What data informed this conclusion; direct observation, documentation, interview, or inference? What is assumed rather than verified?
- **Ask: Representation?** Whose experience is reflected in this analysis, and whose is missing? Does the narrative reflect work-as-done across roles, shifts, and contexts?
- **Ask: Counterfactual?** What alternative explanation could also fit the facts? If one condition had been different, would this conclusion still hold?

Used consistently, these three questions pause helps teams slow down just enough to restore human judgment to AI-assisted analysis. It reinforces that AI can support safety learning, but it cannot replace the disciplined curiosity, contextual awareness, and professional skepticism that make improvement work credible and safe.

## The Risk of "Checklist Completion" Thinking

One of the first training challenges is helping new leaders move beyond checklist thinking. AI can generate RCAs or FMEAs that appear polished and comprehensive, but safety work has never been about producing a document that looks right. It is about asking uncomfortable questions:

- Whose perspective is absent?
- Which assumptions went unchallenged?
- What conditions made this failure more likely *for this patient*?
- What does the data not explain?

AI systems are trained on historical patterns. If past analyses underrepresented certain patient populations, minimized social context, or normalized unsafe work-arounds, those patterns may reappear in AI-generated output. Without the ability to recognize these gaps, new leaders may unintentionally reinforce existing inequities or system blind spots.

## Teaching Validation Before Acceptance

Training should emphasize a simple but critical principle: AI output must be validated, not accepted. New leaders need to learn how to interrogate AI-assisted analyses the same way they would question a junior analyst or consultant.

Effective validation training includes teaching leaders to ask:

- **Source questions:** What data informed this conclusion? Is it event specific or generalized?
- **Representation questions:** Does the analysis account for patient characteristics that affect risk (e.g., race, language, disability, home environment)?
- **Process questions:** Does this explanation reflect how work actually happens, or how policy says it should happen?
- **Equity questions:** Would this analysis look different if the patient or staff involved belonged to a different group?
- **Counterfactual questions:** What alternative explanations were not explored?

These questions help leaders detect algorithmic bias not by understanding code, but by applying safety thinking.

## Grounding New Leaders in Pre-AI Safety Skills

One of the most effective safeguards against overreliance on AI is ensuring that new leaders are trained first in *manual* event review skills. This includes:

- Conducting interviews without pre-populated cause lists
- Mapping timelines from raw data and firsthand accounts
- Facilitating multidisciplinary RCA discussions

- Distinguishing between human error, at-risk behavior, and system design issues
- Identifying latent conditions without relying on templates

When leaders understand how to build an analysis from the ground up, they are better equipped to recognize when AI output is helpful and when it is misleading. AI should accelerate analysis, not replace the analyst.

## Normalizing Skepticism as a Leadership Skill

New quality and safety leaders often hesitate to challenge AI output, especially when it appears more "complete" than their own early analyses. Training programs should explicitly normalize skepticism as a professional skill. Questioning AI is not resistance to innovation; it is responsible oversight.

Organizations can reinforce this by:

- Requiring human-authored executive summaries alongside AI-assisted analyses
- Incorporating bias checks into RCA and FMEA review processes
- Encouraging leaders to document where AI output was modified or rejected
- Reviewing AI-assisted cases in peer forums focused on learning, not performance

This approach reinforces that accountability remains human, even when tools are digital.

## From AI Assistance to Informed Judgment

Ultimately, training new quality and safety leaders is not about teaching them how to use AI, it is about teaching them how to think with it. AI can surface patterns, suggest contributing factors, and organize information. It cannot replace contextual understanding, ethical judgment, or responsibility for harm prevention.

When leaders learn to validate AI output against lived experience, equity considerations, and system realities, AI becomes a powerful ally rather than a silent authority. In this model, safety analysis remains what it has always been: a disciplined practice of curiosity, humility, and accountability; now applied to both human and algorithmic systems.

As illustrated in Figure 17.3, the structured validation process for AI-assisted case reviews highlights several critical checkpoints designed to ensure accuracy, fairness, and alignment with real-world practice. The figure shows how reviewers systematically assess underlying assumptions, interrogate data sources for completeness and relevance, examine outputs for potential bias, and verify whether the narrative reflects actual clinical workflows rather than idealized models. Together, these steps provide a disciplined approach to validating AI-generated conclusions before they are incorporated into safety analyses, reinforcing that human judgment remains essential in interpreting and contextualizing algorithmic insights.

*Figure 3. A structured validation process for AI-assisted case reviews, highlighting key checkpoints for accuracy, bias, and real-world alignment*

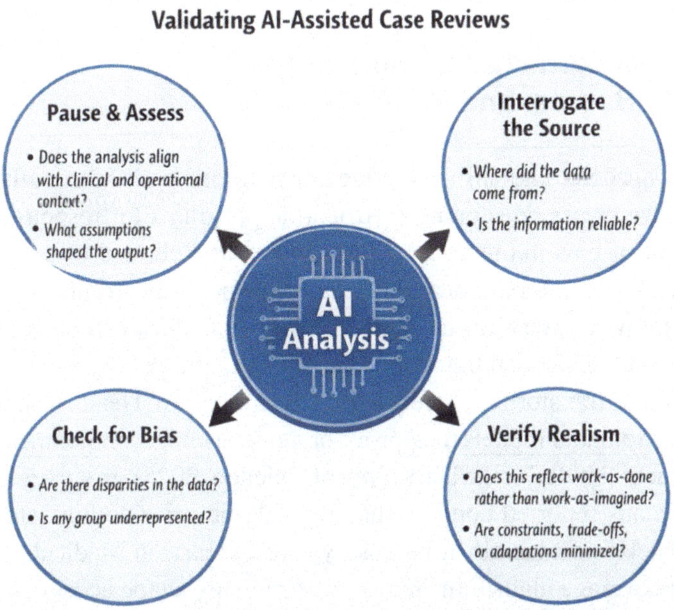


## The Next Horizon of Safety: Patients, Algorithms, and Oversight

The next frontier of safety will extend far beyond hospitals, laboratories, or dashboards, it will emerge wherever data meets human judgment. Artificial intelligence is no longer the exclusive domain of clinicians or engineers. Patients, regulators, insurers, and accreditation bodies are now building and deploying algorithms of their own. Each brings new visibility, and new vulnerability to the system of care.

## Patient Empowered AI and the Challenge to Clinical Authority

Patients are increasingly arriving at the point of care equipped with AI-generated insights, symptom predictions, wearable data, or personalized treatment forecasts. While this democratization of data can empower patients, it also shifts traditional power dynamics. When a patient's AI tool disagrees with a clinician's recommendation, how do we ensure that *disagreement itself* remains safe? Safety governance must evolve to include patient facing algorithm awareness, documenting when patient supplied outputs influence decision-making and ensuring clinicians are trained to respond constructively (Tun et al. 2025)

## External Oversight via AI: Regulators, Accrediting Bodies, and Payors

Oversight agencies are also adopting algorithmic tools. Accrediting bodies like URAC have begun developing certification programs for responsible AI use, requiring proof of bias mitigation, fairness audits, and clinical oversight (URAC, 2025). Similarly, regulators such as the U.S. Food and Drug Administration (FDA) now treat many AI-driven tools as "high-risk" medical devices, subject to ongoing performance monitoring and bias audits (U.S. FDA, 2024).

Even payors are transforming safety indirectly through AI. Health insurers increasingly rely on automated models to approve or deny coverage, sometimes overriding clinical judgment (NORC at the University of Chicago, 2025). In surveys, more than 60% of physicians reported concern that algorithmic prior authorization systems contribute to delays or denials of necessary care (American Medical Association, 2024). These coverage algorithms may unintentionally shape access and therefore safety long before a clinician intervenes.

## Algorithmic Governance in a Global Context

Globally, the European Union AI Act now classifies most healthcare AI as high-risk, requiring transparent data governance, formal risk management, and post-market monitoring (European Commission, 2024). For U.S. hospitals, this means procurement questions will increasingly mirror EU-style high risk due diligence expectations such as documentation of training data, bias testing, and monitoring plans even before FDA classification decisions are finalized.

The World Health Organization (WHO) has issued ethics guidance emphasizing accountability, explainability, and equity in AI-enabled health systems (WHO, 2021). For U.S. organizations, this translates into an expectation that algorithm behavior must be explainable to clinicians and patients, and that equity impacts will be reviewed as part of routine quality and safety governance, not treated as optional research activities.

In the United Kingdom, NICE has integrated AI evaluation standards directly into health technology assessment and procurement processes (NICE, 2023). For U.S. payors and health systems, this signals a future in which reimbursement, contracting, and vendor selection will increasingly depend on evidence of real-world performance, monitoring capability, and safety oversight not just FDA clearance.

Together, these frameworks point to a shared global direction: algorithmic safety is becoming a baseline expectation across regulators, payors, and purchasers, requiring health systems to operationalize governance, monitoring, and accountability well beyond compliance alone.

## A Broader Lens on Accountability

As AI enters every tier of healthcare, safety leaders will move from managing *incidents* to managing *intelligence*. They will be asked not just "What went wrong?" but "Which algorithm flagged it, trained it, or missed it?" The field of safety will expand from tracking harm caused by people or processes to monitoring harm caused or predicted by data itself. No single actor, clinician, coder, regulator, or patient will hold full accountability. Safety will depend on shared transparency and mutual learning. Just as infection prevention became a collective discipline, algorithmic safety will require an ecosystem approach that links human ethics, digital design, and system governance.

## PRACTICE IMPACT

## Building the Learning Loop

The future of safety will depend less on detecting harm and more on learning fast enough to prevent its return. Once AI-related findings bias audits, override logs, version histories, enter event reporting systems, they can fuel a continuous learning loop within the health system. In mature frameworks, every AI interaction becomes a lesson. A clinician override may signal mistrust; repeated false negatives in one subgroup may indicate drift. Aggregated, these signals guide retraining, redesign, and education. One practical indicator is the percentage of AI alerts overridden by clinicians that are later validated as correct or incorrect based on downstream clinical outcomes, providing a direct measure of both algorithm reliability and human AI alignment.

An effective learning loop bridges three levels of intelligence:

1. **Human intelligence**, where clinicians interpret and challenge algorithmic output.
2. **Artificial intelligence**, which adapts through feedback from real-world outcomes.
3. **Organizational intelligence**, which integrates those insights into policy, dashboards, and oversight.

When these layers connect, data silos dissolve. Imagine a dashboard where algorithm performance and fairness metrics sit beside infection and medication error indicators. Each anomaly, algorithmic or clinical, triggers review. Over time, AI safety dashboards may inform board-level oversight, helping leaders balance innovation with accountability. Ultimately, AI should not be seen as a fixed product but as a learning partner, capable of reflection when guided by human ethics. In this symbiosis, clinicians learn from algorithms, algorithms learn from clinicians, and organizations learn from both. What emerges is not only safer AI but a more intelligent, self correcting system of care. As illustrated in Figure 4, the continuous learning loop shows how human, artificial, and organizational intelligence interact to detect emerging risks, adapt systems, and strengthen safety over time. The figure emphasizes the dynamic exchange of insights between clinicians, algorithmic tools, and governance structures, creating an iterative cycle of monitoring, feedback, and system improvement. Through this integrated loop, safety programs evolve alongside AI-enabled workflows, ensuring that both human judgment and machine-generated insights contribute to a more resilient and responsive care environment.

*Figure 4. The future of safety as a learning loop*

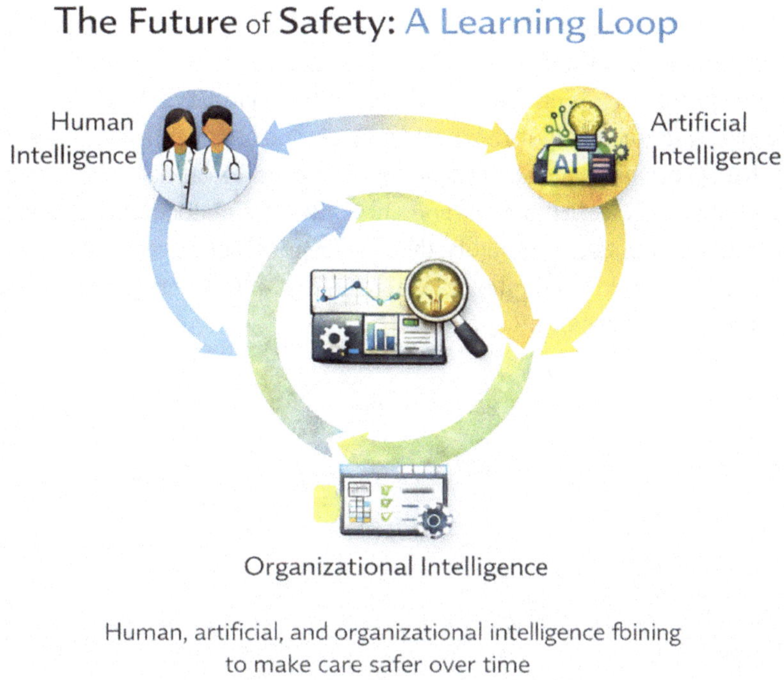


## CONCLUSION

This chapter argues that artificial intelligence introduces a new form of patient harm; algorithmic bias that often remains invisible within traditional safety surveillance. Because AI systems inherit the limitations and inequities embedded in their training data, they can distort clinical risk assessment, misclassify patients, and delay recognition of deterioration without triggering familiar safety signals. The chapter reframes algorithmic bias as a latent safety condition that must be managed with the same rigor applied to medication safety, device safety, and system failures.

It demonstrates how established safety science tools such as Root Cause Analysis, Failure Mode and Effects Analysis, Apparent Cause Analysis, and Just Culture can be adapted to examine model design, data quality, subgroup performance, and real world deployment. The chapter proposes Algorithm Safety Review Committees to oversee algorithm validation, monitor fairness over time, and integrate AI-related events into reporting systems. Transparency and explainability are framed as central to maintaining clinician trust, particularly as AI becomes a routine co-participant in decision making.

The chapter also widens the safety lens to include patient facing AI tools, insurer algorithms that influence access to care, and emerging national and global regulatory expectations. It emphasizes the need for continuous learning loops that connect human judgment, algorithm performance, and organizational governance. It cautions that new quality and safety leaders must learn to validate rather than defer to AI-generated analyses. Human oversight, contextual understanding, and ethical judgment remain essential. Ultimately, the chapter positions algorithmic oversight as core patient safety work in a digital era where equity, transparency, and compassion must remain at the center of innovation.

## REFERENCES


Amann, J., Blasimme, A., Vayena, E., Frey, D., & Madai, V. I. (2020). Explainability for artificial intelligence in healthcare: A multidisciplinary perspective. *BMC Medical Informatics and Decision Making, 20*(1), 310. Advance online publication. DOI: 10.1186/s12911-020-01332-6 PMID: 33256715

American Medical Association. (2024). *How AI is leading to more prior-authorization denials.* https://www.ama-assn.org/practice-management/prior-authorization

Buolamwini, J., & Gebru, T. (2018). Gender shades: Intersectional accuracy disparities in commercial gender classification. *Proceedings of Machine Learning Research, 81*, 1–15. http://proceedings.mlr.press/v81/buolamwini18a.html

European Commission. (2024). *EU Artificial Intelligence Act: Legislative text and implementation guidance.* https://digital-strategy.ec.europa.eu

Friedman, C. P., Rubin, J. C., & Sullivan, K. J. (2017). Toward an information infrastructure for global health improvement. *Yearbook of Medical Informatics, 26*(1), 16–23. DOI: 10.15265/IY-2017-004 PMID: 28480469

Joint Commission. (2025). *Joint Commission and Coalition for Health AI (CHAI) release initial guidance to support responsible AI adoption across U.S. health systems.* https://www.jointcommission.org/en-us/knowledge-library/news/2025-09-jc-and-chai-release-initial-guidance-to-support-responsible-ai-adoption

Martin, D., Johns, C., Sorrell, L., Healy, E., Phull, M., Olusanya, S., Peters, M., & Fabes, J. (2024). Effect of skin tone on the accuracy of the estimation of arterial oxygen saturation by pulse oximetry: A systematic review. *British Journal of Anaesthesia, 132*(5), 945–956. DOI: 10.1016/j.bja.2024.01.023 PMID: 38368234

Marx, D. (2001). *Patient safety and the "Just Culture": A primer for health care executives.* Columbia University.

National Institute for Health and Care Excellence. (2023). *Evidence standards framework for digital health technologies: Update for AI tools.* https://www.nice.org.uk

NORC at the University of Chicago. (2025). *Artificial intelligence in health insurance: The use and regulation of AI in utilization management.* https://www.norc.org

Obermeyer, Z., Powers, B., Vogeli, C., & Mullainathan, S. (2019). Dissecting racial bias in an algorithm used to manage the health of populations. *Science, 366*(6464), 447–453. DOI: 10.1126/science.aax2342 PMID: 31649194

Sjoding, M. W., Dickson, R. P., Iwashyna, T. J., Gay, S. E., & Valley, T. S. (2020). Racial bias in pulse oximetry measurement. *The New England Journal of Medicine, 383*(25), 2477–2478. DOI: 10.1056/NEJMc2029240 PMID: 33326721

The Joint Commission. (2023). *Responsible use of health data certification for hospitals* [Press release]. The Joint Commission.

Tun, H. M., Abdul Rahman, H., Naing, L., & Malik, O. A. (2025). Trust in artificial intelligence–based clinical decision support systems among health care workers: A systematic review. *Journal of Medical Internet Research, 27*, e69678. DOI: 10.2196/69678 PMID: 40772775

URAC. (2025). *Health care AI accreditation: Responding to the industry's call for responsible AI implementation.* https://www.urac.org

U.S. Food and Drug Administration. (2021, October 22). *Pulse oximeter accuracy and limitations: FDA safety communication.* https://www.fda.gov/medical-devices/safety-communications/pulse-oximeter-accuracy-and-limitations-fda-safety-communication

U.S. Food and Drug Administration. (2024). *Artificial intelligence and machine learning software as a medical device (discussion paper).* https://www.fda.gov

Wachter, R. M. (2023). *The digital doctor: Hope, hype, and harm at the dawn of medicine's computer age*. McGraw Hill.

World Health Organization. (2021). *Ethics and governance of artificial intelligence for health: WHO guidance.* https://www.who.int

## KEY TERMS AND DEFINITIONS

**Algorithm Safety Review Committee (ASRC):** A multidisciplinary group overseeing AI fairness and performance.

**Algorithmic Bias:** Systematic error in AI outputs caused by skewed or incomplete data.

**Algorithmic Event:** A safety incident or near miss linked to AI behavior or bias.

**Artificial Intelligence (AI):** Machine systems that perform tasks requiring human-like perception or reasoning.

**Bias Audit:** Structured review of data or outputs to identify performance disparities.

**Data Transparency:** Clear disclosure of how data are collected, processed, and applied in AI systems.

**Drift:** Gradual decline in AI model performance as data inputs evolve over time.

**Ethical AI:** The integration of fairness, accountability, and moral principles in algorithm development.

**Event Analysis:** Systematic study of incidents or near misses to uncover contributing factors.

**Explainable AI (XAI):** Techniques that make algorithm reasoning interpretable for human users.

**High-Risk AI:** Systems regulated for their potential to cause significant harm.

**Patient Generated Intelligence:** Insights created by patients using AI or digital health tools.

**Predictive Analytics:** The use of data models to forecast outcomes or behaviors.

**Safety Intelligence Platform:** A system that integrates traditional and AI-related safety data for real-time monitoring.

## APPENDIX I

## Responsible Use of AI: Executive Alignment Framework

Figure 5 maps the RUAIH elements to event review expectations, reinforcing that responsible AI use is a core safety function, not a technical add-on.

*Figure 5. Executive safety interpretation of RUAIH elements*

Translating Responsible Use of AI in Healthcare to Executive Safety Interpretations

| RUAIH Element | Executive Safety Interpretation |
|---|---|
| AI Policies and Governance Structures | AI oversight is embedded within existing safety governance, with clear leadership accountability and documentation of human decision authority |
| Patient Privacy and Transparency | AI influence on care and analysis is **transparent**, with attention to trust, attribution, and **fairness** |
| Data Security and Data Use Protections | Data completeness, representativeness, and secondary use risks are treated as **safety concerns** |
| Ongoing Quality Monitor | AI performance, drift, and subgroup impact are **continuously monitored** through **learning loops** |
| Voluntary, Blinded Reporting | AI-related safety risks and near misses are **reportable** through established safety channels |
| Risk and Bias Assessment | Bias is treated as a **latent safety condition** requiring **proactive detection** |
| Education and Training | Leaders and reviewers are trained to validate, question, and **contextualize** AI output |

# APPENDIX II

## Validating AI assisted Event Review

As illustrated in Figure 6, the validation process for AI-assisted event reviews presents an executive-level checklist designed to ensure responsible use of AI in safety analysis. The figure highlights the key steps reviewers must take before accepting AI-generated conclusions, including verifying underlying assumptions, examining data sources for completeness, checking outputs for potential bias, and confirming alignment with real-world clinical practice. Together, these actions reinforce the central role of human judgment, maintain clear accountability, and support continuous learning within AI-enabled safety workflows.

*Figure 6. Validating an AI-assisted event review*

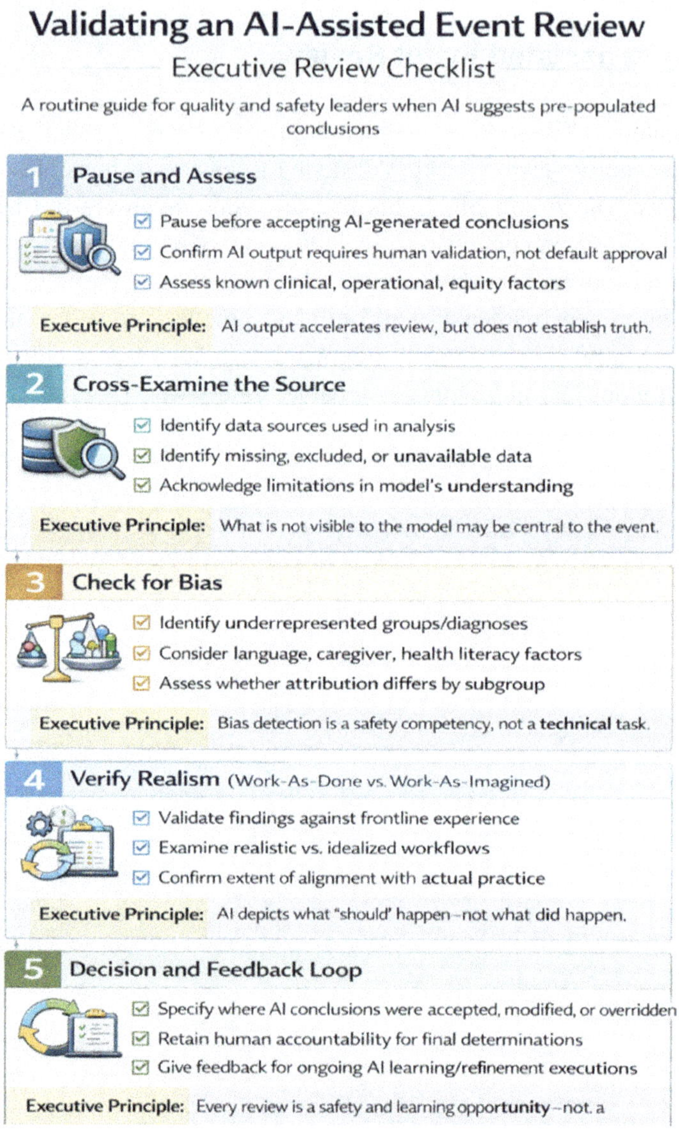
Validating an AI-Assisted Event Review
Executive Review Checklist
A routine guide for quality and safety leaders when AI suggests pre-populated conclusions
1 Pause and Assess
Pause before accepting AI-generated conclusions
Confirm AI output requires human validation, not default approval
Assess known clinical, operational, equity factors
Executive Principle: AI output accelerates review, but does not establish truth.
2 Cross-Examine the Source
Identify data sources used in analysis
Identify missing, excluded, or unavailable data
Acknowledge limitations in model's understanding
Executive Principle: What is not visible to the model may be central to the event.
3 Check for Bias
Identify underrepresented groups/diagnoses
Consider language, caregiver, health literacy factors
Assess whether attribution differs by subgroup
Executive Principle: Bias detection is a safety competency, not a technical task.
4 Verify Realism (Work-As-Done vs. Work-As-Imagined)
Validate findings against frontline experience
Examine realistic vs. idealized workflows
Confirm extent of alignment with actual practice
Executive Principle: AI depicts what "should" happen–not what did happen.
5 Decision and Feedback Loop
Specify where AI conclusions were accepted, modified, or overridden
Retain human accountability for final determinations
Give feedback for ongoing AI learning/refinement executions
Executive Principle: Every review is a safety and learning opportunity–not a

## APPENDIX III

This mock tracer dialogue (Figure 7) illustrates how leaders and frontline teams can clearly articulate responsible use of AI during surveyor conversations by grounding responses in human accountability, real world practice, equity awareness, and sustained learning. Each exchange demonstrates that AI is positioned as a decision support tool rather than an authority, with leaders emphasizing validation against frontline experience, proactive assessment of bias and missing context, and structured reporting into governance systems. Together, the dialogue models how organizations can translate AI governance principles into practical, survey ready explanations that reflect transparency, equity, and continuous improvement in quality and safety oversight.

*Figure 7. Example of mock tracer dialogue related to the use of AI*

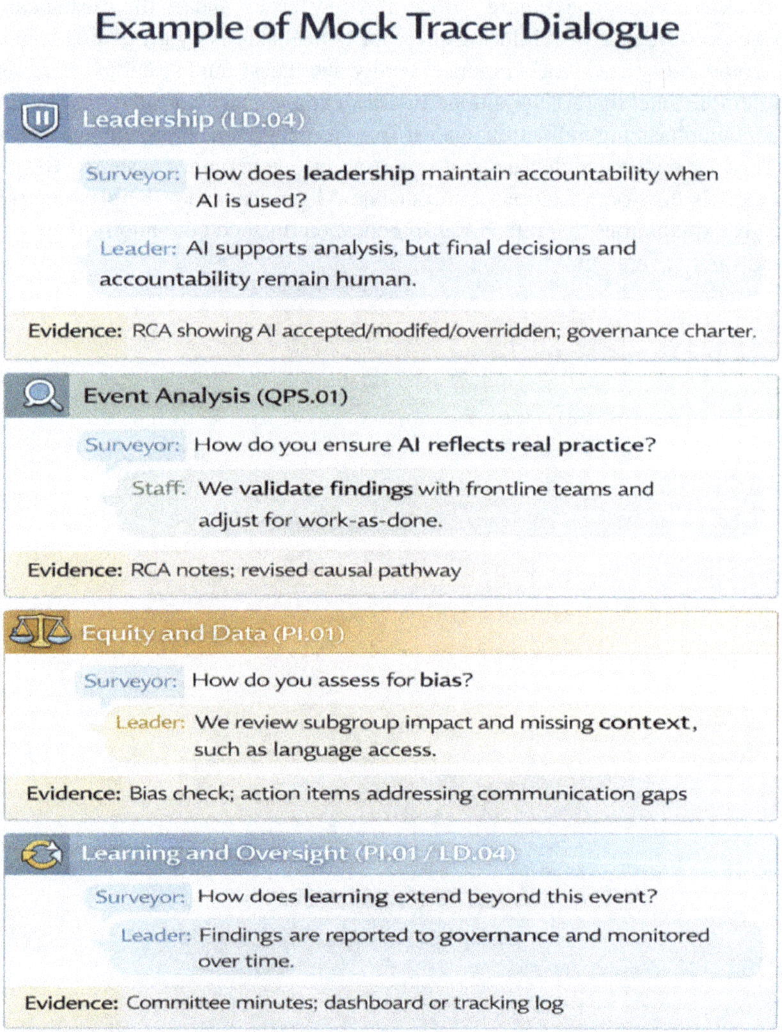
Example of Mock Tracer Dialogue
Leadership (LD.04)
Surveyor: How does leadership maintain accountability when AI is used?
Leader: AI supports analysis, but final decisions and accountability remain human.
Evidence: RCA showing AI accepted/modifed/overridden; governance charter.
Event Analysis (QPS.01)
Surveyor: How do you ensure AI reflects real practice?
Staff: We validate findings with frontline teams and adjust for work-as-done.
Evidence: RCA notes; revised causal pathway
Equity and Data (PI.01)
Surveyor: How do you assess for bias?
Leader: We review subgroup impact and missing context, such as language access.
Evidence: Bias check; action items addressing communication gaps
Learning and Oversight (PI.01 / LD.04)
Surveyor: How does learning extend beyond this event?
Leader: Findings are reported to governance and monitored over time.
Evidence: Committee minutes; dashboard or tracking log

# Chapter 18

# Imagining Care Again: Returning Safety, Quality, and Service to Their Human Roots


## ABSTRACT

*Over time, safety, quality, and service across the continuum of care have become closely linked to metrics, reporting requirements, incentives, and digital systems. These efforts have reduced harm and improved outcomes, while also reshaping how care is understood and practiced. This final chapter reflects on what may have been diminished along the way. Drawing on themes developed throughout the book, including leadership presence, Just Culture, human factors, patient experience, workforce well-being, equity, transitions of care, and artificial intelligence, the chapter considers what safety, quality, and service might look like if guided first by care and responsibility rather than performance and comparison. Using a reflective, practice-based lens grounded in safety science and ethics, the chapter emphasizes that lasting improvement depends on protecting human judgment, relationships, and accountability as care becomes increasingly mediated by technology.*


## INTRODUCTION: REMEMBERING WHY SAFETY AND QUALITY EXIST

Healthcare improvement has long been driven by a basic moral impulse: to protect patients, reduce harm, and deliver care that is both reliable and compassionate. Over time, these aims were translated into systems of measurement, oversight, and accountability. Metrics, dashboards, benchmarks, and digital tools became central to how organizations defined progress. These changes mattered. They brought structure

DOI: 10.4018/979-8-3373-6496-4.ch018

where there had been variation and visibility where there had been silence. Many lives were improved and saved because of them.

At the same time, a quieter shift occurred. As safety, quality, and service became increasingly measured, they also became more distant from the day to day experience of care. What once lived in conversations, judgment calls, and small acts of attention began to live in reports and scores. Improvement slowly moved from something people practiced together to something organizations demonstrated outwardly.

Historically, safety and quality were not treated as separate domains. They were embedded in how clinicians showed care. They appeared in noticing when something felt off, in taking the time to explain, in staying present a moment longer than required. As formal improvement frameworks expanded, these human practices were supplemented and, at times, overshadowed by standardized indicators.

This chapter does not argue against measurement or structure. Instead, it asks a more foundational question: what are these tools meant to serve? As healthcare grows more complex and increasingly digital, how do we ensure that improvement efforts remain grounded in care, responsibility, and trust?

## When Improvement Quietly Shifted Its Focus

The move toward measurement and accountability did not emerge from indifference. It came from urgency. Preventable harm demanded action. Unwarranted variation required attention. Transparency was overdue. Yet as metrics became central to governance and reimbursement, they began to shape attention in powerful ways. What could be counted often became what mattered most. What resisted easy measurement, such as fatigue, moral distress, uncertainty, or erosion of trust, tended to fall to the margins, even though these conditions frequently precede harm (Reason, 2000; Vincent & Amalberti, 2016).

In many organizations, safety discussions gradually migrated away from clinical spaces and into conference rooms. Quality became something reviewed quarterly rather than practiced daily. Service was increasingly reduced to survey results, detached from the context in which care occurred. Care itself did not disappear. But improvement began to feel more like performance than presence. Measurement is not the problem. The problem arises when metrics are treated as ends rather than signals. When numbers become the goal, they risk crowding out the human awareness that makes care safe in the first place.

## Safety as a Human Relationship

At its core, safety is about vulnerability. Patients enter healthcare at moments when they cannot fully protect themselves. They rely on the attention, judgment, and care of others. From their perspective, safety is not experienced through policies or standards. It is experienced through interactions. It shows up in whether someone listens, whether explanations make sense, whether care feels thoughtful rather than rushed. One patient once described feeling safe not after a procedure, but when a nurse paused, sat down, and explained what would happen next. The pause mattered as much as the information.

Leadership presence matters because it reconnects decision making with this reality. When leaders spend time where care happens, listening and observing rather than auditing, they see how safety is actually maintained. They witness the cognitive effort, emotional labor, and trade offs clinicians make every day. Presence alone, however, is not sufficient. People quickly learn whether speaking up leads to action or whether concerns fade into process. Trust grows when issues are addressed and shrinks when they disappear. More than any checklist, trust determines whether risks are raised early enough to prevent harm (Frankel et al., 2017). Safety is not a technical target. It is a relationship built through responsiveness and shared responsibility.

## How Culture Shows Up in Small Moments

Culture is often described in broad terms, yet it is formed in ordinary moments. It is revealed in how leaders respond to mistakes, how questions are received, and how accountability is handled. Just Culture frameworks were developed to support learning while maintaining responsibility by recognizing that systems shape behavior (Marx, 2001). When applied with care, they create space for honesty. When applied rigidly, they risk becoming another compliance exercise.

The most consequential cultural signals tend to surface when something goes wrong. A leader's tone, willingness to listen, and ability to tolerate uncertainty send lasting messages. Over time, these responses shape whether people feel safe telling the truth. Psychological safety plays a central role here. Teams that feel safe to speak up are more likely to identify risks, learn from failure, and improve care (Edmondson, 2018). Without it, even well designed systems struggle to deliver their promise.

## Improvement as Curiosity About Real Work

Throughout this book, improvement methods are treated not as efficiency tools but as ways of seeing. Their value lies in helping teams understand how work actually happens, not just how it is imagined. Observation, process mapping, and dialogue surface interruptions, workarounds, and constraints that remain invisible on paper. They create space for frontline staff to explain why adaptations occur rather than being judged for making them. Workarounds are often signals of commitment, not carelessness. When examined with curiosity, they point directly to system weaknesses that require attention (Reason, 2000). Improvement grounded in curiosity builds resilience. Improvement driven primarily by control tends to produce compliance, but little learning.

## Learning From Harm Without Losing People

When harm occurs, organizations face a choice. They can move quickly toward explanation, or they can slow down long enough to learn. Event review methods were designed to shift attention away from individual blame and toward system conditions. Learning, however, is not purely analytical. Harm carries emotional weight for patients and for staff. Shame and fear can silence insight. When leaders acknowledge the emotional impact of harm, accountability is not weakened. It becomes more meaningful by making honesty possible (NASEM, 2018). This human dimension of learning grows even more important as harm increasingly emerges from complex systems rather than isolated actions.

## Using Measurement Without Letting It Replace Meaning

Data matters. Measurement reveals trends, highlights inequities, and supports improvement. At the same time, dashboards inevitably simplify reality. That simplification is both their strength and their limitation. Patient experience measures such as Likelihood to Recommend reflect trust and perceived safety, not merely satisfaction. They are useful as starting points for conversation rather than definitive conclusions (Doyle et al., 2013). Measurement that supports humane care invites reflection. It raises questions about what may be missing, whose voices are absent, and how numbers align with lived experience. Data becomes meaningful only when paired with listening.

## Patients as Partners in Seeing Risk

Patients and families often notice risks before systems do. They encounter confusion during transitions, conflicting instructions, and gaps in follow up firsthand. Historically, these insights were captured late, if at all. Inviting patient stories into governance and learning processes broadens understanding and strengthens prevention. When patients feel emotionally safe to speak, they become partners in safety rather than passive recipients of care (Khan et al., 2018).

## Workforce Well Being Is Patient Safety

Patient safety cannot exist without workforce well being. Clinicians carry cognitive load, emotional labor, and moral tension every day. When systems demand resilience without providing support, fatigue and error predictably follow. Psychological safety, peer support, and visible leadership engagement are not optional benefits. They function as core safety strategies (WHO, 2021). Designing care environments that acknowledge emotional labor and allow recovery is essential to sustaining safe care over time.

## What Transitions Reveal About Responsibility

Transitions of care expose whether responsibility is clear or fragmented. Patients experience care as a continuous story, even when systems do not. Practices such as warm handoffs, teach back, and proactive follow up work because they communicate something fundamental: someone remains responsible (Coleman et al., 2005). Technology can support coordination, but trust is ultimately built through human connection.

## Equity as a Test of Our Commitments

Equity asks whether safety and quality are working for everyone, not only for those easiest to serve. Improvements that leave some groups behind fail to meet the ethical promise of care. Quality, understood as a moral practice, requires attention to structural disadvantage and unequal risk (Donabedian, 1988). Equity restores safety to its original purpose: protecting those most vulnerable to harm.

## Looking Ahead: Technology Without Stepping Away

Healthcare is entering a period of rapid technological change. Artificial intelligence and automation are increasingly shaping decisions about risk and care. These tools offer significant promise, but they also introduce new responsibilities. Algorithms reflect the data and assumptions that shape them. Without careful oversight, they can reproduce inequities while making accountability harder to see (Obermeyer et al., 2019). The challenge is not whether to use technology, but how to ensure that human judgment remains central. Future safety systems will need to balance innovation with transparency, and efficiency with responsibility (NASEM, 2018).

### Why Stories Still Matter

Stories do more than add narrative texture. They reveal conditions that metrics overlook: the hesitation before a critical decision, the teamwork that prevents escalation, the early instinct that something is not quite right. These accounts illuminate how judgment, context, and emotion shape real care. When shared across teams, stories act as mirrors, helping clinicians see how small choices ripple into safety, trust, and healing. Storytelling is not a soft alternative to data. It is a discipline of meaning that preserves the moral texture of care and reminds organizations why improvement matters.

## CONCLUSION: IMAGINING CARE AGAIN

This book has traced the practical, often imperfect work of strengthening safety, quality, and service across settings where care is delivered, received, and lived. Across the chapters, a consistent lesson emerges. Improvement takes hold only when it remains grounded in real clinical work, attentive to human factors, committed to equity, and sustained through visible leadership and shared learning. Tools matter, but they never stand alone. As introduced in Chapter 1, quality and safety are distinct yet inseparable. Quality organizes care around what should happen. Safety attends to what can go wrong when real people, under real pressures, adapt that work. Throughout this book, that distinction has guided decisions about methods, leadership response, and learning, particularly in moments when protocol and human need collide.

This final chapter returns to the question beneath all improvement efforts: why safety, quality, and service matter in the first place. They are not merely technical achievements or performance indicators. They reflect how responsibility is carried when patients and families are most vulnerable, and how clinicians are supported when judgment matters most. Reimagining care does not require abandoning measurement, technology, or accountability. It asks that these tools remain in service of dignity, trust, and human judgment. When they do, healthcare systems can become not only more effective, but more faithful to the care they exist to provide.

### Author's Closing Reflection

As this book comes to a close, I find myself returning to the same image that shaped how I first began to make sense of this work. Not a framework or a dashboard, but a way of seeing. Years spent watching care unfold in real time, in hospitals, clinics, and homes, taught me that the most meaningful improvements rarely start with mandates or metrics. They start with attention. Someone notices what is happening. Someone listens closely. Someone stays present when the situation resists easy explanation.

Throughout this book, I have described safety, quality, and service as deeply intertwined. I still think of them as complementary forces, much like a yin and yang. Quality and safety are not opposing aims, nor are they interchangeable. Each gives shape to the other. Service flows between them, translating technical reliability into lived experience. When these elements are in balance, trust has room to grow. When one is neglected, the strain shows up everywhere, often first in small moments that are easy to overlook.

The strategies explored in these chapters are grounded in structure, governance, and evidence because those things matter. But experience has made one truth hard to ignore. Beneath every framework sits a human commitment. Safety, quality, and service endure only when people feel accountable to one another. Technology will continue to advance. Incentives will shift. Systems will become more complex. Care, however, remains relational. It depends on judgment, trust, and the willingness to speak up when something does not feel right, even when doing so carries personal risk.

What I have tried to show, from bedside practice to system leadership, is that improvement lives in both the visible and the unseen. It lives in policies and workflows, and in the quiet pause before an action is taken. Leaders shape systems, and systems shape behavior. When presence, fairness, curiosity, and equity guide decisions, reliability becomes possible. When those qualities fade, risk moves in, often silently.

My hope is that this book supports leaders and clinicians not only in improving systems, but in protecting the human commitments that give improvement its meaning. If progress and compassion can be held together, particularly as health care moves deeper into a digital future, safety, quality, and service can remain what they were always meant to be. Expressions of care, practiced with integrity, for those who place their lives in our hands.

Figure 1 synthesizes the central message of the book. Reliable care is not produced by isolated tools, metrics, or policies, but by relationships, presence, and shared accountability across settings. From hospital to home, the figure reflects how leadership, culture, improvement science, patient voice, workforce safety, equity, and emerging digital risks remain connected rather than siloed. As the final image, it is offered not as a roadmap, but as a reminder. Quality, safety, and service endure when they are lived daily, governed thoughtfully, and carried forward through human connection across the continuum of care.

*Figure 1. Reimagining care quality, safety, and service across the continuum*

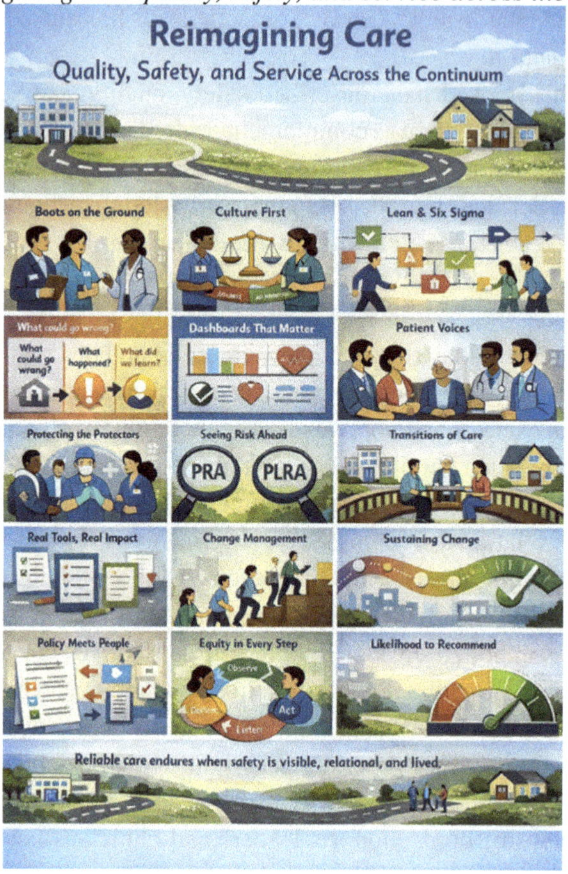

## REFERENCES


Coleman, E. A., Smith, J. D., Raha, D., & Min, S.-J. (2005). Posthospital medication discrepancies: Prevalence and contributing factors. *Archives of Internal Medicine*, *165*(16), 1842–1847. DOI: 10.1001/archinte.165.16.1842 PMID: 16157827

Donabedian, A. (1988). The quality of care: How can it be assessed? *Journal of the American Medical Association*, *260*(12), 1743–1748. DOI: 10.1001/jama.1988.03410120089033 PMID: 3045356

Doyle, C., Lennox, L., & Bell, D. (2013). A systematic review of evidence on the links between patient experience and clinical safety and effectiveness. *BMJ Open*, *3*(1), e001570. DOI: 10.1136/bmjopen-2012-001570 PMID: 23293244

Edmondson, A. C. (2018). *The fearless organization: Creating psychological safety in the workplace for learning, innovation, and growth*. Wiley.

Frankel, A., Haraden, C., Federico, F., & Lenoci-Edwards, J. (2017). *A framework for safe, reliable, and effective care* (White paper). Institute for Healthcare Improvement & Safe & Reliable Healthcare.

Khan, A., Spector, N. D., Baird, J. D., Ashland, M., Starmer, A. J., Rosenbluth, G., Garcia, B. M., Litterer, K. P., Rogers, J. E., Dalal, A. K., Lipsitz, S., Yoon, C. S., Zigmont, K. R., Guiot, A., O'Toole, J. K., Patel, A., Bismilla, Z., Coffey, M., Langrish, K., & Landrigan, C. P. (2018). Patient safety after implementation of a coproduced family-centered communication programme: Multicenter before and after intervention study. *BMJ (Clinical Research Ed.)*, *363*, k4764. DOI: 10.1136/bmj.k4764 PMID: 30518517

Marx, D. (2001). *Patient safety and the "Just Culture": A primer for health care executives*. Trustees of Columbia University.

Obermeyer, Z., Powers, B., Vogeli, C., & Mullainathan, S. (2019). Dissecting racial bias in an algorithm used to manage the health of populations. *Science*, *366*(6464), 447–453. DOI: 10.1126/science.aax2342 PMID: 31649194

Reason, J. (2000). Human error: Models and management. *BMJ (Clinical Research Ed.)*, *320*(7237), 768–770. DOI: 10.1136/bmj.320.7237.768 PMID: 10720363

Vincent, C., & Amalberti, R. (2016). *Safer healthcare: Strategies for the real world*. Springer., DOI: 10.1007/978-3-319-25559-0

World Health Organization. (2021). *Global patient safety action plan 2021–2030: Towards eliminating avoidable harm in health care*. World Health Organization.

## KEY TERMS AND DEFINITIONS

**Adaptive capacity:** the ability of teams to adjust effectively when conditions change.

**Care reliability:** consistent performance of clinical processes to reduce variation and harm.

**Equity informed improvement:** applying safety and quality methods that identify and address disparities.

**Moral distress:** discomfort experienced when clinicians cannot act on what they believe is the right course of care.

**Operational learning:** examining daily work to understand real practices and reveal vulnerabilities.

**Risk sensemaking:** the shared interpretation of signals or concerns that indicate emerging safety risks.

**Safety intelligence:** insights drawn from events, near misses, stories, and data to guide risk reduction.

**System resilience:** the ability of a healthcare system to absorb disruption and continue functioning safely.

**Work system design:** structuring tasks, tools, and environments to support safe and efficient performance.

# APPENDIX I

## BOX A.1 Reflecting on Your Own Journey

A Guided Pause Across Quality, Safety, and Service

Purpose

This boxed appendix offers a structured pause for leaders, clinicians, and anyone engaged in improvement work. Rather than introducing new tools, it invites reflection on how personal experience, relationships, and daily behaviors shape quality, safety, and service across the continuum of care. The prompts may be used individually, in team settings, or as part of leadership development, Gemba walks, or improvement retreats.

1. Where Are You in Your Story?

Reflection Prompt

If your improvement journey were a chapter title today, what would it be?

- Write the first five words that come to mind.
- Circle the word that feels out of place.
- Reflect on why that word stands apart.

Optional:

If this season of work had a soundtrack, what would the title of the first track be?

2. Seeing the Continuum of Care Through Your Lens

Reflection Prompts

- Which part of the continuum feels most familiar (hospital, clinic, home, community)?
- Which part feels most distant or hardest to see?
- Where do you notice the most resilience?
- Where do you notice emerging risk?

Practice Insight

Sketch the continuum as *you* experience it; not as a formal process map, but as a lived view that highlights people, transitions, and moments that matter most.

3. Your Relationship with Measurement

Reflection Prompts

- When did a metric last change your behavior?
- When did a story last change your behavior?
- Which dashboard number do you check most often?
- Which number do you trust least and why?

Sentence Starter
"If I could redesign one measure so it captured the human side of care, I would redesign ________."

4. Culture in Small Moments

Reflection Prompts

- Recall a recent moment when someone spoke up. What made that possible?
- Recall a moment when someone hesitated. What made that hesitation understandable?
- What small behaviors do you model intentionally or not that signal whether honesty is welcome?

Practice Pause
Write one sentence you wish someone had said to you during a difficult moment. Consider offering that sentence to someone else this week.

5. Learning From Real Work

Reflection Prompts

- What workaround have you seen recently that reflects commitment rather than carelessness?
- What question have you stopped asking that deserves to return?
- After a recent harm event or near miss, what did you learn about the system? About yourself?

Practice Insight
Draw two overlapping circles labeled *Work as Imagined* and *Work as Done*. Write one insight in the overlap.

6. Equity as a Daily Practice

Reflection Prompts

- Where do inequities show up most clearly in your setting?
- What inequities do you suspect but cannot yet fully see?
- Whose voices are missing when safety is discussed?
- What is one zero cost change you could make tomorrow to strengthen equity?

7. Your Digital Future

Reflection Prompts

- What aspects of technological change excite you?
- What aspects make you uneasy?
- Which decisions should always require human judgment, regardless of technology?

Quick Reflection
"If technology could remove one frustration from my day, it would be ________."

8. Your Next Small Step

Improvement rarely depends on dramatic leaps. It lives in presence, attention, and small acts of care.

Reflection Prompts

- What is one small act of care you can offer tomorrow that aligns with the system you hope to build?
- What small act would help someone else feel seen?
- What small act would help you feel grounded?

Quiet Commitment
Write down one small commitment.
Keep it private.
Carry it forward quietly.

## How This Box Can Be Used

- As a **leadership reflection** at the end of a chapter or section

- As a **Gemba walk or debrief companion**
- As a **team learning or retreat exercise**
- As a **personal reset during periods of change or fatigue**

# Conclusion

Across healthcare, safety and quality are often framed as outcomes to be achieved or measures to be tracked. The chapters in this book suggest a quieter, more demanding view. Safety is something organizations practice. It takes shape through attention, relationships, and decisions made in conditions that are rarely stable or complete. It strengthens when people feel able to speak, when leaders remain close to the work, and when systems are designed with a clear-eyed understanding of human limits.

The journey traced here begins where care is delivered and gradually widens to include the structures that influence it. Leadership presence emerges not as visibility, but as sustained curiosity and follow-through. Culture shows itself less in statements or policies than in how organizations respond when something feels off, when workarounds appear, or when someone raises a concern. Improvement methods matter, but their value lies less in technical precision than in their ability to help teams see what is actually happening and learn together without losing sight of the people involved.

Listening runs through the book as a steady undercurrent. Patient and family stories, workforce experience, and frontline observation surface risks that formal measures often miss. These signals arrive early, sometimes uncomfortably so. When they are taken seriously, organizations gain time to adapt and intervene. When they are ignored, risk accumulates quietly until it announces itself through harm. In this sense, safety is closely tied to attentiveness and to the willingness to act before certainty is complete.

Several chapters return to the reality that protection extends beyond patients. The safety of those who deliver care shapes reliability in ways that are easy to overlook until strain becomes visible as fatigue, disengagement, or error. Workplace violence, moral distress, and chronic overload are not peripheral concerns. They are central to quality itself. Organizations that attend to workforce safety create conditions for steadier care, clearer judgment, and more durable improvement.

Transitions of care reveal how fragile safety can be at the edges of systems. Responsibility shifts, information thins, and assumptions multiply. The book argues that continuity depends as much on presence and verification as on documentation. Safety improves when transitions are treated as shared moments of accountability rather than procedural endpoints.

Tools and structures appear throughout the chapters, but they are offered with restraint. Dashboards, checklists, scripts, and readiness assessments matter because they support speaking up, closing the loop, and sustaining attention when conditions become unpredictable. Their effectiveness depends on how they are used, not how polished they appear. Change takes hold when people understand why it matters, believe they can carry it, and see reinforcement over time. Resistance, when it surfaces, often points to misalignment rather than unwillingness.

Stories play a distinct role in sustaining improvement. Data remain essential, but they can lose meaning when detached from lived experience. Stories restore context. They influence where leaders look, what teams prioritize, and how learning is preserved across transitions. When used with care, narrative keeps improvement grounded in purpose rather than performance alone.

Later chapters widen the lens to policy, equity, and emerging risk. Policies matter most when work becomes uncertain and guidance is needed quickly. Equity is treated not as an abstract goal, but as a safety signal, revealing where systems fail some people more reliably than others. The discussion of artificial intelligence underscores that new technologies do not remove responsibility. They redistribute it. Algorithmic bias, like other latent conditions, requires governance, transparency, and human accountability if safety is to be preserved.

The book closes by returning to a simple question. What might safety, quality, and service look like if they were guided first by care and responsibility rather than comparison and compliance. Metrics and systems will continue to matter. Technology will continue to shape practice. The challenge for leaders is to ensure that judgment, relationships, and ethical accountability remain intact as care evolves.

This is not a call for perfection. It is an invitation to practice. To stay close to the work, to listen more carefully, to notice weak signals, and to respond with clarity and fairness. When organizations do this consistently, safety becomes less about reacting to harm and more about designing conditions in which people can do their best work. Over time, that practice is where enduring quality takes root.

# Compilation of References


Administration for Strategic Preparedness and Response. (2024). *Workplace violence*. U.S. Department of Health and Human Services, Office of the Assistant Secretary for Preparedness and Response. https://asprtracie.hhs.gov/technical-resources/resource/2791/workplace-violence

Agency for Healthcare Research and Quality Patient Safety Network. (2024). *Patient- and family-centered I-PASS: Family-centered communication program to reduce medical errors*. https://psnet.ahrq.gov

Agency for Healthcare Research and Quality. (2022). *Strategies and approaches for investigating patient safety events (RCA, FMEA, etc.)*. Patient Safety Network (PSNet). https://psnet.ahrq.gov/primer/strategies-and-approaches-investigating-patient-safety-events

Agency for Healthcare Research and Quality. (2023). *Patient safety culture surveys: User guide and resources.* U.S. Department of Health and Human Services. https://www.ahrq.gov/sops

Agency for Healthcare Research and Quality. (2023). *Patient safety culture surveys: User guide and resources.* U.S. Department of Health and Human Services. https://www.ahrq.gov/sops/index.html

Agency for Healthcare Research and Quality. (2024). *Guide to patient and family engagement in hospital quality and safety*. U.S. Department of Health and Human Services.

AHRQ Communication and Optimal Resolution (CANDOR) Toolkit. Rockville, MD: Agency for Healthcare Research and Quality; May 2016.

Amann, J., Blasimme, A., Vayena, E., Frey, D., & Madai, V. I. (2020). Explainability for artificial intelligence in healthcare: A multidisciplinary perspective. *BMC Medical Informatics and Decision Making*, *20*(1), 310. Advance online publication. DOI: 10.1186/s12911-020-01332-6 PMID: 33256715

American Hospital Association / Health Research & Educational Trust. (2013). *Checklists to improve patient safety*. Health Research & Educational Trust.

American Medical Association. (2024). *How AI is leading to more prior-authorization denials.* https://www.ama-assn.org/practice-management/prior-authorization

Anhang Price, R., Elliott, M. N., Zaslavsky, A. M., Hays, R. D., Lehrman, W. G., Rybowski, L., Edgman-Levitan, S., & Cleary, P. D. (2014). Examining the role of patient experience surveys in measuring health care quality. *Medical Care Research and Review : MCRR, 71*(5), 522–554. DOI: 10.1177/1077558714541480 PMID: 25027409

Balasubramanian, I., Andres, E. B., & Malhotra, C. (2025). Outpatient follow-up and 30-day readmissions: A systematic review and meta-analysis. *JAMA Network Open, 8*(11), e2541272. DOI: 10.1001/jamanetworkopen.2025.41272 PMID: 41186947

Bate, P., & Robert, G. (2007). *Bringing user experience to healthcare improvement: The concepts, methods and practices of experience-based design.* Radcliffe Publishing.

Bell, S. (2025, July 25). Eisenhower's urgent/important principle. *Mind Tools.*

Berwick, D. M. (1989). Continuous improvement as an ideal in health care. *The New England Journal of Medicine, 320*(1), 53–56. DOI: 10.1056/NEJM198901053200110 PMID: 2909878

Bilicki, D. J., & Reeves, M. J. (2024). Outpatient follow-up visits to reduce 30-day all-cause readmissions. *Preventing Chronic Disease, 21*, 240138. https://www.cdc.gov/pcd/issues/2024/24_0138.htm. DOI: 10.5888/pcd21.240138 PMID: 39325638

Boulding, W., Glickman, S. W., Manary, M. P., Schulman, K. A., & Staelin, R. (2011). Relationship between patient satisfaction with inpatient care and hospital readmission within 30 days. *The American Journal of Managed Care, 17*(1), 41–48. PMID: 21348567

Broughton, T., Weggelaar, A. M., & Sülz, S. (2025). From data to improvement: Social mechanisms as a key to understanding dashboard adoption. *American Journal of Medical Quality, 40*(2), 31–37. DOI: 10.1097/JMQ.0000000000000225 PMID: 39910757

Brown, T., & Patel, N. (2021). Communicating with data: How meaning drives measurement. *Journal of Healthcare Management, 66*(4), 215–223. DOI: 10.1097/JHM.0000000000000103

Buolamwini, J., & Gebru, T. (2018). Gender shades: Intersectional accuracy disparities in commercial gender classification. *Proceedings of Machine Learning Research, 81*, 1–15. http://proceedings.mlr.press/v81/buolamwini18a.html

Carroll, J. S., & Edmondson, A. C. (2021). *Learning from failure in healthcare: Systems that learn, people who care*. Harvard Business Review Press.

Centers for Medicare & Medicaid Services. (2023). *CAHPS® Hospital Survey (HCAHPS)*. https://www.cms.gov

Centers for Medicare & Medicaid Services. (2023). *Framework for health equity 2022–2032: A 10-year vision to advance equity in the pursuit of improved health outcomes for all people*. U.S. Department of Health and Human Services. https://www.cms.gov/about-cms/agency-information/omh/equity-initiatives/framework-for-health-equity

Centers for Medicare & Medicaid Services. (2023). *Quality Assurance and Performance Improvement (QAPI) and Health Equity Framework: Guidance for Home Health and Post-Acute Settings*. U.S. Department of Health and Human Services.

Centers for Medicare & Medicaid Services. (2023). *Value-based programs overview*. https://www.cms.gov/valuebasedprograms

Centers for Medicare & Medicaid Services. (2024). *Home Health CAHPS Survey (HHCAHPS): Quality reporting and participation requirements*. https://www.cms.gov

Chance, E. A., Shah, N., & Ali, R. (2024). The effectiveness of checklists and error reporting systems on enhancing patient safety and reducing medical errors in hospital settings. *Journal of Patient Safety, 20*(3), 145–153. https://pmc.ncbi.nlm.nih.gov/articles/PMC11329062/ PMID: 39156684

Charon, R. (2006). *Narrative medicine: Honoring the stories of illness*. Oxford University Press. DOI: 10.1093/oso/9780195166750.001.0001

Chosewood, L. C., Nigam, J. A. S., & Cunningham, T. R. (2024). Workplace violence prevention in healthcare: Integrating worker well-being and system safety. *Journal of Occupational and Environmental Medicine, 66*(3), 189–196. DOI: 10.1097/JOM.0000000000003098

Chyon, F. A., Ahmmed, M. S., Shuvo, M. K. A., Suman, M. N. H., & Hossain, M. M. (2020). Measuring process capability in a hospital by using lean tools. *International Journal of Health Care Quality Assurance, 33*(7), 543–555. DOI: 10.1108/IJHCQA-09-2019-0096

Coiera, E., Chan, A., Brooke-Cowden, K., Rahimi-Ardabili, H., Halim, N., & Tufanaru, C. (2025). Clinical and economic impact of digital dashboards on hospital inpatient care: A systematic review. *JAMIA Open*, *8*(4), ooaf078. Advance online publication. DOI: 10.1093/jamiaopen/ooaf078 PMID: 40718761

Coleman, E. A., Smith, J. D., Raha, D., & Min, S.-J. (2005). Posthospital medication discrepancies: Prevalence and contributing factors. *Archives of Internal Medicine*, *165*(16), 1842–1847. DOI: 10.1001/archinte.165.16.1842 PMID: 16157827

Cowie, J., Nicoll, A., Dimova, E. D., Campbell, P., & Duncan, E. A. S. (2020). The barriers and facilitators influencing the sustainability of hospital-based interventions: A systematic review. *BMC Health Services Research*, *20*(1), 588. DOI: 10.1186/s12913-020-05434-9 PMID: 32594912

Crandall, K. M., Sten, M.-B., Almuhanna, A., Fahey, L., & Shah, R. K. (2017). Improving apparent cause analysis reliability: A quality improvement initiative. *Pediatric Quality & Safety*, *2*(3), e025. DOI: 10.1097/pq9.0000000000000025 PMID: 30229162

Cui, Y., Wang, Y., Liu, H., Xu, S., & Zhang, X. (2025). Exploring the correlation between patient safety culture and adverse medical events using failure mode and effect analysis (FMEA). *Risk Management and Healthcare Policy*, *17*, 163–176. DOI: 10.2147/RMHP.S502725 PMID: 40264504

Damberg, C. L., Sorbero, M. E., Lovejoy, S. L., Martsolf, G., Rybowski, L., & Meili, R. (2014). *Measuring success in health care value-based purchasing*. RAND Corporation.

Dashboards, D. (2023).. . *Healthcare Executive*, *38*(6), 24–27.

Davis, T. R., Straatmann, K., Snyder, N., Shiner, D., Evans, A., Caruso, C., & Alton, M. (2025). Promoting a culture of patient safety: Using the principles of just culture to improve transparency and risk reporting in the hospital setting. *Patient Safety*, *7*(2). Advance online publication. DOI: 10.33940/001c.137737

De Haro, T., Papay Ramirez, L., & Garcia Chileme, S. (2024). Failure Mode and Effects Analysis (FMEA) methodology as a strategy to increase patient safety. *Clinical Chemistry*, *70*(Supplement 1), hvae106.186. Advance online publication. DOI: 10.1093/clinchem/hvae106.186

Dekker, S. (2011). *Drift into failure: From hunting broken components to understanding complex systems*. Ashgate.

Dekker, S. (2016). *Just culture: Restoring trust and accountability in your organization*. CRC Press. DOI: 10.4324/9781315251271

Dekker, S. (2020). *Foundations of safety science: A century of understanding accidents and disasters*. CRC Press.

Deming, W. E. (1986). *Out of the crisis*. MIT Press.

Dolan, P., Hallsworth, M., Halpern, D., King, D., & Vlaev, I. (2018). *Influencing behaviour: The MINDSPACE approach*. Cabinet Office Behavioural Insights Team.

Donabedian, A. (1988). The quality of care: How can it be assessed? *Journal of the American Medical Association*, *260*(12), 1743–1748. DOI: 10.1001/jama.1988.03410120089033 PMID: 3045356

Dossey, B. M. (2010). *Florence Nightingale: Mystic, visionary, healer* (2nd ed.). Springer.

Doyle, C., Lennox, L., & Bell, D. (2013). A systematic review of evidence on the links between patient experience and clinical safety and effectiveness. *BMJ Open*, *3*(1), e001570. DOI: 10.1136/bmjopen-2012-001570 PMID: 23293244

Dwidar, M. M., Fakhry, S. F., & Abdel-Hamed, L. A. (2025). Just culture and its influence on nurse interns' willingness to report near-miss events: A cross-sectional study in five Egyptian university hospitals. *BMC Nursing*, *24*(1), 1397. Advance online publication. DOI: 10.1186/s12912-025-03979-w PMID: 41233794

Edmondson, A. C. (2018). *The fearless organization: Creating psychological safety in the workplace for learning, innovation, and growth*. Wiley.

Equity is essential to patient safety. (2023). *The Joint Commission Sentinel Event Alert,* (67), 1–6.

European Commission. (2024). *EU Artificial Intelligence Act: Legislative text and implementation guidance*. https://digital-strategy.ec.europa.eu

Farias, E., & Van de Walle, S. (2025). From dashboards to dialogue: Behavioural approaches to public performance management. *Public Administration Review*, *85*(2), 411–427. DOI: 10.1111/puar.13425

Felice, S. T., Goodwin, S. G., Oliveri, A., Socias-Morales, C., Castillo, D., & Olawoyin, R. (2021). Home health care workers: A growing and diverse workforce at high risk for workplace violence. *Centers for Disease Control and Prevention: NIOSH Science Blog*. https://blogs.cdc.gov/niosh-science-blog/2021/09/02/hhc-violence

Foster, M., Edwards, A., . . .. (2023). Impact of leadership walkarounds on operational, cultural, and clinical outcomes: A systematic review. *Journal of Patient Safety*. https://pmc.ncbi.nlm.nih.gov/articles/PMC10582976/

Foster, M., Shultz, B. M. A., & Mazur, Ł. (2023). Impact of leadership walkarounds on operational, cultural, and clinical outcomes: A systematic review. *Journal of Patient Safety*, *19*(6), 455–462. DOI: 10.1097/PTS.0000000000000992 PMID: 37827728

Frankel, A., Haraden, C., Federico, F., & Lenoci-Edwards, J. (2017). *A framework for safe, reliable, and effective care* (White paper). Institute for Healthcare Improvement & Safe & Reliable Healthcare.

Frankel, A., Haraden, C., Federico, F., & Lenoci-Edwards, J. (2017). *A framework for safe, reliable, and effective care.* Institute for Healthcare Improvement. https://www.ihi.org/resources/Pages/IHIWhitePapers/AFrameworkforSafeReliableandEffectiveCare.aspx

Frankel, A. S., Leonard, M. W., & Denham, C. R. (2006). Fair and just culture, team behavior, and leadership engagement: The tools to achieve high reliability. *Health Services Research*, *41*(4 Pt 2), 1690–1709. DOI: 10.1111/j.1475-6773.2006.00572.x PMID: 16898986

Frankel, A., Grillo, S. P., Baker, E. G., Huber, C. N., Abookire, S., Grenham, M., Console, P., O'Quinn, M., Thibault, G., & Gandhi, T. K. (2003). Patient safety leadership walkrounds at Partners HealthCare. *Joint Commission Journal on Quality and Safety*, *29*(1), 16–26. https://pubmed.ncbi.nlm.nih.gov/12520830. DOI: 10.1016/S1549-3741(03)29003-1 PMID: 12528570

Friedman, C. P., Rubin, J. C., & Sullivan, K. J. (2017). Toward an information infrastructure for global health improvement. *Yearbook of Medical Informatics*, *26*(1), 16–23. DOI: 10.15265/IY-2017-004 PMID: 28480469

Ghosh, S., Chawla, N., & Sinha, S. (2021). Communication failures and patient safety: A systematic review. *Journal of Patient Safety*, *17*(3), 157–165. DOI: 10.1097/PTS.0000000000000798 PMID: 29994818

Glasgow, R. E., Vogt, T. M., & Boles, S. M. (1999). Evaluating the public health impact of health promotion interventions: The RE-AIM framework. *American Journal of Public Health*, *89*(9), 1322–1327. DOI: 10.2105/AJPH.89.9.1322 PMID: 10474547

Goleman, D. (2022). *Emotional intelligence: Why it can matter more than IQ* (25th anniversary ed.). Bantam.

Grailey, K. E., Murray, E., Reader, T., & Brett, S. J. (2021). The presence and potential impact of psychological safety in the healthcare setting: An evidence synthesis. *BMC Health Services Research*, *21*(1), 773. DOI: 10.1186/s12913-021-06740-6 PMID: 34353319

Hatfield, E., Cacioppo, J. T., & Rapson, R. L. (1994). *Emotional contagion*. Cambridge University Press.

Health Quality & Safety Commission New Zealand. (2016). *Checklists, briefings, debriefings, and huddles: Evidence summary*. https://www.hqsc.govt.nz

Health Service Executive. (2025). *Dashboards & data visualisation in healthcare: International best practices and design pillars*. https://www.hse.ie

Hiatt, J. (2006). *ADKAR: A model for change in business, government, and our community*. Prosci.

Holden, R. J., Carayon, P., Gurses, A. P., Hoonakker, P., Hundt, A. S., Ozok, A. A., & Rivera-Rodriguez, A. J. (2013). SEIPS 2.0: A human factors framework for studying and improving the work of healthcare professionals and patients. *Ergonomics, 56*(11), 1669–1686. DOI: 10.1080/00140139.2013.838643 PMID: 24088063

Ilin, M., & Bohlen, J. (2023). Six sigma method. In *StatPearls*. StatPearls Publishing.

Institute for Healthcare Improvement. (2017). *Achieving health equity: A guide for health care organizations*. Institute for Healthcare Improvement.

Institute for Healthcare Improvement. (2022). *Establishing measures: The Model for Improvement*. https://www.ihi.org/library/model-for-improvement/establishing-measures

Institute for Healthcare Improvement. (2022). *Improving health equity through patient safety: The intersection of social determinants and harm prevention*. Institute for Healthcare Improvement.

Institute for Healthcare Improvement. (2022). *Partnering with patients and families to design a better health care system*. Institute for Healthcare Improvement.

Institute for Healthcare Improvement. (n.d.). *4 steps to sustaining improvement in health care*. https://www.ihi.org/library/publications/four-steps-sustaining-improvement-health-care

Institute for Healthcare Improvement. (n.d.). *Care transitions: Key strategies from evidence to implementation*. https://www.ihi.org/resources/Pages/ImprovementStories/Care-Transitions.aspx

Institute of Medicine. (2000). *To err is human: Building a safer health system*. National Academies Press.

Joint Commission Resources. (2025). *Health care worker safety checklists: Protecting those who serve* (2nd ed.). Joint Commission Store.

Joint Commission. (2019). *High reliability in healthcare: Creating the culture and improving the process.* Joint Commission Resources.

Joint Commission. (2024). *Comprehensive Accreditation Manual for Home Care (CAMHC): The official handbook.* Joint Commission Resources.

Joint Commission. (2024). *Comprehensive Accreditation Manual for Hospitals (CAMH): The official handbook.* Joint Commission Resources.

Joint Commission. (2025). *Joint Commission and Coalition for Health AI (CHAI) release initial guidance to support responsible AI adoption across U.S. health systems.* https://www.jointcommission.org/en-us/knowledge-library/news/2025-09-jc-and-chai-release-initial-guidance-to-support-responsible-ai-adoption

Kam, A. W., Gunja, N., & Seow, C. H. (2021). Using lean six sigma techniques to improve efficiency in outpatient clinics: Root cause analysis and clinic flow redesign. *BMC Health Services Research, 21*, 1105. DOI: 10.1186/s12913-020-06034-3

Keller, S. C., Salinas, A., Williams, D., McGoldrick, M., Gorski, L. A., Alexander, M., Norris, A., Charron, J., Stienecker, R. S., Passaretti, C. L., Maragakis, L. L., & Cosgrove, S. E. (2020). Reaching consensus on a home infusion central line–associated bloodstream infection surveillance definition via a modified Delphi approach. *American Journal of Infection Control, 48*(9), 993–1000. DOI: 10.1016/j.ajic.2019.12.015 PMID: 31982215

Khan, A., Furtak, S. L., Melvin, P., Rogers, J. E., Schuster, M. A., & Landrigan, C. P. (2017). Parent-reported errors and adverse events in hospitalized children. *JAMA Pediatrics, 171*(4), 372–381. DOI: 10.1001/jamapediatrics.2016.4812 PMID: 28241211

Khan, A., Spector, N. D., Baird, J. D., Ashland, M., Starmer, A. J., Rosenbluth, G., Garcia, B. M., Litterer, K. P., Rogers, J. E., Dalal, A. K., Lipsitz, S., Yoon, C. S., Zigmont, K. R., Guiot, A., O'Toole, J. K., Patel, A., Bismilla, Z., Coffey, M., Langrish, K., & Landrigan, C. P. (2018). Patient safety after implementation of a coproduced family-centered communication programme: Multicenter before and after intervention study. *BMJ (Clinical Research Ed.), 363*, k4764. DOI: 10.1136/bmj.k4764 PMID: 30518517

Khan, A., Spector, N. D., Baird, J. D., Starmer, A. J., Rosenbluth, G., Simon, J. L., O'Toole, J. K., Yu, C. E., & Landrigan, C. P. (2018). Patient-centered I-PASS: Family-centered rounds to improve communication and safety. *Pediatrics, 142*(1), e20171873.

Kim, S., Kitzmiller, R., Baernholdt, M., Lynn, M. R., & Jones, C. B. (2022). Patient safety culture: The impact on workplace violence and health-worker burnout. *Workplace Health & Safety*, *71*(2), 78–88. DOI: 10.1177/21650799221126364 PMID: 36476112

Kumah, A. (2025). Adverse event reporting and patient safety: The role of a just culture. *Frontiers in Health Services*, *5*, 1581516. Advance online publication. DOI: 10.3389/frhs.2025.1581516 PMID: 40910122

Lanctôt, N., & Guay, S. (2014). The aftermath of workplace violence among healthcare workers: A systematic literature review of consequences. *Aggression and Violent Behavior*, *19*(5), 492–501. DOI: 10.1016/j.avb.2014.07.010

Lennox, L., Antonacci, G., Harris, M., & Reed, J. (2023). Unpacking the 'process of sustaining'—identifying threats to sustainability and the strategies used to address them: A longitudinal multiple case study. *Implementation Science Communications*, *4*(1), 68. DOI: 10.1186/s43058-023-00445-z PMID: 37337274

Liker, J. K. (2004). *The Toyota way: 14 management principles from the world's greatest manufacturer*. McGraw-Hill.

Martin, D., Johns, C., Sorrell, L., Healy, E., Phull, M., Olusanya, S., Peters, M., & Fabes, J. (2024). Effect of skin tone on the accuracy of the estimation of arterial oxygen saturation by pulse oximetry: A systematic review. *British Journal of Anaesthesia*, *132*(5), 945–956. DOI: 10.1016/j.bja.2024.01.023 PMID: 38368234

Marx, D. (2001). *Patient safety and the "Just Culture": A primer for health care executives*. Trustees of Columbia University.

Marx, D. (2001). *Patient safety and the "just culture."*. Columbia University.

Marx, D. (2001). *Patient safety and the "Just Culture."*. Columbia University.

Marx, D. (2001). *Patient safety and the "Just Culture": A primer for health care executives*. Columbia University.

McMartin, K. (2013). Discharge planning in chronic conditions: Effects on readmissions and length of stay. *Canadian Journal of Respiratory Therapy*. https://pmc.ncbi.nlm.nih.gov/articles/PMC3804053/

Mello, M. M., Boothman, R. C., McDonald, T., Driver, J., Lembitz, A., Bouwmeester, D., Dunlap, B., & Gallagher, T. (2014). Communication-and-resolution programs: The challenges and lessons learned from six early adopters. *Health Affairs*, *33*(1), 20–29. DOI: 10.1377/hlthaff.2013.0828 PMID: 24395931

Menendez, C. C., Arespacochaga, E., Begley, R., Bhatnagar, M., Ross, P., Schaefer, M. E., Spring, C., & Tisdale-Pardi, J. (2024, May 29). *Prioritizing our healthcare workers: The importance of addressing the intersection of workplace violence and mental health and wellbeing*. †NIOSH Science Blog.‡ Centers for Disease Control and Prevention. https://blogs.cdc.gov/niosh-science-blog/2024/05/29/hcw_violence_mh/

Murray, J. S., Clifford, J., Scott, D., Kelly, S., & Hanover, C. (2024). Leader rounding for high reliability and improved patient safety. *Federal Practitioner : for the Health Care Professionals of the VA, DoD, and PHS*, *41*(1), 16–21. DOI: 10.12788/fp.0444 PMID: 38835357

National Academies of Sciences, Engineering, and Medicine. (2018). *Crossing the global quality chasm: Improving health care worldwide*. National Academies Press.

National Committee for Quality Assurance. (2024). *Health Equity Accreditation 2024 Standards*. NCQA.

National Institute for Health and Care Excellence. (2023). *Evidence standards framework for digital health technologies: Update for AI tools*. https://www.nice.org.uk

National Patient Safety Foundation. (2015). *Free from harm: Accelerating patient safety improvement fifteen years after To Err Is Human*.

National Patient Safety Foundation. (2015). *Free from harm: Accelerating patient safety improvement fifteen years after To Err Is Human*. National Patient Safety Foundation.

National Patient Safety Foundation. (2015). *RCA$^2$: Improving root cause analyses and actions to prevent harm*. Author.

NORC at the University of Chicago. (2025). *Artificial intelligence in health insurance: The use and regulation of AI in utilization management*. https://www.norc.org

O'Donovan, R., De Brún, A., & McAuliffe, E. (2021). Healthcare professionals' experience of psychological safety, voice, and silence. *Frontiers in Psychology*, *12*, 626689. DOI: 10.3389/fpsyg.2021.626689 PMID: 33679547

Obermeyer, Z., Powers, B., Vogeli, C., & Mullainathan, S. (2019). Dissecting racial bias in an algorithm used to manage the health of populations. *Science*, *366*(6464), 447–453. DOI: 10.1126/science.aax2342 PMID: 31649194

Occupational Safety and Health Administration. (2015). *Guidelines for preventing workplace violence for health care and social service workers* (OSHA Publication 3148). U.S. Department of Labor. https://www.osha.gov/sites/default/files/publications/osha3148.pdf

Ohno, T. (1988). *Toyota production system: Beyond large-scale production*. Productivity Press.

Paine, L. A., Holzmueller, C. G., Elliott, R., Kasda, E., Pronovost, P. J., Weaver, S. J., Sutcliffe, K. M., & Mathews, S. C. (2018). Latent risk assessment tool for health care leaders. *Journal of Healthcare Risk Management*, *38*(2), 36–46. DOI: 10.1002/jhrm.21316 PMID: 29631323

Paine, L. A., Rosenstein, A. H., & Sexton, J. B. (2018a). Safety culture and handoff communication: Implications for patient safety. *Journal of Nursing Care Quality*, *33*(3), 213–220. DOI: 10.1097/NCQ.0000000000000333 PMID: 29035906

Paine, L. A., Rosenstein, B. J., Pronovost, P. J., & Bagian, J. P. (2018b). Safety as a system property: Lessons from high-reliability organizations. *Joint Commission Journal on Quality and Patient Safety*, *44*(7), 377–384. DOI: 10.1016/j.jcjq.2018.02.006 PMID: 30008350

Patient Safety Learning. (2024). *The missed bilirubin test: Cal Sheridan's story*. https://www.pslhub.org/learn/patient-safety-in-health-and-care/diagnosis/diagnostic-error/the-missed-bilirubin-test-cal-sheridans-story-r11885/

Performance Health. (2025). *Metrics that matter: Enhancing safety with healthcare dashboards*. https://www.performancehealthus.com

Press Ganey. (2023). *Human experience in healthcare: 2023 performance insights report*. Press Ganey Associates. https://www.pressganey.com

Press Ganey. (n.d.). *The HPI SEC® and SSER® patient safety measurement system for healthcare*. https://www.pressganey.com

Pronovost, P. J., Berenholtz, S. M., & Needham, D. M. (2016). Translating evidence into practice: A model for large-scale knowledge translation. *BMJ (Clinical Research Ed.)*, *333*(7565), 1210–1212. DOI: 10.1136/bmj.333.7565.1210 PMID: 18838424

Pronovost, P. J., & Paine, L. (2019). Creating learning health systems to improve patient care and safety. *BMJ Quality & Safety*, *28*(5), 389–392. DOI: 10.1136/bmjqs-2018-008726 PMID: 30337498

Reader, T. W., Gillespie, A., & Roberts, J. (2014). Patient complaints in healthcare systems: A systematic review and coding taxonomy. *BMJ Quality & Safety*, *23*(8), 678–689. DOI: 10.1136/bmjqs-2013-002437 PMID: 24876289

Reason, J. (2000). Human error: Models and management. *BMJ (Clinical Research Ed.)*, *320*(7237), 768–770. DOI: 10.1136/bmj.320.7237.768 PMID: 10720363

Reason, J. (2008). *The human contribution: Unsafe acts, accidents and heroic recoveries*. Ashgate.

Reason, J. (2016). *Managing the risks of organizational accidents* (2nd ed.). Routledge. DOI: 10.4324/9781315543543

Scott, S. D., Hirschinger, L. E., Cox, K. R., McCoig, M., Hahn-Cover, K., Epperly, K. M., Phillips, E. C., & Hall, L. W. (2009). The natural history of recovery for the healthcare provider "second victim" after adverse patient events. *Quality & Safety in Health Care*, *18*(5), 325–330. DOI: 10.1136/qshc.2009.032870 PMID: 19812092

Sexton, J. B., Adair, K. C., Leonard, M. W., Frankel, T. C., Proulx, J., Watson, S. R., Magnus, B., Bogan, B., Jamal, M., Schwendimann, R., & Frankel, A. S. (2018). Providing feedback following Leadership WalkRounds is associated with better patient safety culture, higher employee engagement and lower burnout. *BMJ Quality & Safety*, *27*(4), 261–270. DOI: 10.1136/bmjqs-2016-006399 PMID: 28993441

Shahid, S., & Thomas, S. (2018). Situation, background, assessment, recommendation (SBAR) communication tool for handoff in health care: A narrative review. *Safety in Health*, *4*(1), 7. DOI: 10.1186/s40886-018-0073-1

Singer, S. J., & Tucker, A. L. (2014). The evolving literature on safety WalkRounds: Emerging themes and practical messages. *BMJ Quality & Safety*, *23*(10), 789–800. DOI: 10.1136/bmjqs-2014-003416 PMID: 25228779

Sjoding, M. W., Dickson, R. P., Iwashyna, T. J., Gay, S. E., & Valley, T. S. (2020). Racial bias in pulse oximetry measurement. *The New England Journal of Medicine*, *383*(25), 2477–2478. DOI: 10.1056/NEJMc2029240 PMID: 33326721

Somani, R., Murnane, A., & Pinto, S. (2021). Effectiveness of interventions to decrease workplace violence toward emergency department nurses: A systematic review. *Journal of Emergency Nursing: JEN*, *47*(4), 620–632.

Starmer, A. J., Spector, N. D., Srivastava, R., West, D. C., Rosenbluth, G., Allen, A. D., Noble, E. L., Tse, L. L., Dalal, A. K., Keohane, C., Lipsitz, S. R., Rothschild, J. M., Wien, M. F., Yoon, C. S., Zigmont, K., Wilson, K. M., O'Toole, J. K., Wayne, D. B., & Landrigan, C. P. (2014). Changes in medical errors after implementation of a handoff program. *The New England Journal of Medicine*, *371*(19), 1803–1812. DOI: 10.1056/NEJMsa1405556 PMID: 25372088

Symplr. (2024). *From pressure to progress: Healthcare operations & the path forward for clinical, operational & IT leaders (2024 Compass Survey Report)*. Symplr. https://www.symplr.com/press-releases/symplr-2024-compass-survey-shows-how-lack-of-alignment-impacts-us-healthcare-organizations

Szanton, S. L., Wolff, J. W., Leff, B., Thorpe, R. J., Tanner, E. K., Boyd, C., Xue, Q., Guralnik, J., Bishai, D., & Gitlin, L. N. (2011). CAPABLE trial: A randomized controlled trial of nurse, occupational therapist, and handyman to reduce disability among older adults: Rationale and design. *Contemporary Clinical Trials*, *32*(6), 1–9. DOI: 10.1016/j.cct.2011.05.003 PMID: 24685996

Szanton, S. L., Wolff, J. W., Leff, B., Thorpe, R. J., Tanner, E. K., Boyd, C., Xue, Q., Guralnik, J., Bishai, D., & Gitlin, L. N. (2016). CAPABLE program: Outcomes of a randomized trial of community aging in place. *Health Affairs*, *35*(9), 1558–1565. DOI: 10.1377/hlthaff.2016.0140 PMID: 27605633

Tawfik, D. S., Adair, K. C., Palassof, S., Sexton, J. B., Levoy, E., Frankel, A., Leonard, M., Proulx, J., & Profit, J. (2023). Leadership behavior associations with domains of safety culture, engagement, and healthcare worker well-being. *Joint Commission Journal on Quality and Patient Safety*, *49*(3), 156–165. DOI: 10.1016/j.jcjq.2022.12.006 PMID: 36658090

Tervalon, M., & Murray-García, J. (1998). Cultural humility versus cultural competence: A critical distinction in defining physician training outcomes in multicultural education. *Journal of Health Care for the Poor and Underserved*, *9*(2), 117–125. DOI: 10.1353/hpu.2010.0233 PMID: 10073197

The Joint Commission. (2017). *Improving handoff communications: Meeting National Patient Safety Goal 02.05.01.* https://www.jointcommission.org

The Joint Commission. (2021, June 18). *Workplace violence prevention standards* ($R^3$ Report, Issue 30). https://www.jointcommission.org/standards/r3-report

The Joint Commission. (2023). *Health care equity standards*. The Joint Commission.

The Joint Commission. (2023). *Responsible use of health data certification for hospitals* [Press release]. The Joint Commission.

The Joint Commission. (2023). *Root cause analysis in health care: A Joint Commission guide to analysis and corrective action of sentinel and adverse events* (7th ed.). Joint Commission Resources.

Treadwell, J. R., Lucas, S., & Tsou, A. Y. (2013). Surgical checklists: A systematic review of impacts and compliance. *BMJ Quality & Safety*, *22*(4), 299–314. DOI: 10.1136/bmjqs-2012-001797 PMID: 23322751

Tronier, R. (2025, December 29). The Eisenhower Matrix: How to prioritize your to-do list. *Asana Resources*.

Tufte, E. R. (1997). *Visual explanations: Images and quantities, evidence and narrative*. Graphics Press.

Tun, H. M., Abdul Rahman, H., Naing, L., & Malik, O. A. (2025). Trust in artificial intelligence–based clinical decision support systems among health care workers: A systematic review. *Journal of Medical Internet Research*, *27*, e69678. DOI: 10.2196/69678 PMID: 40772775

U.S. Food and Drug Administration. (2021, October 22). *Pulse oximeter accuracy and limitations: FDA safety communication*. https://www.fda.gov/medical-devices/safety-communications/pulse-oximeter-accuracy-and-limitations-fda-safety-communication

U.S. Food and Drug Administration. (2024). *Artificial intelligence and machine learning software as a medical device (discussion paper)*. https://www.fda.gov

URAC. (2025). *Health care AI accreditation: Responding to the industry's call for responsible AI implementation*. https://www.urac.org

Van der Kolk, B. (2014). *The body keeps the score: Brain, mind, and body in the healing of trauma*. Viking.

Vehviläinen, E., Charles, A., Sainsbury, J., Stacey, G., Field-Richards, S. E., & Westwood, G. (2024). Influences of leadership, organizational culture, and hierarchy on raising concerns about patient deterioration: A qualitative study. *Journal of Patient Safety*, *20*(5), e73–e77. DOI: 10.1097/PTS.0000000000001234 PMID: 39028433

Vélez Díaz Pallarés, M., Delgado Silveira, E., Carretero Accame, M. E., & Bermejo Vicedo, T. (2013). Using Healthcare Failure Mode and Effect Analysis to reduce medication errors in the process of drug prescription, validation and dispensing in hospitalized patients. *BMJ Quality & Safety*, *22*(1), 42–52. https://qualitysafety.bmj.com/content/22/1/42. DOI: 10.1136/bmjqs-2012-000983 PMID: 22976504

Vincent, C., & Amalberti, R. (2016). *Safer healthcare: Strategies for the real world*. Springer., DOI: 10.1007/978-3-319-25559-0

Vincent, C., Burnett, S., & Carthey, J. (2014). *The measurement and monitoring of safety*. Health Foundation.

Vincent, C., Burnett, S., & Carthey, J. (2023). *The measurement and monitoring of safety: A new framework for improvement*. Health Foundation.

Wachter, R. M. (2023). *The digital doctor: Hope, hype, and harm at the dawn of medicine's computer age*. McGraw Hill.

Waseem, H. M., Ul Islam, S., Harrison, S., Epiphaniou, G., Matragkas, N., Arvanitis, T. N., & Maple, C. (2025). Data driven FMEA approach for hazard identification and risk evaluation in digital health. *Scientific Reports, 15*(1), 11929. DOI: 10.1038/s41598-025-11929-4 PMID: 40702036

Wears, R. L., Hollnagel, E., & Braithwaite, J. (2015). *Resilient healthcare (Vol. 2): The resilience of everyday clinical work.* CRC Press.

Weggelaar-Jansen, A. M. J. W. M., Broekharst, D. S. E., & de Bruijne, M. (2018). Developing a hospital-wide quality and safety dashboard: A qualitative research study. *BMJ Quality & Safety, 27*(12), 1000–1007. DOI: 10.1136/bmjqs-2018-007784 PMID: 29950323

Weick, K. E., & Sutcliffe, K. M. (2015). *Managing the unexpected: Sustained performance in a complex world* (3rd ed.). Wiley. DOI: 10.1002/9781119175834

Weiner, B. J., Amick, H., & Lee, S. Y. D. (2020). Conceptualization and measurement of organizational readiness for change: A review of the literature. *Medical Care Research and Review : MCRR, 77*(4), 379–392. DOI: 10.1177/1077558708317802 PMID: 18511812

Wolf, J. A., Niederhauser, V., Marshburn, D., & LaVela, S. L. (2021). Defining patient experience. *Patient Experience Journal, 8*(1), 10–14. DOI: 10.35680/2372-0247.1594

World Health Organization. (2021). *Ethics and governance of artificial intelligence for health: WHO guidance.* https://www.who.int

World Health Organization. (2023). *Global patient safety action plan 2021–2030: Towards eliminating avoidable harm in health care.* WHO Press.

World Health Organization. (2023). *Social determinants of health: Key concepts.* World Health Organization.

World Health Organization. (n.d.). *Safe surgery: Tools and resources (WHO surgical safety checklist and adaptations).* https://www.who.int/teams/integrated-health-services/patient-safety/research/safe-surgery

Wu, A. W., & Connors, C. (2018). Supporting clinicians after adverse events: The second victim phenomenon. *BMJ (Clinical Research Ed.), 363*, k4149. DOI: 10.1136/bmj.k4149

Wu, A. W., Shapiro, J., Harrison, R., Scott, S. D., Connors, C., Kenney, L., & Etchegaray, J. (2017). The impact of adverse events on clinicians: What's needed to support second victims. *BMJ Quality & Safety*, *26*(11), 878–882. DOI: 10.1136/bmjqs-2016-005987

# About the Author

**Badia Faddoul**, DNP, RN, CPHQJohns Hopkins Care at Home in Baltimore, Maryland. For more than three decades, she has worked across hospital, ambulatory, and home based settings, advancing patient safety, workforce safety, quality improvement, and regulatory readiness. Dr. Faddoul is known for translating complex systems and standards into meaningful practice at the point of care. Her work blends analytic rigor with close attention to the human conditions under which care is delivered, with a particular focus on creating environments where accountability, learning, and psychological safety can coexist. She has led multidisciplinary initiatives spanning patient safety, workforce protection, infection prevention, transitions of care, and organizational resilience. Her leadership philosophy is grounded in presence, showing up where care happens, listening to those delivering and supporting care, and translating what is observed into sustainable improvement. The perspective reflected in this book draws from her lived experience as a nurse, quality and safety leader, and mentor, and from a core belief that quality begins with connection.

# Index

## A



## B



## C



## D

## E



## F



## H



## I

## L



## M



## O

## P



## Q



## R

# S



# T

## V



## W

www.ingramcontent.com/pod-product-compliance
Lightning Source LLC
LaVergne TN
LVHW080905300926
849162LV00003B/563